MEDICARE: I GET IT NOW!

Master Framework: Systemic Mechanics, Regulatory Timelines, and Cross-Household Financial Interfaces

ROBERT BONNER

Independent Licensed Agent & Healthcare Educator

Published by

People Will Read Again Book Publishing

Atlanta, Georgia

MEDICARE: I GET IT NOW!

Master Framework: Systemic Mechanics, Regulatory Timelines, and Cross-Household Financial Interfaces

---

Copyright and Publication Information

Published by People Will Read Again Book Publishing

Atlanta, Georgia

Paperback ISBN:	979-8-9972025-0-7
Hardcover ISBN:	979-8-9972025-1-4
EPUB ISBN:	979-8-9972025-2-1
Library of Congress Control Number:	2026918990

INDEPENDENT EDUCATIONAL AND NON-GOVERNMENT AFFILIATION NOTICE

This publication is an independent educational resource. It is not affiliated with, endorsed by, or connected to Medicare, the Centers for Medicare & Medicaid Services, the Social Security Administration, the U.S. Department of Health and Human Services, or any other federal, state, or local government agency.

The information presented is general educational information and does not constitute individualized legal, tax, actuarial, medical, fiduciary, financial, or insurance advice. This book does not rank, recommend, market, or solicit enrollment in any insurance carrier or plan. Medicare rules, costs, thresholds, and administrative guidance may change. Readers should verify current information with Medicare.gov, the Social Security Administration, the Internal Revenue Service, or another appropriate official source before making decisions.

Printed in the United States of America.

Source Reference Convention

This publication uses short parenthetical institutional source markers, such as (CMS), (IRS), (SSA), (Social Security), (eCFR), (Medicare.gov), and (HealthCare.gov), to identify the controlling federal or institutional source category supporting the adjacent sentence, paragraph, data point, or regulatory explanation. These parenthetical markers are not intended to function as individualized legal citations, Bluebook footnotes, formal tax opinions, actuarial certifications, or legal memoranda. They are reader-navigation signals designed to preserve source transparency while maintaining the instructional flow of the manuscript.

The formal source architecture, statutory cross-reference structure, and federal document registries appear in the back matter under the Primary Source Compliance Matrix, the Glossary of Federal Systemic Terms and Medical-Legal Nomenclature, and the Institutional Resource Guide and Federal Document Registries. Where a parenthetical marker references a legal database, code compilation, or public regulatory mirror, the governing authority remains the underlying statute, regulation, official handbook, agency publication, or federal administrative guidance, not the database label itself. Readers should verify current rules through the official federal source applicable to the relevant plan year before executing enrollment, tax, legal, or household liquidity decisions.

Primary federal reference architecture includes the official United States government Medicare handbook, *Medicare & You 2026*, identified by CMS as the official government Medicare handbook and organized around Medicare Parts A, B, C, and D, enrollment, coverage, rights, and federal assistance resources.

EDUCATIONAL COMPLIANCE NOTICES AND NON-GOVERNMENT AFFILIATION DISCLOSURES

Non-Government Affiliation Statement

Compliance Reference: 42 CFR § 422.2262

This publication is an independent educational text and reference manual. It is not affiliated with, endorsed by, or connected to the federal Medicare program, the Centers for Medicare & Medicaid Services (CMS), the Social Security Administration

(SSA), the Department of Health and Human Services (HHS), or any other municipal, state, or federal government agency.

The preceding statement operates as a structural compliance boundary. Its function is not merely reputational; it prevents institutional confusion in a policy environment where federal program names, benefit terminology, enrollment windows, and official seals may create an erroneous impression of governmental sponsorship. Under the Medicare Advantage communications framework, organizations may not mislead, confuse, or provide materially inaccurate information to current or potential enrollees, and communications may not misrepresent the identity, authority, or institutional character of the communicating entity (42 CFR § 422.2262). The non-government affiliation statement therefore preserves the separation between federal program administration and independent educational commentary.

Independent Medicare scholarship occupies a necessary space between statutory enactment and operational execution. Federal source documents state governing rules, define benefit categories, and establish enrollment procedures; however, the practical household consequences of those rules often arise only after multiple federal systems intersect. A beneficiary may encounter Medicare entitlement, Social Security claiming, employer group health plan coordination, Health Savings Account eligibility, Marketplace premium tax credit reconciliation, and prescription drug cost-sharing redesign within the same chronological period. The statutory text supplies the controlling legal architecture, but the household implementation problem requires a disciplined interpretive framework capable of sequencing those rules without carrier promotion, plan steering, or locality-specific benefit inducement.

The educational function of this textbook is therefore analytic rather than transactional. Medicare Part A, Part B, Part C, and Part D are examined as federal institutional mechanisms. Enrollment periods are treated as legal time structures. Premiums, penalties, and tax interfaces are treated as statutory and actuarial consequences. The official CMS handbook identifies the major federal categories of Medicare coverage and enrollment, including Original Medicare, Medicare Advantage, Medigap, and Medicare drug coverage; this publication extends that architecture into an academic framework for evaluating how those categories interact across households, employment status, tax accounts, and insurance dependency structures.

This publication consequently avoids the defining features of proprietary marketing. It does not rank private insurance carriers, describe local provider networks, quote plan-specific premiums, compare proprietary formularies, or assert suitability for any individual enrollment election. Medicare Advantage marketing is defined by federal regulation as a subset of communications that both intends to draw attention to, influence selection of, or influence retention in a Medicare Advantage plan and includes or addresses plan benefits, benefit structures, premiums, cost sharing, ranking standards, or rewards and incentives (42 CFR § 422.2260). The absence of plan-specific benefit claims is therefore not a stylistic choice; it is the structural condition that maintains the work as generic educational communication rather than a plan-selection instrument. (eCFR)

The federal review structure reinforces that distinction. Medicare Advantage marketing materials and election forms are subject to CMS review, deemed approval after forty-five days absent CMS disposition, a ten-day deemed-approval period for certain model or standardized materials, or file-and-use treatment for designated categories; non-marketing communications materials generally are not subject to pre-use CMS submission and approval, except for designated critical communications or materials selected for additional oversight (42 CFR § 422.2261). Thus, a generic textbook that does not advertise a specific Medicare Advantage plan, solicit enrollment into a specific plan, or present proprietary plan benefits is analytically distinguishable from the marketing materials contemplated by the forty-five-day CMS review mechanism. (eCFR)

Third-Party Marketing Organization Standardized Disclaimer Notice

Compliance Reference: 42 CFR § 422.2267

The following standardized TPMO disclaimer may apply in separate regulated sales or marketing communications when a licensed professional or third-party marketing organization does not represent all available plans in a service area. "We do not offer every plan available in your area. Any information we provide is limited to those plans we do offer in your area. Please contact Medicare.gov or 1-800-MEDICARE to get information on all of your options." This textbook itself does not offer, rank, sell, or solicit enrollment in any Medicare Advantage, Medicare Prescription Drug Plan, or other private Medicare product.

The quoted notice is reproduced as a conservative omnidirectional compliance perimeter. Federal regulation requires standardized third-party marketing organization disclaimer content when a third-party marketing organization does not sell for all Medicare Advantage organizations in a service area. Current Medicare Advantage regulatory text identifies the standardized disclaimer and requires qualifying TPMOs to use it in specified contexts, including sales calls, electronic communications, TPMO websites, and marketing materials developed, used, or distributed by the TPMO (42 CFR § 422.2267(e)(41)). (eCFR)

The statutory intent behind the TPMO disclosure regime is institutional transparency. Medicare beneficiaries encounter a fragmented communication environment composed of federal agencies, private insurers, licensed agents, brokers, lead generators, call centers, public educators, nonprofit counselors, and digital comparison platforms. The regulatory architecture therefore attempts to prevent a commercial intermediary from appearing to represent the complete Medicare market when the intermediary's actual contractual access may be narrower than the full universe of available plan sponsors. The disclaimer directs the public record back to Medicare.gov and 1-800-MEDICARE as federal baseline sources for comprehensive plan information, thereby preserving the distinction between official plan-finder infrastructure and partial private distribution channels.

This textbook's inclusion of the TPMO notice does not convert the work into a marketing instrument. Rather, the disclosure establishes a broader institutional boundary: any later encounter between a reader and a licensed professional, agency, call center, website, or enrollment channel must be understood as a separate regulated communication context. This manuscript remains a generic educational framework. It does not present plan-specific carrier inventory, does not identify the number of organizations represented in a locality, and does not ask a household to enroll in, retain, or leave any private plan. The notice is included to prevent any reasonable confusion between academic instruction and complete-market representation.

The regulation also preserves legitimate independent education. Federal communications rules do not prohibit licensed independent professionals from authoring neutral educational materials that explain Medicare entitlement, enrollment sequencing, primary-payer ordering, prescription drug architecture, or tax interactions. Instead, the rules police the transition point at which education becomes marketing: the introduction of specific plans, benefit structures, premiums, cost sharing, Star Ratings comparisons, rewards, incentives, or enrollment persuasion. Under 42 CFR § 422.2260, the marketing analysis depends on objective context, including audience, timing, surrounding information, and content, rather than merely the author's stated intent. (eCFR)

The definitive baseline for localized benefit allocation remains the official federal infrastructure, including Medicare.gov, 1-800-MEDICARE, and official state exchange marketplaces where Marketplace eligibility and premium tax credit rules are implicated. The Medicare handbook itself directs beneficiaries to Medicare.gov plan comparison tools, 1-800-MEDICARE, and State Health Insurance Assistance Program resources for personalized counseling and plan comparison assistance. This textbook therefore functions as a pre-decisional academic map: it explains the governing machinery before any localized plan inventory, tax filing reconciliation, or enrollment action enters the analysis.

This specific disclosure structure also aligns with the front-facing Household Medicare Diagnostic Matrix. The matrix frames Medicare not as a single enrollment event, but as a multi-variable statutory transition involving household dependency, employer status, tax accounts, prescription drug exposure, and secondary coverage architecture. The notices in preceding parts of the book perform the same analytic function at the institutional level: they separate government program administration from private authorship, generic education from plan marketing, and federal baseline resources from partial private distribution channels.

The Household Medicare Diagnostic Matrix functions as a front-facing analog search engine. Rather than forcing linear consultation of a chronological table of contents, the matrix begins with household configuration, isolates the governing operational anxiety, and directs the analysis immediately toward the controlling Medicare, Marketplace, managed-care, prescription-drug, hospice, and federal tax frameworks. Each row treats Medicare not as a single beneficiary event, but as a statutory transition embedded inside employment law, tax eligibility, household dependency, administrative review rights, and federal benefit sequencing.

If Your Current Household Scenario Is...	...And Your Primary Operational or Financial Concern Is...	...Then Turn Instantly to These Verified Primary Source Analysis Pages:	Referenced Primary Source Clusters & Regulatory Frameworks
Active corporate employment continues beyond age sixty-five, with employer group health coverage based on current employment and a workforce count at or above the federal twenty-employee threshold.	The central risk is erroneous primary-payer sequencing: whether the employer group health plan remains primary, whether Medicare is secondary, and whether Part B deferral creates later enrollment exposure.	Module III, Chapter 5: "Active Employment, TEFRA Twenty-Employee Thresholds, and COBRA Boundary Failures"; Module II, Chapter 3: "Worker Special Enrollment Periods"; CMS 2026 handbook, Section 1	CMS 2026 handbook primary-payer matrix: employer group health coverage based on current employment generally pays first for age-sixty-five-or-older workers when the employer has twenty or more employees, while Medicare pays first below that threshold; the same source distinguishes primary and secondary payer functions. Regulatory architecture: Medicare Secondary Payer aged-worker rules, TEFRA employer-size logic, and 42 CFR § 411.170.
Employment has ended, but COBRA continuation coverage, retiree coverage,	The central risk is mistaking COBRA for "coverage based on current employment" and thereby allowing	Module III, Chapter 5: "Separation from Employment and the COBRA Non-Creditable Trap";	CMS 2026 enrollment guidance states that the Part A/Part B Special Enrollment Period extends during current-

If Your Current Household Scenario Is...	...And Your Primary Operational or Financial Concern Is...	...Then Turn Instantly to These Verified Primary Source Analysis Pages:	Referenced Primary Source Clusters & Regulatory Frameworks
severance-related coverage, or former-employer coverage remains available.	the eight-month Part B Special Enrollment Period clock to expire while continuation coverage persists.	Module II, Chapter 3: "Eight-Month Worker SEP Mechanics"; CMS 2026 handbook, Section 1	employment group health coverage and for the eight-month period beginning after employment or coverage ends, whichever occurs first; COBRA is expressly excluded from current-employment coverage status for that SEP. Framework: CMS Part A/B enrollment guidance, COBRA continuation doctrine, and Medicare late-enrollment penalty administration.
An active Health Savings Account contributor delays Medicare enrollment while remaining covered by a high-deductible health plan, then later applies for premium-free Part A.	The central risk is the retroactive Part A entitlement period disqualifying HSA contributions for prior months and creating excise-tax exposure under the HSA eligibility rules.	Module III, Chapter 7: "HSA Disqualification, Six-Month Retroactive Part A Entitlement, and Form 8889 Correction Mechanics"; Module II, Chapter 3: "Delayed Part A Enrollment"; CMS 2026 handbook, Section 1	CMS states that HSA contributions are not permitted after Medicare begins and that premium-free Part A may go back retroactively six months from Part A enrollment or Social Security/Railroad Retirement Board benefit application, but no earlier than the first Medicare-eligible month. Framework: IRS Publication 969, Internal Revenue Code § 223, Form 8889 excess-contribution correction

If Your Current Household Scenario Is...	...And Your Primary Operational or Financial Concern Is...	...Then Turn Instantly to These Verified Primary Source Analysis Pages:	Referenced Primary Source Clusters & Regulatory Frameworks
			logic, and CMS Part A retroactivity guidance.
A high-income Medicare household has modified adjusted gross income above the applicable statutory threshold and receives an Income-Related Monthly Adjustment Amount determination.	The central risk is whether the two-year MAGI lookback correctly reflects current income capacity, and whether a recognized life-changing event supports Social Security administrative reconsideration through Form SSA-44.	Module III, Chapter 6: "IRMAA MAGI Brackets, Two-Year Lookback Math, and SSA-44 Administrative Appeals"; Module III, Chapter 6: "The High-Income Surcharge: IRMAA Mechanics"; CMS 2026 handbook, Section 1, p. 23 and Section 6, p. 82.	CMS states that Medicare uses modified adjusted gross income from the IRS return filed two years earlier to determine IRMAA, and that 2026 IRMAA exposure begins above $109,000 for individual filing status or $218,000 for joint filing status; CMS also identifies income-reduction life events as grounds to seek review through Social Security. Framework: Social Security Act § 1839(i), Part B IRMAA, Part D IRMAA, MAGI lookback administration, and Form SSA-44.
A Marketplace household contains one person transitioning into Medicare while a younger spouse, minor children, or other tax dependents remain	The central risk is simultaneous Medicare activation, Marketplace termination timing, dependent re-enrollment, Special Enrollment Period access, and year-end	Module VI, Chapter 14: "Household Dependency Separations and Market Re-Entry"; Module III, Chapter 7: "Part A Retroactivity and Marketplace Overlap"; CMS Product No. 11694;	CMS Marketplace guidance states that once Medicare Part A or Part C exists, Marketplace financial help ends, excess help may have to be repaid at tax filing, and non-Medicare household members may need separate re-

If Your Current Household Scenario Is...	...And Your Primary Operational or Financial Concern Is...	...Then Turn Instantly to These Verified Primary Source Analysis Pages:	Referenced Primary Source Clusters & Regulatory Frameworks
in qualified health plan coverage.	premium tax credit reconciliation.	IRS ACA/PTC materials.	enrollment to preserve coverage. IRS guidance further requires Form 8962 reconciliation when advance premium tax credits were paid and identifies repayment on Form 8962 when advance payments exceed the allowable credit. Framework: 45 CFR § 155.420, Form 1095-A, Form 8962, Internal Revenue Code § 36B, and Marketplace dependency SEP administration.
A chronologically standard Medicare enrollee reaches age sixty-five without active-employment deferral, disability-based alternative entitlement, ESRD sequencing, or exceptional-circumstance relief.	The central risk is executing the seven-month Initial Enrollment Period without misunderstanding the first-of-month birthday rule, delayed effective dates, or Part B penalty exposure.	Module II, Chapter 3: "Initial Enrollment Period Architecture"; Module I, Chapter 1: "Federal Entitlement Foundations"; CMS 2026 handbook, Section 1.	CMS defines the Initial Enrollment Period as the seven-month period beginning three months before the month of the sixty-fifth birthday and ending three months after that month; if the birthday falls on the first day of a month, the period begins four months before the birthday month and ends two months after it. Framework: 42 CFR § 406.13, CMS Part A/B entitlement guidance, Social Security

If Your Current Household Scenario Is...	...And Your Primary Operational or Financial Concern Is...	...Then Turn Instantly to These Verified Primary Source Analysis Pages:	Referenced Primary Source Clusters & Regulatory Frameworks
			enrollment administration, and Part B effective-date rules.
Historic Medicare enrollment windows were missed, and no active-employment SEP, Medicaid-loss SEP, disaster SEP, employer-error SEP, incarceration SEP, or other exceptional circumstance applies.	The central risk is reliance on the General Enrollment Period, the next-month effective-date rule, and permanent actuarial late-enrollment penalty exposure.	Module II, Chapter 3: "General Enrollment Period Modernization"; Module II, Chapter 4: "Part B Actuarial Penalty Construction"; CMS 2026 handbook, Section 1.	CMS states that the General Enrollment Period runs January 1 through March 31 each year for missed Part B enrollment when no SEP applies, and coverage begins the first day of the month after enrollment; CMS separately states that the Part B late-enrollment penalty may increase the monthly premium by ten percent for each full twelve-month period of delayed enrollment. Framework: CMS GEP modernization, Part B late-enrollment penalty statute, Medicare Savings Program penalty relief, and exceptional-circumstance SEP rules.
A chronically ill beneficiary evaluates standardized Medigap risk transfer against Part C managed-	The central risk is comparing uncapped Original Medicare cost exposure plus supplemental standardization against Medicare	Module IV, Chapter 9: "The Standardized Supplemental (Medigap) Architecture"; Module IV, Chapter 10: "The Managed Care	CMS describes Original Medicare as permitting use of any Medicare-accepting provider nationwide while lacking an annual out-of-pocket maximum absent

If Your Current Household Scenario Is...	...And Your Primary Operational or Financial Concern Is...	...Then Turn Instantly to These Verified Primary Source Analysis Pages:	Referenced Primary Source Clusters & Regulatory Frameworks
care structures such as HMO or PPO designs.	Advantage network use, prior authorization, referral requirements, and annual maximum out-of-pocket protection.	Paradigm: Medicare Advantage (Part C)"; CMS 2026 handbook.	supplemental coverage; CMS describes Medicare Advantage as an alternative Part C structure that may require networks, referrals, prior authorization, and includes an annual limit on Part A and Part B out-of-pocket costs. Medigap source material states that policies are standardized by plan letters A–D, F, G, and K–N in most states, with identical basic benefits inside the same letter category. Framework: 42 CFR Part 422, Medigap federal standardization, guaranteed issue, open enrollment, underwriting, MOOP, and utilization-management governance.
Catastrophic prescription drug utilization produces high Part D spending early in the calendar year.	The central risk is mapping deductible exposure, formulary cost-sharing, TrOOP accumulation, the 2026 annual out-of-pocket cap, and whether the Medicare Prescription Payment	Module V, Chapter 11: "Actuarial Flow of the Part D Benefit Design," especially Sections 11.1 through 11.3; Module V, Chapter 12: "Formulary Architecture and Utilization	CMS states that yearly out-of-pocket costs for covered Part D drugs are capped at $2,100 in 2026 and that, after the cap is reached, no copayment or coinsurance is owed for covered Part D drugs for the rest of the

If Your Current Household Scenario Is...	...And Your Primary Operational or Financial Concern Is...	...Then Turn Instantly to These Verified Primary Source Analysis Pages:	Referenced Primary Source Clusters & Regulatory Frameworks
	Plan changes cash-flow timing without reducing total liability.	Governance"; CMS 2026 handbook, Section 6.	calendar year; CMS also states that the Medicare Prescription Payment Plan spreads covered out-of-pocket drug costs across the calendar year but does not lower drug costs. Framework: Part D TrOOP, formulary tiers, utilization management, Inflation Reduction Act redesign, Medicare Prescription Payment Plan, and creditable coverage rules.
A beneficiary, representative, clinician, supplier, or plan enrollee receives a denial, termination notice, adverse organization determination, coverage determination, or unfavorable payment decision.	The central risk is selecting the correct administrative appeal channel, preserving deadlines, distinguishing Original Medicare from Part C and Part D review paths, and escalating through independent adjudicatory layers.	Module V, Chapter 12: "Formulary Architecture and Utilization Governance," especially Section 12.2; Module IV, Chapter 10: "The Managed Care Paradigm: Medicare Advantage (Part C)," especially Section 10.3; Appendix & Reference Manual: "Primary Source Compliance Matrix"; CMS 2026 handbook, Section 8.	CMS defines an appeal as the action available when Medicare or a Medicare plan issues an unfavorable coverage or payment decision, including denial of services, supplies, items, drugs, payment, or continued coverage; CMS also describes Original Medicare appeal initiation through the Medicare Summary Notice and review by the Medicare Administrative Contractor, generally within sixty days. Framework: Medicare Administrative

If Your Current Household Scenario Is...	...And Your Primary Operational or Financial Concern Is...	...Then Turn Instantly to These Verified Primary Source Analysis Pages:	Referenced Primary Source Clusters & Regulatory Frameworks
			Contractor redetermination, Qualified Independent Contractor reconsideration, Independent Review Entity review, Administrative Law Judge hearing, Medicare Appeals Council review, and federal judicial review thresholds.
Serious illness reaches terminal prognosis and hospice election becomes the governing federal benefit decision, including situations in which Medicare Advantage enrollment already exists.	The central risk is isolating the hospice benefit from ordinary plan administration, determining which system pays for terminal-illness care, and preserving coverage for unrelated conditions, supplemental benefits, and non-hospice drugs.	Module V, Chapter 13: "Serious Illness Transitions and Hospice Care Integration," especially Section 13.1; Module V, Chapter 13: "Serious Illness Transitions and Hospice Care Integration," especially Section 13.2; CMS 2026 handbook, Section 2; CMS hospice booklet, "Medicare Hospice Benefits".	CMS hospice guidance states that, once hospice care begins, Original Medicare covers services related to the terminal illness even when Medicare Advantage enrollment continues; the Medicare Advantage plan may still cover extra benefits, unrelated medically necessary services, and non-terminal-illness drugs when applicable. Framework: Medicare hospice benefit, CMS Product No. 11303 hospice framework, Part A palliative-care allocation, Part C hospice carveout, attending professional election,

If Your Current Household Scenario Is...	...And Your Primary Operational or Financial Concern Is...	...Then Turn Instantly to These Verified Primary Source Analysis Pages:	Referenced Primary Source Clusters & Regulatory Frameworks
			respite care, and terminal-illness-related drug segregation.

Questions About This Book or Medicare Education Seminars?

Visit www.medicareigetitnow.com

to submit a general question, request information about an upcoming Medicare educational seminar, or inquire about hosting a seminar for your library, church, community, employer, or organization.

TABLE OF CONTENTS

MODULE I: FOUNDATIONS OF THE AMERICAN SOCIAL INSURANCE INFRASTRUCTURE

Chapter 1: The Bicameral and Agency Governance of Social Insurance

1.1 Jurisdictional Splits in Administrative Oversight

The American Medicare system is not administered through a single institutional command center. It operates through a divided administrative structure in which entitlement intake, wage-record verification, premium collection, benefit design, claims adjudication, managed-care contracting, and regulatory enforcement are allocated across distinct federal agencies and downstream administrative contractors. This chapter characterizes that structure as bicameral in the administrative rather than legislative sense: two governing chambers of operational authority process the same beneficiary life event through different legal instruments. The Social Security Administration functions as the primary federal intake and entitlement gatekeeper for most Part A and Part B enrollment events, while the Centers for Medicare & Medicaid Services functions as the program administrator responsible for coverage architecture, claims operations, managed-care oversight, drug-benefit regulation, contractor supervision, and beneficiary-rights enforcement. The official 2026 Medicare handbook reflects this separation by directing Part A and Part B enrollment activity toward Social Security or the Railroad Retirement Board while directing coverage comparison, Medicare account administration, claims review, benefits coordination, plan information, and rights enforcement toward Medicare and CMS-administered channels.

This split is not merely bureaucratic ornamentation. It reflects the historical layering of American social insurance. Social Security began as an earnings-related retirement and disability income system grounded in wage records, payroll taxation, and Title II benefit administration. Medicare, added later as a health-insurance entitlement, necessarily borrowed Social Security's age, disability, wage-history, and benefit-payment infrastructure. As a result, Medicare eligibility does not begin as a hospital claim or physician bill. It begins as an entitlement determination resting on age, disability status, lawful presence, Railroad Retirement Board status, Social Security benefit receipt, and Medicare-tax work history. The official CMS-facing handbook states that premium-free Part A generally depends on whether the beneficiary or spouse paid Medicare taxes while working for the required amount of time, while federal tax source material identifies social security and Medicare taxes as employment taxes reported through employer filing systems, including W-2 and W-3 reporting to the SSA.

The advantage of this divided architecture is institutional specialization. SSA retains the labor-record, earnings-credit, disability-benefit, retirement-benefit, and premium-withholding machinery. CMS retains the health-program machinery: coverage manuals, plan contracts, claims-payment systems, Medicare Administrative Contractors, Medicare Advantage organizations, Part D sponsors, quality oversight, appeals channels, privacy notices, and beneficiary protections. Such specialization reduces the risk that a single federal office will simultaneously define entitlement, adjudicate all claims, collect all premiums, police all private contractors, and control all beneficiary communications. The same division, however, creates friction. A household moving from employer-sponsored coverage into Medicare does not experience the transition as two clean institutional lanes. The household experiences a single event: employment status changes, group health plan status changes, Social Security claiming may or may not begin, Medicare Part A may become retroactive, Part B may require active enrollment, Part D creditable coverage must be evaluated, and Marketplace or HSA tax rules may be triggered. This is the precise interlocking dilemma anticipated by the front-facing Household Medicare Diagnostic Matrix. The matrix exists because the administrative structure divides authority, while household financial exposure combines consequences.

The Social Security Administration's first Medicare function is legal intake. Under the official 2026 Medicare handbook, an individual already receiving Social Security or Railroad Retirement Board benefits is automatically enrolled in Medicare Part A and Part B beginning the first day of the month of the sixty-fifth birthday; when the birthday falls on the first day of the month, coverage begins the first day of the prior month. The same handbook states that disability-based automatic enrollment occurs after twenty-four months of Social Security disability benefits or certain Railroad Retirement Board disability benefits, and that ALS produces automatic Part A and Part B entitlement when Social Security disability benefits begin. The Puerto Rico exception confirms the limits of automation: Social Security or Railroad Retirement Board beneficiaries residing in Puerto Rico receive Part A automatically but must actively enroll in Part B.

The automatic-enrollment rule demonstrates SSA's role as a trigger-based administrative engine. Social Security benefit receipt is not merely a monthly income event; it also functions as a Medicare enrollment signal. When Title II benefit status already exists, Medicare entitlement can be generated without a separate affirmative Medicare application for the ordinary age-sixty-five case. Conversely, when Social Security or Railroad Retirement Board benefits are not already being paid near age sixty-five, the same official source states that an individual must sign up for Medicare and identifies Social Security's Medicare sign-up portal as the Part A and Part B application channel, with Railroad Retirement Board contact procedures for railroad cases. Thus, SSA's jurisdiction is neither incidental nor advisory. It is the legal front door through which baseline Part A and Part B entitlement is commonly established.

That intake role also explains the importance of enrollment-period architecture. The Initial Enrollment Period, Special Enrollment Period, and General Enrollment Period are not merely educational labels. They are time-coded legal permissions that determine whether SSA may establish Part B without delay, whether a late-enrollment penalty attaches, and whether CMS downstream systems receive an entitlement file compatible with subsequent plan enrollment. Under the official 2026 Medicare handbook, the Initial Enrollment Period generally spans seven months, beginning three months before the month of the sixty-fifth birthday and ending three months after that month; for first-day-of-month birthdays, the period begins four months before the birthday month and ends two months after that month.

SSA's enrollment gatekeeping becomes even more consequential after the Initial Enrollment Period closes. Under CMS enrollment guidance reflected in the official handbook, a worker Special Enrollment Period may permit Part A and Part B enrollment during coverage under a group health plan based on current employment or during the eight-month period beginning after employment ends or that employment-based coverage ends, whichever occurs first. The same source states that COBRA, retiree coverage, Veterans Affairs coverage, Marketplace individual coverage, and severance-related former-employer coverage do not constitute coverage based on current employment for this Special Enrollment Period. This distinction is jurisdictionally important because SSA must process the Medicare enrollment request, while CMS benefit-coordination logic determines whether the underlying coverage is current-employment group coverage or merely continuation, retiree, individual, or post-employment coverage.

The General Enrollment Period illustrates the penalty side of the same intake framework. The official handbook states that the General Enrollment Period runs from January 1 through March 31 each year for individuals who missed the Initial Enrollment Period and lack a Special Enrollment Period, with coverage beginning the first day of the month after enrollment. The same handbook states that the Part B late-enrollment penalty may increase the monthly Part B premium by ten percent for each full twelve-month period in which Part B could have been held but was not, and that the penalty may last for as long as Part B remains in force. This rule transforms enrollment timing into an actuarial premium multiplier. SSA processes the enrollment and premium obligation, but the penalty arises from Medicare's statutory enrollment design.

SSA's second jurisdictional domain is baseline eligibility verification. In common Medicare administration, premium-free Part A is associated with sufficient Medicare-tax work history. The 2026 handbook expresses that concept in beneficiary-facing terms: Part A usually has no monthly premium when the beneficiary or spouse paid Medicare taxes while working for a sufficient period; when that work-tax history is insufficient, Part A may be purchased, and the 2026 premium is either $311 or $565 per month depending on the length of Medicare-tax work history. The deeper actuarial structure is that Medicare Part A entitlement is financed through payroll-tax participation and recorded work history rather than through a purely residence-based national health card. SSA's recordkeeping function thereby links historical labor-market attachment to current hospital-insurance entitlement.

The employment-tax record is not a peripheral tax artifact. IRS source material identifies social security and Medicare taxes as employment taxes, requiring employer filings such as Forms 941 or 944 and wage-reporting forms W-2 and W-3 to the SSA. In practical administrative terms, the wage record becomes the entitlement ledger. Payroll taxation, employer reporting, SSA wage posting, and Medicare Part A premium status are separate legal moments in time, but they are causally connected. A household may perceive Medicare entitlement as an age-sixty-five event, while the federal system treats that event as the present consequence of decades of reported earnings and Medicare-tax contributions.

SSA's third jurisdictional domain is premium collection and federal financial clearinghouse administration. Under the official 2026 handbook, the standard Part B premium for 2026 is $202.90 per month, and Medicare uses modified adjusted gross income from the IRS tax return filed two years earlier to determine whether the Income-Related Monthly Adjustment Amount applies. The same source identifies the 2026 IRMAA threshold as modified adjusted gross income above $109,000 for individual filing status or $218,000 for joint filing status, and it directs income-related disputes arising from life events to Social Security channels. The Part B premium is therefore not merely a flat insurance charge. It is an administratively collected federal premium that can incorporate income-tested surcharges imported from IRS tax data and administered through Social Security premium protocols.

Premium collection further illustrates the mechanical connection between SSA benefit payment and Medicare financing. The official handbook states that Part B premiums are deducted from monthly Social Security or Railroad Retirement Board benefit payments when those benefits are being received. For beneficiaries not receiving Social Security or Railroad Retirement Board benefits, Medicare bills the premium directly, generally on a quarterly basis; monthly billing may occur when Part A, Part D IRMAA, or Medicare Easy Pay is involved. This structure creates two beneficiary classes for premium administration: benefit-receipt households whose Medicare premiums are netted against federal income benefits, and non-benefit-receipt households whose Medicare premiums are civil-billed through Medicare premium billing channels.

The Centers for Medicare & Medicaid Services assumes a different institutional role. Once entitlement has been established, CMS governs the operational health-insurance structure into which that entitlement flows. The official handbook divides Medicare into Part A Hospital Insurance, Part B Medical Insurance, and Part D drug coverage. Part A helps cover inpatient hospital care, skilled nursing facility care, hospice care, and home health care; Part B helps cover services from doctors and other providers, outpatient care, home health care, durable medical equipment, and preventive services; Part D helps cover prescription drugs, including many recommended vaccines, and is delivered through private companies that follow Medicare rules.

CMS also defines the beneficiary's delivery architecture. Original Medicare includes Part A and Part B, with the option to add separate Part D coverage and, where applicable, supplemental coverage. Medicare Advantage, also known as Part C, is described by CMS as a Medicare-approved private-plan alternative that bundles Part A, Part B, and usually Part D, may require network use and approval for certain drugs or services, and includes an annual out-of-pocket limit for covered services. This is the central administrative transition from entitlement to delivery model: SSA may establish Part A and Part B entitlement, but CMS defines whether that entitlement is used through Original Medicare claims administration or through a Medicare Advantage contract structure regulated under Part C.

CMS's operational responsibility is visible in claims, privacy, contractor usage, and beneficiary-rights administration. The official Medicare privacy notice states that Medicare Administrative Contractors use Medicare information to pay or deny claims, collect premiums, coordinate benefit payments with other insurers, and prepare Medicare Summary Notices. The same notice states that Medicare may use information for customer service, complaint resolution, research, quality care, federal and state payment oversight, Medicaid program coordination, public health activities, fraud and abuse oversight, and judicial or administrative proceedings. CMS therefore functions as the operational hub that converts entitlement into claim adjudication, payment decisions, coordination-of-benefits records, privacy notices, and administrative accountability.

National coverage administration belongs to the CMS side of the divide. The 2026 handbook states that Original Medicare covers most medically necessary services and supplies in hospitals, doctors' offices, and other health care facilities, while Medicare Advantage plans must cover all medically necessary services that Original Medicare covers and may also offer extra benefits. It further states that Original Medicare generally does not require prior authorization for covered services or supplies, while Medicare Advantage may require approval before certain services or supplies are covered. In doctrinal terms, CMS coverage governance establishes the federal baseline of medical necessity, while private delivery models operate inside regulatory boundaries that do not erase the underlying Medicare entitlement.

The source packet's visible materials ground the coverage system in medical necessity, contractor adjudication, and appeal rights rather than providing a complete National Coverage Determinations manual. Within those grounded limits, the operational conclusion is clear: CMS sets the federal coverage architecture, and Medicare Administrative Contractors execute Original Medicare payment determinations within that architecture. When a coverage or payment decision is disputed under Original Medicare, the official handbook states that the Medicare Summary Notice identifies the item or service at issue, and the appeal is sent to the Medicare Administrative Contractor listed on the notice; a decision is generally issued within sixty days after receipt of the appeal request. Thus, CMS coverage governance is not abstract policy alone. It is manifested in claim-line adjudication, contractor notices, appeal deadlines, and beneficiary-review rights.

CMS's managed-care authority is more explicitly regulatory. The Part C and Part D enrollment guidance in the source packet defines a Medicare Advantage Organization as a public or private risk-bearing entity, licensed by a state where applicable, and certified by CMS as meeting Medicare Advantage contract requirements. The same guidance defines a Medicare Advantage plan as health-benefits coverage offered under a policy or contract by a Medicare Advantage Organization, with a specific set of benefits offered at a uniform premium and uniform cost-sharing level to Medicare beneficiaries residing in the plan service area. This definition is the hinge between federal entitlement and private delivery. The private organization does not own Medicare entitlement; it administers a CMS-approved delivery structure under federal contract.

CMS also polices the mechanics of Part C and Part D enrollment. Under CMS enrollment guidance citing 42 CFR §§ 422.50(a)(3), 422.60, 423.30, and 423.32, a Medicare Advantage Organization or Part D sponsor must accept enrollment requests from eligible individuals during a valid election period and must process the request to determine enrollment eligibility. Processing begins with acceptance of the request and ends with written communication stating whether the request has been accepted or denied by the plan or by CMS. The same guidance requires plans to verify Medicare entitlement through the Batch Eligibility Query process or the MARx online query, and it requires permanent-residence analysis for service-area eligibility.

The enrollment file is therefore an administrative object that must satisfy both beneficiary intent and federal eligibility data. CMS guidance states that a completed enrollment request requires a completed and signed request mechanism, evidence of Medicare Part A entitlement or Part B enrollment as applicable, authorized-representative attestation where relevant, and any required Special Needs Plan eligibility verification. Once complete, the plan must transmit the enrollment to CMS. The system is intentionally documentary. Enrollment is not merely oral interest, nor merely private plan acceptance, nor merely possession of a Medicare card. It requires a valid election period, a complete request, verified entitlement, and successful CMS processing.

Time discipline is central to CMS oversight. CMS guidance requires plans to submit information necessary for CMS to add an individual to Medicare Advantage or Part D enrollment records within seven calendar days after receipt of a completed enrollment request, with the receipt date counted as day zero and the following day counted as day one. CMS guidance also states that enrollment requests must be processed chronologically by date of receipt and encourages early transaction submission to resolve data issues arising from late submissions. These rules are designed to protect the integrity of the federal enrollment file, but they also reveal how easily households can be harmed by late data, incomplete files, or mismatched eligibility records.

CMS's communication and marketing oversight is likewise embedded in the Part C and Part D regulatory structure. The source packet states that electronic enrollment mechanisms must be submitted to and approved by CMS, must comply with HIPAA privacy and security requirements, must advise applicants that an enrollment request is being completed, must capture electronic intent and timestamps, and must provide required CMS marketing-rule information under 42 CFR Parts 422 and 423, Subpart V. In addition, CMS guidance identifies enrollment materials as subject to CMS marketing requirements, including 42 CFR §§ 422.2261(b), 422.2267, 423.2261(b), and 423.2267. This regulatory apparatus preserves the line between federal entitlement and private plan solicitation.

CMS enforcement extends beyond process formality. Under CMS guidance citing 42 CFR §§ 422.62(b)(3) and 423.38(c)(8), an SEP may arise when CMS determines that a Medicare Advantage Organization or Part D sponsor substantially violated a material plan-contract provision or materially misrepresented the plan in communications, failed to provide medically necessary services on a timely basis, or failed to provide medical services according to applicable quality standards. Under related guidance, a separate SEP applies when an enrollee disenrolls in connection with a CMS sanction, and CMS may require notice to affected enrollees under 42 CFR §§ 422.111(g) and 423.128(f). The enforcement point is doctrinally significant: CMS does not merely approve plan entry into the Medicare marketplace; it retains authority to police contract conduct, communications, service access, and sanction-related election relief.

The most consequential failures occur at the interface between SSA and CMS, rather than wholly inside either agency. CMS enrollment guidance defines a system error as an unintended error or delay in enrollment-request processing clearly attributable to a specific federal government system, such as an SSA or Railroad Retirement Board system, and related to Medicare entitlement information or other information required to process an enrollment request. This definition confirms that the federal structure anticipates inter-agency data vulnerabilities. Entitlement status may exist in one system, plan enrollment may be pending in another, premium withholding may depend on a monthly cutoff, and coverage materials may arrive after the effective date even though coverage legally begins on that date.

Premium withholding illustrates the timing problem with unusual clarity. CMS guidance states that when an enrollment request includes SSA or Railroad Retirement Board premium withholding and the CMS enrollment transaction is processed after the monthly payment cutoff, the plan must submit the premium-withholding request separately; the plan must inform the enrollee that withholding may begin in one to two months, that withholding will not be retroactive, that direct payment is required for premiums due before withholding begins, and that nonpayment may result in disenrollment. A household may believe premium withholding has been elected, while the administrative file has not yet synchronized payment implementation. The legal election and the financial debit do not necessarily begin simultaneously.

Employer and union group health plan transactions create an additional layer of vulnerability. CMS guidance allows retroactive employer/union group health plan transactions when a delay exists between completion of an enrollment request through the employer group and plan receipt, or when the employer group fails to forward a valid enrollment or disenrollment request within required timeframes. Repeated errors may be escalated to the CMS account manager for compliance monitoring. Retroactive employer-group enrollments may be processed up to, but not beyond, ninety days from the date the organization received the employer or union group request, consistent with 42 CFR §§ 422.66(f), 422.308(f)(2), 423.32(i), and 423.343(a). Such rules are remedial, not merely administrative. They exist because a beneficiary's intended election can be separated from the federal enrollment record by employer, union, plan, or system latency.

The same friction appears in erroneous incarceration or unlawful-presence data. CMS guidance states that where disenrollment arises from erroneous incarceration or unlawful-presence information, the plan must check CMS systems, and if CMS systems still reflect the erroneous status, the individual is referred to SSA so that SSA may review and correct records; if SSA determines the information is erroneous, CMS systems are updated, the plan receives confirmation through the Daily Transaction Reply Report, and coverage resumes seamlessly as though disenrollment had not occurred. This is a paradigmatic example of divided sovereignty within a single program. CMS administers plan enrollment consequences, but SSA may control the correction of the underlying federal status record.

The household impact of these inter-agency seams is most severe during the transition out of active employment. The official handbook's primary-payer framework states that for age-sixty-five-or-older individuals with group health plan coverage based on current employment, the group health plan pays first when the employer has twenty or more employees, while Medicare pays first when the employer has fewer than twenty employees. It further states that the primary payer pays up to its coverage limits, the secondary payer pays only if uncovered costs remain, and the secondary payer may not pay all remaining costs. The same source states that if group health plan coverage ends, Medicare's records should be updated, and the Benefits Coordination & Recovery Center may be contacted for insurance changes.

This interface directly corresponds to the Household Medicare Diagnostic Matrix. The matrix's active-worker row, COBRA row, HSA row, Marketplace-dependency row, and General Enrollment Period row all arise from the same structural fact: SSA controls enrollment and premium mechanics, CMS controls coverage and coordination mechanics, IRS-administered tax rules may attach to Medicare status, and household coverage may include dependents who are not themselves Medicare eligible. An error in one file can generate effects in another domain. An uncorrected primary-payer record can misdirect claims. An unrecognized end of employment can produce Part B delay. A mistaken assumption that COBRA equals current-employment coverage can allow the eight-month Special Enrollment Period to expire. A late CMS transaction can create temporary direct-bill exposure despite intended premium withholding. A federal-system error can require retroactive correction. The statutory framework therefore dictates that Medicare literacy must be file-based, timeline-based, and agency-specific.

The central analytic conclusion of Section 1.1 is that Medicare is not merely a health-insurance card issued at age sixty-five. It is a coordinated social-insurance file passing through distinct federal institutions. SSA establishes and maintains the legal and financial gateway: age, disability, earnings record, Medicare-tax history, enrollment intake, premium withholding, and income-related premium administration. CMS governs the operational health system: coverage categories, claims contractors, coordination-of-benefits records, privacy administration, appeals, plan-contract certification, Part C and Part D enrollment processing, communications regulation, and enforcement remedies. A household that fails to understand the jurisdictional split may mistake a Social Security enrollment event for a CMS coverage decision, a CMS plan notice for an SSA premium determination, a private enrollment form for a completed federal transaction, or a continuation policy for current-employment coverage. The actuarial reality is that these distinctions have monetary value: they determine premiums, penalties, payer order, claims payment, drug access, coverage continuity, and household tax exposure.

1.2 Actuarial Financing of the Federal Trust Funds

Medicare's governance cannot be understood solely through the vocabulary of eligibility, enrollment, and medical coverage. Beneath the visible entitlement structure lies a bifurcated financing architecture in which distinct trust funds perform different macroeconomic functions. The Hospital Insurance Trust Fund finances Part A, principally through payroll taxation and related statutory income streams. The Supplementary Medical Insurance Trust Fund finances Part B and Part D through a radically different structure, one that combines beneficiary premiums with annually reset federal general-revenue transfers. The 2026 Medicare Trustees Report states that the Hospital Insurance and Supplementary Medical Insurance trust funds are separate and distinct, each with its own revenue sources and mandated expenditures, and that no statutory mechanism permits the use of HI revenues to finance SMI expenditures, the use of SMI revenues to finance HI expenditures, or lending between the two funds. (CMS)

This separation produces the central actuarial contrast of Medicare finance. The Hospital Insurance Trust Fund resembles a wage-tax social-insurance reserve; its income stream depends primarily on taxable payroll, the number of covered workers, wage growth, statutory tax rates, and supplemental sources such as the taxation of certain Social Security benefits. The Supplementary Medical Insurance Trust Fund resembles an annually recalibrated public-finance account; its Part B and Part D accounts are designed so that premiums and general-fund transfers are set prospectively to cover expected expenditures. The Trustees state that current law provides for annual determination of Part B and Part D beneficiary premiums and government contributions to cover expected costs for the following year, while HI tax rates do not automatically adjust to match expenditures absent new legislation. (CMS)

The Hospital Insurance Trust Fund constitutes the fiscal base of Medicare Part A. Under CMS's 2026 beneficiary-facing structure, Part A helps cover inpatient hospital care, skilled nursing facility care, hospice care, and home health care; the same federal handbook states that most persons do not pay a monthly Part A premium when the beneficiary or spouse paid Medicare taxes while working for the required period. This premium-free status is not a gratuity. It is the household-facing expression of a payroll-tax social-insurance model. The payroll tax is paid during working years and later supports entitlement to hospital-insurance coverage without a monthly premium for those with sufficient Medicare-tax work history. When that work-tax history is insufficient, Part A may be purchased, and CMS states that the 2026 premium is either $311 or $565 per month depending on the duration of Medicare-tax work history.

The payroll-tax foundation is imposed through the Federal Insurance Contributions Act for employees and through parallel self-employment tax rules under the Self-Employment Contributions Act for self-employed persons. The Internal Revenue Service states that the current Medicare tax rate is 1.45 percent for the employer and 1.45 percent for the employee, producing a combined 2.9 percent Medicare tax rate for covered wages; the IRS further states that no wage-base limit applies to Medicare tax, so all covered wages remain subject to Medicare tax. (IRS) For the self-employed population, IRS Publication 334 states that the self-employment tax rate includes a 2.9 percent Medicare component, that all combined wages, tips, and net earnings are subject to the Medicare portion, and that self-employment tax rules apply regardless of age or receipt of Social Security or Medicare benefits.

The absence of a Medicare wage cap is actuarially decisive. Social Security payroll taxation has a wage base limit, while Medicare's basic tax reaches all covered wages. The HI Trust Fund therefore captures revenue from the full covered wage distribution rather than only the lower and middle portions of earnings. This structure links Part A financing to aggregate labor compensation and the size of the covered workforce. It also makes the HI Trust Fund sensitive to labor-market composition, wage growth, employment participation, and the ratio of active workers to beneficiaries. When the number of beneficiaries grows faster than taxable payroll, the tax base becomes less able to support the expenditure base. The Trustees define the ratio of HI income to taxable payroll as the income rate and the ratio of expenditures to taxable payroll as the cost rate, thereby placing the solvency analysis directly inside the relationship between covered employment and Part A outlays. (CMS)

The Additional Medicare Tax supplies a second statutory layer. The IRS states that a 0.9 percent Additional Medicare Tax applies to Medicare wages, self-employment income, and railroad retirement compensation above filing-status thresholds:

$250,000 for married filing jointly, $125,000 for married filing separately, and $200,000 for all other taxpayers. (IRS) IRS withholding guidance further states that employers must withhold the 0.9 percent Additional Medicare Tax on wages paid to an individual in excess of $200,000 in a calendar year, without regard to filing status, beginning in the pay period in which wages exceed that amount, and that no employer match applies to the Additional Medicare Tax. (IRS)

This surcharge performs two distinct functions. At the individual tax-compliance level, it creates an additional liability that may require Form 8959 computation when wages, self-employment income, or railroad retirement compensation exceed the statutory thresholds. IRS Publication 334 states that a 0.9 percent Additional Medicare Tax may apply when self-employment earnings exceed the filing-status threshold, and that when both wages and self-employment income exist, the self-employment threshold is reduced by wages subject to the Additional Medicare Tax, but not below zero. At the macro-finance level, the surcharge increases the HI revenue stream on high earnings. The 2026 Trustees Report states that high-income workers pay an additional 0.9 percent of earnings above $200,000 for single workers or $250,000 for married couples filing jointly, and because the thresholds are not indexed, an increasing proportion of workers and earnings is projected to become subject to the higher HI tax rate over time. (CMS)

The non-indexed design of the Additional Medicare Tax is one of the more subtle fiscal mechanisms in Medicare finance. A nominal threshold that does not rise with wage growth gradually captures a larger share of the earnings distribution. The Trustees project that by the end of the long-range projection period, an estimated 80 percent of workers would become subject to the additional tax. (CMS) The result is not an immediate transformation of HI solvency, but a gradual broadening of effective tax exposure. This mechanism partially offsets demographic pressure, yet does not eliminate the long-range financial imbalance. The Trustees project a 75-year HI actuarial deficit of 0.56 percent of taxable payroll under current law, calculated from a summarized income rate of 4.06 percent and a summarized cost rate of 4.63 percent. (CMS)

Solvency analysis therefore begins with the dependency ratio. The HI Trust Fund receives revenue from the covered labor force and pays claims for a beneficiary population that is aging, medically heterogeneous, and increasingly expensive to serve. The Trustees report that Medicare expenditures represented 3.9 percent of gross domestic product in 2025, are projected to increase to 6.5 percent of GDP by 2050, and are projected to reach 7.5 percent of GDP by 2100 under current law. (CMS) That expenditure trajectory is driven by beneficiary growth, demographic composition, health-cost growth per beneficiary, service volume, service intensity, and statutory payment-update rules. This is why the Hospital Insurance Trust Fund cannot be evaluated simply by asking whether a payroll tax exists. The actuarial question is whether scheduled tax income, supplemental income, interest income, and accumulated reserves remain sufficient to pay scheduled Part A obligations when due.

The Trustees' annual reporting process supplies the formal risk-management apparatus. CMS states that the Medicare Boards of Trustees report annually to Congress on the financial operations and actuarial status of the Medicare program, and that the Office of the Actuary in CMS prepares the combined report under the direction of the Boards. (CMS) The 2026 Trustees Report states that the Social Security Act established the Medicare Board of Trustees to oversee the financial operations of the HI and SMI trust funds; the Board includes the Secretary of the Treasury as Managing Trustee, the Secretary of Labor, the Secretary of Health and Human Services, the Commissioner of Social Security, and two public trustees, while the CMS Administrator serves as Secretary of the Board. (CMS) The same report states that the Board must report annually to Congress on the financial and actuarial status of the HI and SMI trust funds, and that the 2026 report is the sixty-first such report. (CMS)

The 2026 actuarial findings describe a trust fund under measurable pressure. The Trustees state that after a small projected surplus in 2026, HI deficits are projected to return in 2027 and persist for the remainder of the projection period, requiring redemption of trust fund assets until depletion in 2033. (CMS) The Trustees further state that the HI asset ratio stood at 53 percent of annual expenditures at the beginning of 2026, down from 150 percent since 2007, and that the Board recommends an asset level at least equal to annual expenditures as an adequate contingency reserve. (CMS) Under the intermediate assumptions, assets are projected to decline steadily as a percentage of annual expenditures until depletion in the second quarter of 2033, one quarter earlier than projected in the preceding report. (CMS)

The consequences of depletion must be interpreted with precision. The Trustees state that if HI assets were depleted, Medicare could pay health plans and providers of Part A services only to the extent allowed by ongoing tax revenues, and those revenues would be inadequate to fully cover costs. (CMS) The report further notes that after asset depletion in 2033, no provision exists to use transfers from the general fund of the Treasury or any other means to cover the HI deficit. (CMS) This is the defining difference between a finite payroll-financed trust fund and an annually financed SMI account. The HI fund contains reserves and receives statutory income, but it does not possess an automatic general-fund draw sufficient to guarantee full scheduled payments after depletion.

The Supplementary Medical Insurance Trust Fund operates on a different fiscal premise. SMI consists of Part B and Part D, with separate accounts inside the SMI Trust Fund. The Trustees state that SMI is composed of two parts, Part B and Part D, and that each has its own separate account within the SMI Trust Fund; they also state that the financial status of each account must be evaluated separately because the law provides no transfer of assets or income between Part B and Part D accounts. (CMS) This internal separation mirrors the larger separation between HI and SMI. Medicare's financing architecture is therefore not a single pool, but a set of legally constrained accounts with distinct inflows and payment obligations.

Part B is the physician, outpatient, durable medical equipment, home health, preventive-services, and medical-insurance arm of Medicare's federal coverage structure. CMS's 2026 handbook identifies Part B as Medical Insurance that helps cover services from doctors and other health care providers, outpatient care, home health care, durable medical equipment, and many preventive services. The cost of this benefit is financed through beneficiary premiums and federal general-revenue transfers. The Trustees state that both Part B and Part D are voluntary and are mostly financed by participant premiums and contributions from the general fund of the Treasury, while HI is generally compulsory and primarily financed from payroll taxes. (CMS)

The standard Part B premium embodies the beneficiary-financed portion of the SMI model. CMS states that the standard Part B premium amount in 2026 is $202.90 per month, and that most beneficiaries pay that standard amount. The Trustees state that under current law, the standard Part B premium is set at about 25 percent of average expenditures for beneficiaries aged sixty-five and over. (CMS) This statutory ratio is central to Part B pricing. A premium does not arise from local plan design, carrier discretion, or underwriting. It arises from a national actuarial projection of program cost, adjusted through statutory rules, reserve requirements, prior legislative repayment mechanisms, and income-related premium obligations.

The remaining Part B cost is supplied principally through federal general revenues. The Trustees explain that financing for 2026 was set to maintain Part B assets at a fully sufficient level, and that total revenues from premiums, matching government contributions, and allocated drug-manufacturer fees must equal the level needed for program financing. (CMS) In practical fiscal shorthand, this means that beneficiary premiums finance approximately one quarter of standard Part B program cost, while federal contributions and related statutory receipts finance the remainder. This is the source of the conventional assertion that general revenue subsidizes approximately three quarters of Part B operational outlays, although high-income beneficiary premiums modify the distribution for affected households.

Part D follows the same general SMI principle, but with a different percentage composition. CMS's 2026 handbook states that Medicare drug coverage helps cover prescription drugs, including many recommended vaccines, and that drug plans are run by private companies that follow Medicare rules. For Part D, premiums are plan-related at the household-facing level, but the national financing system includes beneficiary premiums, state payments, and federal government contributions. The Trustees project, on an infinite-horizon present-value basis, that beneficiary premiums would finance approximately 18 percent of Part D expenditures, state payments about 9 percent, and government contributions the remaining 73 percent. (CMS) Part D is therefore not financed by a simple 25 percent premium rule like standard Part B, but it remains dependent on federal general-fund contributions and annual recalibration.

SMI's structural insulation arises from its financing mechanism. The Trustees state that the law establishes a mechanism under which Part B premiums, Part D premiums, and corresponding general-fund transfers are sufficient to cover the following year's estimated expenditures, making each SMI account automatically in financial balance under current law. (CMS) The 2026 Trustees Report also states that both accounts of the SMI Trust Fund are automatically in financial balance, whereas the HI Trust Fund is not. (CMS) The distinction is not semantic. HI can face depletion because income does not automatically adjust to expenditure. SMI does not face insolvency in the same manner because income is reset to expected costs, although the resulting burden is shifted to beneficiaries through premiums and to taxpayers through general revenues.

This insulation does not mean fiscal harmlessness. It means that the SMI financing problem appears as federal budget pressure and beneficiary premium pressure rather than as a trust-fund depletion date. The Trustees state that SMI premiums and transfers from the general fund of the Treasury are expected to grow at the same rate as SMI expenditures, while HI revenue does not; consequently, SMI revenues are expected to represent a growing share of total Medicare revenues as HI sources become increasingly inadequate. (CMS) CMS's 2026 handbook confirms the household-facing effect: Medicare uses modified adjusted gross income from the IRS return filed two years earlier to determine whether a beneficiary owes an Income-Related Monthly Adjustment Amount, and in 2026 IRMAA exposure begins above $109,000 for individual filing status or $218,000 for joint filing status.

IRMAA is therefore not merely an administrative surcharge. It is a statutory cost-allocation instrument that moves a greater portion of SMI cost onto higher-income beneficiaries. CMS states that higher-income beneficiaries may also pay an extra amount for Part D, and that the 2026 Part D IRMAA threshold uses the same $109,000 individual and $218,000 joint-income trigger. The Trustees state that high-income beneficiaries have paid an income-related premium for Part B since 2007 and for Part D since 2011. (CMS) This policy mechanism links federal solvency pressure, beneficiary premium pricing, and household tax-return data. It also explains why the Household Medicare Diagnostic Matrix treats IRMAA as a systemic household-finance issue rather than as a simple monthly bill.

Part D cost sharing supplies a parallel cost-containment interface. CMS states that out-of-pocket costs for covered Part D drugs are capped at $2,100 in 2026, and that once this cap is reached, no copayment or coinsurance is owed for covered Part D drugs for the rest of the calendar year. The Trustees state that the Part D catastrophic threshold is set at $2,100 in 2026 and indexed annually thereafter. (CMS) These drug-benefit mechanics change household cash-flow exposure, but they also alter program financing obligations. When beneficiary exposure is capped, remaining costs must be allocated through plan liability, manufacturer obligations, federal reinsurance or subsidy structures, premium pricing, and government contributions. Thus, the cap is simultaneously a household protection device and a macro-financing variable.

The trust-fund architecture ultimately shapes federal policy through different forms of constraint. HI constraint is visible as depletion risk. SMI constraint is visible as budgetary absorption and premium growth. The Trustees state that the Board believes solutions are necessary to ensure HI financial integrity and reduce Medicare cost growth, and that earlier reforms allow more flexible and gradual implementation while giving providers, beneficiaries, and taxpayers more time to adjust expectations and behavior. (CMS) This is the actuarial foundation for policy tools such as payroll-tax adjustments, payment-update constraints, fraud and abuse control activity, IRMAA surcharges, premium recalibration, cost-sharing redesign, and drug-price mechanisms.

The Household Medicare Diagnostic Matrix later in this book therefore operates as more than a navigational index. It reflects the financing architecture of the program itself. The high-income household row corresponds to SMI premium recapture through IRMAA. The catastrophic drug-spend row corresponds to Part D's cost-sharing redesign and general-revenue dependence. The active-worker and HSA rows correspond to the payroll-tax and entitlement foundations of Part A. The Marketplace-to-Medicare dependency row corresponds to the boundary between federal entitlement, tax credits, and household coverage allocation. The matrix's purpose is to expose the economic logic behind household-level rules: the same statutory machinery that prices Part B premiums, caps Part D drug exposure, and finances Part

A through payroll taxation also determines when families encounter penalties, surcharges, benefit coordination, and tax reconciliation.

The actuarial reality is that Medicare's stability depends on dual insulation. The HI Trust Fund requires sufficient payroll-tax and related income to maintain timely payment for Part A benefits. The SMI Trust Fund requires annual political and budgetary capacity to absorb rising Part B and Part D expenditures through premiums and general revenues. These structures do not eliminate cost growth; they distribute it across workers, beneficiaries, taxpayers, providers, plans, and future legislative sessions. A serious academic treatment of Medicare must therefore reject the superficial view that the program is financed by a single "Medicare premium." The program is funded through a layered statutory apparatus: 2.9 percent baseline HI payroll taxation, the 0.9 percent Additional Medicare Tax on high earnings, taxation of certain Social Security benefits, Part A premiums for voluntary enrollees, Part B standard premiums, Part B and Part D IRMAA, Part D beneficiary premiums, state payments for Part D, federal general-fund contributions, and Treasury trust-fund securities. Each layer is governed by a separate legal logic. Each layer produces distinct household consequences. Each layer explains why Medicare is not only a health entitlement, but a central component of the American social-insurance balance sheet.

1.3 Statutory Distinctions: Entitlement vs. Voluntary Eligibility

The statutory grammar of Medicare requires a sharp distinction between entitlement and voluntary eligibility. Entitlement describes a legally matured right to Medicare coverage produced by age, disability, End-Stage Renal Disease, Amyotrophic Lateral Sclerosis, Railroad Retirement Board status, or sufficient covered employment. Voluntary eligibility describes a narrower legal permission to purchase coverage after the individual fails to satisfy the insured-status rules that normally produce premium-free Hospital Insurance. The distinction is not semantic. It determines whether Part A arrives without a monthly premium, whether Part B may be declined and later reacquired only through time-limited enrollment machinery, whether a household must expect quarterly premium billing, whether an employer group health plan remains primary or secondary, and whether other tax-subsidized health coverage terminates or becomes financially unrecoverable. As established by the official 2026 Medicare handbook, most persons do not pay a Part A premium when the beneficiary or spouse paid Medicare taxes while working for the required period, but persons lacking premium-free status may purchase Part A, with 2026 monthly premiums specified at either \$311 or \$565 depending on covered-work history.

The controlling work-history standard is forty quarters of coverage, commonly expressed as forty Social Security and Medicare credits. A contrary formulation of forty-two quarters is not the governing federal standard. The Social Security Administration explains that in 2026 one Social Security and Medicare credit is earned for each $1,890 of covered earnings, with a maximum of four credits available in a calendar year; therefore, forty credits generally represent ten years of covered employment rather than forty calendar quarters in a literal chronological sense. (Social Security) The monetary value of the credit is not frozen. The SSA quarter-of-coverage table explains that after 1978 the earnings amount required for one quarter of coverage changes automatically each year with changes in the national average wage index; in 2026, the required amount is $1,890. (Social Security) The actuarial importance of this indexing mechanism is that Medicare insured status remains tied to covered labor-market participation while the monetary threshold for earning credit adjusts to wage growth.

Premium-free Part A is the most concrete household manifestation of the FICA track. The official Social Security description of Medicare parts states that Part A is free when the worker paid Medicare taxes for at least ten years, and that eligibility may also arise from the work record of a current or former spouse. (Social Security) The 2026 Medicare handbook states the same rule in Medicare-administrative form: Part A usually carries no monthly premium when the beneficiary or spouse paid Medicare taxes for the required period. This framework reveals why Part A differs from commercial insurance. The relevant capitalization event is not the purchase of coverage at age sixty-five, but the long-run accumulation of covered wages and Medicare-tax contributions. A beneficiary who satisfies insured status has already capitalized the Hospital Insurance system through payroll taxation; a beneficiary who lacks that status enters a voluntary premium-buyer channel.

Spousal crossover entitlement is an essential feature of this social-insurance design. A spouse's work record may supply the required Medicare-tax foundation where the applicant's own record is insufficient, thereby converting what would otherwise be premium-buyer status into premium-free Part A. SSA's public Medicare description recognizes eligibility based on a current or former spouse's work, while SSA family-benefit materials separately recognize ex-spouse eligibility when the prior marriage lasted at least ten years. (Social Security) For Medicare-specific premium-Hospital Insurance administration, SSA Program Operations Manual System material identifies divorced-spouse premium reduction status when the divorced spouse was married to the number holder for at least ten years immediately before the divorce became final and the number holder had at least thirty quarters of coverage at the time of divorce. (Social Security Administration) The crossover rule is therefore not a courtesy doctrine; it is a derivative insured-status framework embedded in the same wage-record system that supports retirement, disability, survivor, and Medicare determinations.

The premium-buyer matrix imposes a different legal and financial posture. CMS's 2026 premium update states that voluntary enrollees may qualify for a reduced Part A premium when they have thirty to thirty-nine quarters of covered employment, and it specifies the 2026 Part A base premium at $565 per month, the forty-five percent reduced premium at $311 per month for those with thirty to thirty-nine quarters of coverage, the ten percent surcharge on the base premium at $621.50, and the reduced premium with surcharge at $342.10. (CMS) The official 2026 Medicare handbook also states that, in most cases, a person who chooses to buy Part A must also have Part B and must pay monthly premiums for both, while a person who does not buy Part A may still buy Part B if otherwise eligible. The legal consequence is that voluntary Part A eligibility produces a bundled premium problem: Hospital Insurance may no longer be costless, Medical Insurance still requires a monthly premium, and delayed purchase may attach a late-enrollment surcharge.

The Part A late-enrollment penalty illustrates the distinction between entitlement and purchase. As established by the official 2026 Medicare handbook, an individual not eligible for premium-free Part A who does not buy Part A when first eligible may face a ten percent monthly premium increase, and that higher premium applies for twice the number of years during which Part A could have been held but was not purchased. This penalty does not apply to the ordinary premium-free Part A beneficiary in the same way because the entitlement itself is not priced as a voluntary monthly purchase. The penalty attaches to the elective failure to purchase premium Part A when statutory opportunity exists. Thus, Medicare law stratifies households into three materially different categories: those with premium-free entitlement through sufficient covered employment or derivative record status, those with partial work history who face a reduced premium, and those with inadequate work history who face the full premium.

Disability-based entitlement follows a separate chronology. Under the official 2026 Medicare handbook, individuals under age sixty-five who have a disability receive Part A and Part B automatically after receiving twenty-four months of Social Security disability benefits or certain Railroad Retirement Board disability benefits. SSA disability materials state the same core rule: the first twenty-four months of disability benefit entitlement are the Medicare qualifying period, and SSA counts one month for each month of disability benefit entitlement. (Social Security) SSA Program Operations Manual System material frames the rule with greater technical precision: disabled Hospital Insurance entitlement generally begins after the person has been entitled or deemed entitled to disability benefits for twenty-four months, meaning Hospital Insurance begins with the first day of the twenty-fifth month of disability-benefit entitlement. (Social Security Administration)

The twenty-four-month disability rule produces a file-based, not merely medical, enrollment event. A clinical impairment does not automatically produce Medicare. The Social Security disability determination must first establish Title II entitlement, and the Medicare waiting period is then measured by months of disability-benefit entitlement rather than by the day a diagnosis was received. The official 2026 Medicare handbook confirms that automatic enrollment materials arrive before the coverage event: a person enrolled automatically receives the Medicare card three months before the sixty-fifth birthday or before the twenty-fifth month of disability benefits, and Part B premiums are retained through Social Security or Railroad Retirement Board benefits if Part B is not rejected before the coverage start date. This creates a two-stage administrative pipeline. SSA establishes disability-benefit entitlement and monthly payment status, then the Medicare enrollment record matures into Part A and Part B entitlement at the twenty-fifth month unless a recognized exception alters the sequence.

Retroactive disability determinations complicate the chronology. CMS program-policy material explains that persons entitled to SSDI benefits become entitled to premium-free Medicare Part A after twenty-four months, and that a favorable SSDI award issued years after the initial application may make Part A entitlement retroactive where the SSDI start date is more than twenty-four months in the past. (CMS) CMS Part C and Part D enrollment guidance also recognizes retroactive Medicare entitlement determinations by SSA, stating that when SSA makes a Medicare entitlement determination for a retroactive date, Part D eligibility begins in the month of notification and continues for three additional months. The interaction is crucial. A retroactive disability onset or entitlement date can shift the effective date of Part A and Part B backward, while drug-plan and managed-care election rights may operate from the notification month or from specific election-period rules. The file does not merely record history; it reorganizes the legal calendar.

The disability pathway has a further household effect because Medicare can arrive before age sixty-five and before the ordinary Medigap and retirement assumptions embedded in many household plans. The 2026 Medicare source packet notes that persons under age sixty-five may have Medicare due to disability or ESRD, but federal law generally does not require insurers to sell Medigap policies to persons under age sixty-five, while some states impose additional rights. In generic federal analysis, this means that disability-based entitlement solves the federal Medicare eligibility problem but may not solve the supplemental risk-transfer problem. A younger disabled beneficiary may receive Original Medicare while facing a distinct secondary-coverage environment from the age-sixty-five enrollee. This distinction later becomes central in the manuscript's treatment of standardized Medigap, Part C managed-care enrollment, and household dependency separation.

End-Stage Renal Disease forms a separate statutory exception because it is not restricted to age sixty-five and does not require the ordinary twenty-four-month SSDI Medicare waiting period. The official Medicare handbook states that a person with ESRD who wants Medicare must sign up, and that the dialysis facility can assist with the End Stage Renal Disease Medical Evidence Report, Form CMS-2728, in the ESRD Quality Reporting System; once completed, the facility may give a copy or help submit it to Social Security. Medicare's ESRD public guidance defines ESRD eligibility as operating differently from other Medicare eligibility pathways, including potential retroactive coverage up to twelve months before the application month where the person was already eligible. (Medicare) The administrative architecture is therefore medical-evidence driven, but still mediated through Social Security intake and Medicare file creation.

For dialysis, the baseline rule is a three-month waiting period with coverage beginning the first day of the fourth month of continuous dialysis treatments. Medicare's kidney-dialysis and transplant publication states that when Medicare is elected because of ESRD and the person is on dialysis, coverage usually starts on the first day of the fourth month of continuous dialysis treatments; the publication illustrates the sequence as first, second, and third months of dialysis followed by Medicare coverage in the fourth month. (Medicare) Medicare's online ESRD guidance states the same rule and adds that the four-month waiting period begins even if Medicare has not yet been elected. (Medicare) This distinction matters because group health coverage may be the only payer during the first three months unless another coverage source exists.

The home-dialysis training exception accelerates entitlement. Medicare ESRD guidance states that coverage may begin as early as the first month of a regular dialysis course when the individual participates in a home dialysis training program offered by a Medicare-certified training facility during the first three months, the physician expects completion of training and capacity for home dialysis, and the individual maintains a regular dialysis course during the otherwise applicable waiting period. (Medicare) The ESRD booklet likewise states that coverage can begin in the first month of dialysis if a Medicare-certified training facility offers home dialysis training during the first three months and the physician expects the person to finish training and perform home dialysis. (Medicare) The statutory logic is evident: federal law rewards early home-dialysis training participation by advancing Medicare entitlement to the clinical start point of dialysis rather than waiting until the fourth month.

Kidney-transplant timing follows a different set of entitlement accelerators. Medicare's ESRD guidance states that Medicare coverage can begin the month of admission to a Medicare-certified hospital for a kidney transplant, or for services needed before the transplant, if the transplant takes place in that same month or within the next two months. If the transplant is delayed more than two months after admission for transplant-related services, coverage can begin two months before the transplant. (Medicare) This rule recognizes that transplant preparation can itself be part of the Medicare-covered ESRD episode. It also reveals that the entitlement month is not simply the surgery month. Admission timing, transplant scheduling, delay duration, and hospital certification status all control the federal coverage date.

The ESRD coordination period is one of the most technical payer-order rules in Medicare. The official 2026 handbook states that where Medicare eligibility is based on ESRD and group health plan coverage exists through employment or former employment, the group health plan pays first for the first thirty months after Medicare eligibility, and Medicare pays first after that thirty-month period. Medicare's ESRD booklet explains the same coordination structure in more granular terms: once Medicare eligibility begins because of permanent kidney failure, an employer or union group health plan continues to pay first during a coordination period, Medicare pays second, and that coordination period lasts thirty months. The same source states that the thirty-month period begins the first month the person would be eligible for ESRD Medicare, usually the fourth month of dialysis, even if the person has not enrolled; if home dialysis training or transplant occurs during the initial three-month waiting period, the coordination period starts earlier. (Medicare)

The regulatory foundation for this structure appears in 42 CFR Part 411, Subpart F. The eCFR states that Subpart F sets special rules for individuals eligible for or entitled to Medicare on the basis of ESRD while also covered under group health plans, and that group health plans may not take into account ESRD-based Medicare eligibility or entitlement during the coordination period specified in § 411.162. (eCFR) Section 411.162 provides that Medicare is secondary to a group health plan with respect to benefits payable to an ESRD-entitled individual for services furnished during the coordination period, and it states that the employer-size and current-employment requirements applicable to aged and disabled Medicare Secondary Payer rules do not apply to ESRD beneficiaries. (eCFR) Consequently, the ESRD coordination rule is not merely another version of the twenty-employee aged-worker rule. It is a pathology-specific payer-order regime that can preserve group-plan primary liability without regard to employer size or active employment status.

ALS occupies the opposite end of the disability waiting-period spectrum. The official 2026 Medicare handbook states that a person with Amyotrophic Lateral Sclerosis automatically receives Part A and Part B in the month Social Security disability benefits begin. SSA's ALS policy material states that, effective July 1, 2001, a disability beneficiary diagnosed with ALS is not required to serve the twenty-four-month Medicare waiting period, and that the Medicare entitlement date is the date of disability-benefit entitlement or July 1, 2001, whichever is later. (Social Security Administration) SSA POMS further states that since July 1, 2001 the twenty-four-month Medicare waiting period is waived for disabled claimants with ALS, and that for a person diagnosed with ALS the Medicare entitlement date is the date of entitlement to disability insurance benefits, disabled widow or widower benefits, or childhood disability benefits based on the ALS diagnosis. (Social Security Administration)

The ALS acceleration reflects a legislative judgment that the ordinary two-year disability Medicare waiting period is incompatible with the disease trajectory. The Social Security Administration separately notes that there is no SSDI cash-benefit waiting period when disability results from ALS for approvals on or after July 23, 2020, while Medicare entitlement for ALS already bypasses the twenty-four-month Medicare waiting period under earlier Medicare-specific legislation. (Social Security) The resulting file logic is compressed: SSA disability entitlement and Medicare entitlement are brought into temporal proximity rather than separated by twenty-four months. This produces immediate household consequences for premium billing, Part B acceptance, drug coverage timing, employer coverage coordination, and the termination of other subsidies dependent on not having Medicare.

The foregoing entitlement pathways explain why the Household Medicare Diagnostic Matrix must begin with household fact pattern rather than age alone. A premium-free Part A beneficiary with forty credits enters Medicare through a wage-record entitlement. A voluntary premium buyer enters through a purchase channel and may incur Part A surcharges if enrollment is delayed. A divorced spouse may derive Medicare status or premium reduction from another wage record, but only after the relevant marital-duration and record-based criteria are satisfied. A disabled beneficiary under age sixty-five may be enrolled automatically at the twenty-fifth month of disability-benefit entitlement, while a retroactive SSDI award may convert what appeared to be a future Medicare issue into a past-dated entitlement block. An ESRD beneficiary may face a dialysis waiting period, home-training acceleration, transplant-related entitlement, and a thirty-month group-plan coordination period. An ALS beneficiary may bypass the ordinary twenty-four-month Medicare waiting period altogether.

The financial stakes are severe because each pathway has external effects beyond Medicare. The official handbook states that once an individual is considered eligible for premium-free Part A, or already has Part A with a premium, Marketplace financial help for Marketplace premiums and other medical costs generally ends, and continuation of such help may require repayment at federal income tax filing. IRS premium tax credit regulation similarly states that government-sponsored coverage such as Medicare generally removes the covered person from the premium tax credit coverage family for months of government-program eligibility, subject to the rule that eligibility must exist for every day of the month. Thus, a retroactive disability, ESRD, or Part A entitlement date can alter not only medical claims responsibility, but also household premium tax credit reconciliation, Form 1095-A reporting, and Form 8962 repayment exposure.

The same cross-coupling appears in employer-sponsored secondary systems. The 2026 handbook states that if group health plan or retiree coverage is secondary, Part B may be required before that secondary coverage will pay; the handbook also states that the primary payer pays up to the limits of coverage, the secondary payer pays only if uncovered costs remain, and the secondary payer may not pay all remaining costs. In the ESRD context, the thirty-month coordination period can cause the group health plan to remain primary even while Medicare eligibility has matured. In the disability context, an automatic Medicare record may change payer order and premium obligations before the household has reorganized existing coverage. In the premium-buyer context, failure to purchase Part A and Part B when required may cause retiree or continuation coverage to pay little or nothing.

Section 1.3 therefore establishes a controlling proposition for the remainder of the manuscript: Medicare entitlement is not a single statutory doorway. It is a set of separate legal channels tied to covered employment, derivative family records, disability-benefit entitlement, renal-failure evidence, transplant timing, ALS diagnosis, and voluntary premium purchase rules. Each channel has its own effective-date grammar. Each effective date can change premium liability, Part D election timing, Marketplace tax-credit eligibility, employer-plan payer order, Medigap access, and family coverage stability. The Household Medicare Diagnostic Matrix is designed precisely for this reason: it forces the household file to be audited by entitlement source, credit count, marital record, disability month, ESRD eligibility month, and payer-order period before any downstream coverage structure is evaluated.

Chapter 2: Structural Anatomy of Core Federal Entitlements (Parts A & B)

2.1 Part A Inpatient Institutional Architecture

Part A is the institutional core of Medicare's original federal benefit design. It does not merely reimburse a hospital bill; it organizes acute illness, post-acute stabilization, skilled rehabilitation, and home-based recovery into a sequence of legally defined coverage environments. The 2026 Medicare handbook identifies Part A as Hospital Insurance that helps cover inpatient hospital care, skilled nursing facility care, hospice care, and home health care, thereby placing institutional risk at the foundation of Medicare's federal social-insurance architecture. The actuarial structure is not built around a simple calendar-year deductible analogous to ordinary commercial insurance. It is built around the benefit period, a statutory operational unit historically associated with the "spell-of-illness" model, under which coverage liability attaches to an episode of institutional need and then resets only after a specified period without inpatient hospital care or skilled nursing facility skilled care. CMS's 2026 definitions state that a benefit period begins the day an individual is admitted as an inpatient in a hospital or skilled nursing facility and ends only after no inpatient hospital care or skilled care in a skilled nursing facility has been received for sixty consecutive days.

The benefit period is therefore the central temporal grammar of Part A. It begins with formal inpatient institutional admission, not with the first medical symptom, the first emergency-room encounter, the first outpatient observation hour, or the first physician consultation. CMS states that inpatient status requires formal hospital admission with a physician's order, while outpatient status can include emergency services, observation services, outpatient clinic services, laboratory tests, and X-rays without formal inpatient admission, even where the patient remains overnight inside the hospital building. This distinction is doctrinally important because Part A institutional liability is not activated merely by physical presence inside a hospital. The legal status of the encounter controls whether inpatient hospital cost-sharing, skilled nursing facility qualification, and post-acute sequencing become available under the Part A architecture.

The operational logic differs fundamentally from a calendar-year deductible. A commercial medical policy commonly accumulates cost sharing during a January-to-December annual measurement period. By contrast, the Part A benefit period can begin, close, and begin again within the same calendar year. CMS states that once a benefit period ends after sixty consecutive days out of inpatient hospital care, a new benefit period starts upon later readmission, and the Part A deductible must be paid each time a new benefit period begins; CMS further states that this can occur multiple times in a calendar year. The definition section reinforces the same premise by stating that the inpatient hospital deductible is owed for each benefit period and that there is no limit to the number of benefit periods.

The financial consequence is a cyclical risk-transfer mechanism rather than an annual maximum-exposure design. A household may encounter a full Part A deductible in January, satisfy the institutional cost-sharing requirements of that benefit period, remain out of inpatient hospital or skilled nursing facility skilled care for sixty consecutive days, and then face another full Part A deductible after a later readmission within the same calendar year. Under CMS Part A benefit specifications for 2026, each new inpatient hospital benefit period requires a $1,736 deductible before Medicare begins paying for the covered inpatient stay. The statutory architecture therefore imposes a reset risk: clinical recovery sufficient to close the benefit period can also restore the household's exposure to a new full institutional deductible.

The days 1 through 60 tier represents the initial acute-care stabilization layer. During this tier, the beneficiary owes the Part A inpatient hospital deductible for the benefit period, and after that deductible has been satisfied, no daily coinsurance is owed for days 1 through 60 of covered inpatient hospital care. CMS states that in 2026, days 1 through 60 require payment of the $1,736 Part A deductible followed by $0 per day during the first sixty days of the benefit period. This is not an annual entrance fee. It is a per-benefit-period liability that attaches to each new spell of institutional illness. The same dollar amount may therefore be encountered repeatedly if the patient's institutional episodes are separated by the required sixty-day break in inpatient hospital or skilled nursing facility skilled care.

The deductible's per-benefit-period character transforms readmission timing into a capital-preservation variable. A readmission before the sixty-day closure point continues the same benefit period; a readmission after the sixty-day closure point opens a new benefit period with a new deductible. CMS's statement that the benefit period ends once the beneficiary has been out of the hospital for sixty consecutive days, and that admission after those sixty days begins a new benefit period requiring a new Part A deductible, gives the timing rule its operative financial force. This structure is the statutory basis for the readmission problem introduced in the Household Medicare Diagnostic Matrix: an unexpected return on day 59 and an unexpected return on day 61 can produce different cost-sharing consequences even where the clinical facts appear nearly identical to the family unit.

The days 61 through 90 tier introduces a daily per-diem liability. CMS states that in 2026, days 61 through 90 of a hospital inpatient benefit period require payment of

$434 per day. The mathematical relationship is visible from the 2026 inpatient deductible: $434 is one-fourth of the $1,736 Part A deductible. This proportional design reflects a statutory indexing structure in which extended inpatient utilization above the initial sixty-day window produces daily cost-sharing rather than a second full deductible. The actuarial meaning is that Medicare continues to bear most covered institutional risk, but the beneficiary assumes a measurable daily share as the hospital stay moves beyond the ordinary acute-stabilization interval.

The days 61 through 90 tier is also where the institutional episode begins to diverge from common household expectations. A beneficiary may believe that a deductible has already been paid and that the remainder of the hospital stay is therefore fully covered. Part A does not operate that way. The deductible covers the entrance into the benefit period, while the extended-stay tier creates a separate daily copayment. CMS identifies copayments as fixed amounts owed as a share of benefit cost after deductibles, and the 2026 Part A schedule fixes the extended-stay inpatient amount at $434 per day for days 61 through 90. The legal distinction between deductible and copayment is therefore essential: the household's first liability is episodic, while the second liability is daily.

The lifetime reserve matrix governs catastrophic inpatient hospital stays beyond day 90. CMS defines lifetime reserve days as additional days Original Medicare will pay for when a beneficiary remains in a hospital for more than ninety days, with a total of sixty reserve days available during the beneficiary's lifetime; for each reserve day, Medicare pays covered costs except for a daily coinsurance amount. In 2026, the lifetime reserve day amount is $868 per day for days 91 through 150, and those days draw from the finite lifetime pool of sixty non-renewable reserve days. The mathematical relationship is exact within the published 2026 cost structure: $868 is twice the day 61 through 90 per-diem amount of $434, and it is one-half of the $1,736 inpatient deductible.

Lifetime reserve days differ from ordinary benefit-period days in legal character. Days 1 through 90 renew with each new benefit period. Lifetime reserve days do not. Once a reserve day has been used, it is consumed permanently from the federal lifetime allocation. CMS states that the beneficiary has a total of sixty reserve days that can be used once during the lifetime. The actuarial consequence is that a prolonged hospitalization can deplete a finite reserve account that no future benefit period restores. A beneficiary who uses twenty lifetime reserve days during one catastrophic stay retains forty for all future inpatient hospital episodes. A beneficiary who uses all sixty has no remaining federal reserve-day cushion for any later stay exceeding ninety days in a benefit period.

The exhaustion threshold produces the sharpest liability shift in Part A inpatient design. CMS states that after day 150 of the benefit period, the beneficiary pays all costs. This rule reflects the outer boundary of Original Medicare inpatient hospital coverage under the benefit-period model: sixty ordinary inpatient days after the deductible, thirty extended-stay coinsurance days, sixty lifetime reserve days with a higher daily coinsurance, and then full cost exposure after the statutory hospital-day allocation has been exhausted. The phrase "all costs" is not a modest copayment category. It marks the termination of Medicare payment for the inpatient hospital day under that Part A benefit-period sequence, subject only to other coverage that may exist outside Original Medicare.

The catastrophic hospital-stay sequence also demonstrates why Original Medicare's institutional architecture cannot be analyzed solely by premium price. The financial risk is embedded in the cost-sharing tiers and in the absence of a general annual maximum out-of-pocket limit for Original Medicare. CMS states elsewhere in the 2026 handbook that Original Medicare has no yearly out-of-pocket limit unless supplemental coverage such as Medigap, Medicaid, employer, retiree, or union coverage exists. The inpatient matrix is therefore a principal location where capital protection becomes a structural issue rather than a discretionary preference. A household exposed only to the federal Original Medicare cost-sharing schedule faces episodic deductibles, extended-stay per-diem liabilities, finite lifetime reserve days, and potential full liability beyond day 150.

Skilled nursing facility care is the post-acute companion to the inpatient hospital architecture, but it is not a long-term custodial care benefit. CMS states that Medicare covers short-term skilled nursing facility care after a three-day minimum medically necessary inpatient hospital stay, excluding the day of discharge, for an illness or injury related to the hospital stay. CMS also states that covered skilled nursing facility services include semi-private rooms, meals, skilled nursing and therapy services, and other medically necessary services and supplies for a limited time. The institutional requirement is clinical and legal: a physician must certify the need for daily skilled care, such as intravenous medications or physical therapy, that as a practical matter can be received only as a skilled nursing facility inpatient.

The three-day inpatient rule makes hospital status decisive. Observation time does not satisfy the same requirement merely because the patient stayed overnight in the hospital. CMS states that inpatient status depends on formal admission with a physician's order, while observation status remains outpatient even when it includes an overnight stay. Therefore, the hospital-to-SNF pathway depends not only on clinical need after discharge, but also on whether the preceding hospital episode was legally inpatient for the required duration. The Medicare Outpatient Observation Notice, issued when observation exceeds twenty-four hours, exists precisely because outpatient observation status affects payment and post-hospital care rights.

The skilled nursing facility benefit follows a 100-day benefit-period matrix. CMS states that each skilled nursing facility benefit period requires the same $1,736 Part A deductible before Medicare starts to pay, but no additional Part A deductible applies to skilled nursing facility care when the deductible already was paid for hospital care in the same benefit period. Days 1 through 20 of covered skilled nursing facility care require $0 per day after satisfaction of the Part A deductible, while days 21 through 100 require $217 per day in 2026. The amount of $217 is one-eighth of the $1,736 Part A deductible and one-half of the inpatient extended-stay amount of $434, reflecting a lower but still substantial post-acute daily exposure.

The termination point is absolute within the federal skilled nursing facility benefit-period structure. CMS states that days 101 and beyond require payment of all costs. This is not a reduction in payment level; it is the exhaustion of covered skilled nursing facility days in that benefit period. The benefit renews only after the benefit period closes under the sixty-day rule. CMS states that the skilled nursing facility benefit period ends when the beneficiary stops getting skilled nursing facility care for sixty consecutive days; after readmission following those sixty days, a new benefit period starts, and a new Part A deductible must be paid. The post-acute rule therefore mirrors the inpatient hospital rule: time outside skilled institutional care can restore a new benefit period, but restoration also resets deductible exposure.

The skilled nursing facility benefit contains an important clinical-protection principle. CMS states that skilled nursing care or therapy may be covered when necessary to improve or maintain the current condition, and that a discharge may be appealed where skilled care or therapy remains necessary to keep the condition from worsening. This statement rejects a simplistic improvement-only model. The skilled benefit may be implicated where maintenance therapy prevents deterioration, provided the statutory and administrative requirements are otherwise satisfied. In actuarial terms, the SNF benefit protects a defined rehabilitative or skilled-maintenance interval, not indefinite residence, custodial supervision, or general non-medical long-term care. CMS expressly states that Medicare does not cover non-medical long-term care.

Limited waiver environments complicate the three-day rule without dissolving it. CMS states that a beneficiary may not need the three-day minimum inpatient hospital stay if the physician participates in an Accountable Care Organization approved for a Skilled Nursing Facility Three-Day Rule Waiver, and that Medicare Advantage plans may also waive the three-day minimum hospital stay. For the purposes of a generic federal textbook, this exception must be treated structurally rather than commercially. The baseline federal Original Medicare rule is the three-day medically necessary inpatient stay; authorized waiver models and alternative federally regulated delivery structures may alter the pathway, but those variations do not erase the default Original Medicare standard.

Home health services occupy a different post-acute location because they are not measured by the same 100-day institutional stay schedule. CMS states that Medicare covers home health services under Part A and Part B, including medically necessary part-time or intermittent skilled nursing care, physical therapy, speech-language pathology services, or continued occupational therapy services. Covered home health services may also include medical social services, part-time or intermittent home health aide services, durable medical equipment, and medical supplies for home use. The coverage structure is therefore function-based: skilled or therapy need, medical necessity, homebound status, provider certification, physician or eligible practitioner order, and Medicare-certified agency delivery.

The homebound requirement is a legal status, not an informal description of limited mobility. CMS states that Medicare covers home health services as long as the beneficiary needs part-time or intermittent skilled services and remains homebound. Homebound status means difficulty leaving home without help such as a cane, wheelchair, walker, crutches, special transportation, or another person because of illness or injury; it also includes situations where leaving home is not recommended because of the condition, or where leaving home is normally impossible without major effort. The statutory premise is that home health substitutes for medically necessary skilled intervention in the home where ordinary access to outpatient care is functionally constrained.

The "part-time or intermittent" requirement imposes a quantitative ceiling on the delivery model. CMS states that part-time or intermittent skilled nursing care and home health aide services may be available up to eight hours per day combined, for a maximum of twenty-eight hours per week, or up to thirty-five hours per week in some limited situations. A physician or other eligible practitioner, such as a nurse practitioner, clinical nurse specialist, or physician assistant, must assess the patient face to face before certifying the need for home health services, must order the care, and a Medicare-certified home health agency must provide it. These requirements distinguish home health from domestic assistance, private-duty custodial support, household maintenance, or indefinite personal care.

The cost-sharing architecture of home health differs from inpatient hospital and skilled nursing facility care. CMS states that the beneficiary pays nothing for covered home health services, but Medicare-covered durable medical equipment used in the home requires payment of 20 percent of the Medicare-approved amount, and the Part

B deductible applies. This bifurcation reinforces the mixed Part A and Part B character of home health. Skilled services may have no direct cost-sharing when covered, while equipment carries standard Part B cost-sharing logic. A household evaluating post-acute recovery cannot therefore treat all home-based care as free, all home equipment as included, or all non-institutional services as outside Medicare. The relevant question is whether the service is a covered home health service, a durable medical equipment item, or non-covered custodial support.

The institutional architecture of Part A ultimately forces an actuarial audit of time, status, and care setting. Acute hospitalization produces a per-benefit-period deductible, an extended-stay daily liability, a finite lifetime reserve account, and possible full liability after day 150. Skilled nursing facility care requires a qualifying inpatient hospital stay unless a recognized waiver pathway applies, covers a limited 100-day post-acute interval per benefit period, imposes daily liability beginning on day 21, and terminates federal payment after day 100. Home health requires homebound status, intermittent skilled need, face-to-face assessment, practitioner certification, and delivery through a Medicare-certified home health agency. These are not isolated benefit descriptions. They are legal levers determining whether federal dollars, household assets, supplemental coverage, or secondary payers bear the next increment of care.

This specific interface addresses the exact multi-variable dilemma outlined in the Household Medicare Diagnostic Matrix. A readmission on day 59 after discharge from inpatient hospital care preserves the existing benefit-period frame because the sixty-day closure rule has not matured. A readmission on day 61 can initiate a new benefit period, impose a new $1,736 Part A deductible, and restart the hospital-day count. CMS's rule that a benefit period ends after sixty consecutive days out of inpatient hospital care or skilled nursing facility skilled care, combined with the rule that each new benefit period requires a new Part A deductible and may occur multiple times in a calendar year, supplies the controlling federal arithmetic. The financial difference between day 59 and day 61 is therefore not a clinical metaphor. It is the statutory hinge on which repeated household exposure to Part A institutional cost sharing can turn.

2.2 Part B Outpatient Supplementary Infrastructure

Part B is the federal medical-insurance counterpart to Part A's institutional hospital architecture. Where Part A organizes inpatient hospitalization, skilled nursing facility recovery, hospice, and certain home health services around benefit periods and institutional episodes, Part B organizes outpatient medical risk around an annual deductible, assignment-based reimbursement, medically necessary professional services, outpatient diagnostics, durable medical equipment, limited outpatient drugs, preventive interventions, and structured access to clinical research costs. CMS's 2026 Medicare handbook defines Part B as Medical Insurance that helps cover medically necessary doctors' services, outpatient care, some home health services, durable medical equipment, mental health services, limited outpatient prescription drugs, other medical services, and many preventive services. This division makes Part B the primary federal gateway for the continuous medical management of chronic illness, diagnostic surveillance, outpatient surgery, professional encounters, ambulatory therapeutics, medical equipment, and prevention-oriented screening. Its fiscal exposure is not episodic in the same manner as Part A. It is recurrent, distributed, claim-line driven, and actuarially open-ended.

The annual Part B deductible supplies the first layer of outpatient cost sharing. Under CMS Part B outpatient specifications for 2026, when the Part B deductible applies under Original Medicare, the beneficiary must pay all costs up to the Medicare-approved amount until the yearly deductible has been met; after satisfaction of the deductible, Medicare pays its share and the beneficiary typically pays 20 percent of the Medicare-approved amount when the physician or other provider accepts assignment. The 2026 deductible is $283, and the official 2026 Medicare cost fact sheet states that the deductible is paid once each year before Original Medicare starts to pay. CMS's 2026 Part B premium and deductible fact sheet further states that Medicare Part B premium, deductible, and coinsurance rates are determined each year according to provisions of the Social Security Act, and that the 2026 Part B deductible rose to $283 from $257 in 2025. (CMS)

The Part B deductible is structurally unlike the Part A inpatient deductible. The Part A deductible is assessed per benefit period, which can recur multiple times in one calendar year when the statutory benefit-period closure rule is satisfied. The Part B deductible is a calendar-year deductible. The 2026 CMS cost fact sheet states expressly that the $283 deductible is paid once each year before Original Medicare begins payment. This annual structure makes Part B more familiar to households accustomed to calendar-year insurance accounting; however, that superficial similarity should not obscure the deeper risk. The deductible is comparatively small relative to the major outpatient exposures that may follow, and the federal design does not terminate cost sharing after a conventional commercial maximum has been reached.

The 20 percent coinsurance layer is the central actuarial hazard. CMS states that, after satisfaction of the Part B deductible, Medicare pays its share and the beneficiary typically pays 20 percent of the Medicare-approved amount when the provider accepts assignment. CMS also states that Original Medicare has no yearly limit on out-of-pocket spending, although supplemental coverage such as Medigap, Medicaid, employer, retiree, or union coverage may impose different limits or absorb some liabilities. The phrase "typically pays 20 percent" carries technical meaning. It describes the ordinary assigned-claim structure for most Part B-covered professional and supplier services. It does not erase special copayment rules for certain hospital outpatient settings, excess-charge exposure where assignment is not accepted, or service-specific statutory exceptions. Nevertheless, the baseline financial architecture remains stark: Original Medicare does not contain a built-in annual maximum out-of-pocket ceiling for Part B services.

This absence of a built-in maximum out-of-pocket limit produces a theoretically uncapped liability stream under Original Medicare. In commercial insurance, an annual maximum out-of-pocket amount often terminates cost sharing for covered in-network care after the insured reaches a defined annual ceiling. Under Original Medicare, no such universal Part B ceiling exists. CMS's Original Medicare comparison material states that, for Part B-covered services, the ordinary liability is 20 percent of the Medicare-approved amount after the deductible, while the same comparison states that there is no yearly limit on Original Medicare out-of-pocket spending unless supplemental coverage exists. The actuarial consequence is not that every household will experience catastrophic outpatient spending, but that the federal baseline does not itself close the 20 percent liability pipeline. Repeated chemotherapy, dialysis-related services, advanced diagnostic imaging, durable medical equipment rental, physician-administered drugs, radiation therapy, outpatient surgery, and chronic disease management can create compounding exposure.

Provider assignment controls the legal amount against which the 20 percent liability is calculated. CMS defines the Medicare-approved amount as the payment amount that Original Medicare sets for a covered service or item, with Medicare paying its share and the beneficiary paying the remaining share of that amount. Where a physician, supplier, or other provider accepts assignment, the provider agrees to accept the Medicare-approved amount as payment for the covered service. CMS warns that use of providers that do not accept assignment can produce higher costs, and the definitions section identifies an excess charge as the difference between the Medicare-approved amount and the higher amount a legally permitted provider may charge under Original Medicare. Therefore, the outpatient liability analysis must distinguish three separate amounts: the deductible, the 20 percent coinsurance of the Medicare-approved amount, and any excess charge permitted when assignment is not accepted.

Durable medical equipment constitutes one of the most regulated Part B benefit gates because it converts clinical necessity into reusable physical capital deployed in the home. CMS's 2026 handbook states that Medicare covers medically necessary items such as oxygen and oxygen equipment, walkers, and hospital beds when a physician or other health care provider orders them for use in the home; most such items must be rented, some can be purchased, and higher-cost equipment such as wheelchairs and hospital beds becomes the beneficiary's property after 13 months of rental payments. The beneficiary pays 20 percent of the Medicare-approved amount, and the Part B deductible applies. Federal regulation defines durable medical equipment as equipment furnished by a supplier or home health agency that can withstand repeated use, has an expected life of at least three years, is primarily and customarily used to serve a medical purpose, generally is not useful to an individual absent illness or injury, and is appropriate for use in the home (42 CFR § 414.202). (eCFR)

The DME coverage gate therefore has multiple documentary elements. The item must be medically necessary. It must be ordered by a treating physician or other recognized health care provider. It must be intended for use in the home. It must satisfy the regulatory durability, medical-purpose, non-utility-without-illness, and home-use criteria. It must be furnished through a Medicare-enrolled supplier or qualifying home health agency under applicable payment rules. CMS's 2026 handbook also makes assignment central to DME liability: participating suppliers must accept assignment, thereby limiting the beneficiary to the Part B deductible and coinsurance on the Medicare-approved amount, while non-participating suppliers may create additional charges or require full upfront payment for unassigned claims, followed by later Medicare reimbursement after claim processing. For rented DME, assignment must be verified for all rental months because a supplier's refusal to assign a rental claim can shift immediate cash-flow risk onto the beneficiary.

The DMEPOS Competitive Bidding Program adds a purchasing and price-discipline layer to this equipment economy. CMS states that not all DMEPOS items are subject to competitive bidding; for selected products, suppliers submit bids through a web-based application, CMS evaluates bids based on factors including enrollment eligibility, financial stability, and bid price, and contracts are awarded to qualified suppliers that offer competitive pricing sufficient to meet beneficiary demand. CMS further states that contract suppliers must accept assignment on all claims for bid items and that Medicare pays a single payment amount for those items. (CMS) The program's statutory and administrative purpose is to protect the Medicare Trust Funds and lower beneficiary copayments by using regulated supplier competition rather than purely historical fee-schedule pricing. (CMS)

Part B immunization protocols demonstrate another form of outpatient benefit engineering. CMS's 2026 handbook identifies Part B as covering many preventive services, including shots or vaccines. Within that category, certain immunizations are financed as Part B preventive benefits rather than through the ordinary Part D drug pathway. CMS's 2026 handbook states that hepatitis B shots are covered when specified conditions exist, including incomplete vaccination history, unknown vaccination history, or a medium or high-risk condition or circumstance such as diabetes, End-Stage Renal Disease, or household exposure to hepatitis B; the beneficiary pays nothing for the shot when the provider accepts assignment. The same source identifies flu and pneumococcal vaccination as preventive interventions addressed within the Welcome to Medicare preventive visit, and plan summary material in the packet lists Medicare-covered vaccines including flu, Hepatitis B, pneumonia, and COVID-19 among covered preventive services.

The policy logic behind the Part B vaccine carveout is preventive capitalization. A vaccine that prevents high-cost hospitalization, respiratory compromise, renal infection complications, or avoidable infectious disease exposure reduces downstream utilization of Part A institutional resources and Part B acute medical services. CMS's 2026 Part B materials state that most covered preventive services cost nothing when furnished by a provider accepting assignment, although deductible, coinsurance, or both may apply to some preventive services or when a preventive service occurs in the same visit as a non-preventive service. Thus, immunization cost sharing is not governed by a universal vaccine maxim; it depends on the vaccine category, preventive-service status, assignment, and whether the encounter includes additional non-preventive clinical work. The federal architecture uses zero cost sharing to remove friction from selected immunizations while preserving ordinary Part B cost sharing for other medical components of the encounter.

Clinical research coverage represents a different outpatient frontier because the clinical object may be investigational while routine medical costs remain federally reimbursable. CMS's 2026 handbook states that clinical research studies test whether different types of medical care are safe and effective, and that for certain clinical research studies Medicare covers some costs, such as office visits and tests; depending on the treatment received, the beneficiary may pay 20 percent of the Medicare-approved amount, and the Part B deductible may apply. CMS's National Coverage Determination 310.1 states that Medicare covers the routine costs of qualifying clinical trials, together with reasonable and necessary items and services used to diagnose and treat complications arising from participation in clinical trials, for items and services furnished on or after September 19, 2000. (CMS)

The clinical-trial distinction is legally exacting. Medicare does not adopt an unrestricted obligation to finance every experimental intervention. The NCD covers routine costs of qualifying clinical trials, not all costs associated with research participation. CMS's NCD language ties coverage to qualifying trials, routine costs, and reasonable and necessary complication-related items and services. (CMS) The 2026 handbook's 20 percent and deductible warning reinforces that research participation does not neutralize ordinary Part B cost sharing for covered routine services. Medicare Advantage enrollment does not fully displace this Original Medicare research architecture because CMS's definitions in the source packet state that certain aspects of clinical trials may remain covered by Original Medicare even while a beneficiary remains enrolled in a Medicare Advantage plan.

Preventive medicine is the philosophical counterweight to reactive outpatient reimbursement. Part B began as supplementary medical insurance for physician and outpatient care, but the modern CMS landscape increasingly deploys Part B as a risk-detection and disease-interruption instrument. CMS's 2026 handbook states that Part B covers many preventive services and that most covered preventive services cost nothing when furnished by a provider accepting assignment. The Affordable Care Act accelerated this preventive orientation by removing cost sharing for specified Medicare preventive services, including services rated A or B by the United States Preventive Services Task Force when statutory and coverage criteria are met; CMS materials implementing the ACA preventive provisions describe the Act's elimination of the Part B deductible and coinsurance for many preventive services. (CMS)

The one-time Welcome to Medicare preventive visit is the entry-level preventive mapping event. CMS's 2026 handbook states that during the first 12 months of Part B enrollment, Medicare covers a Welcome to Medicare preventive visit; the visit is not a physical exam, and it includes review of medical and social history related to health, education and counseling regarding preventive services, certain screenings, shots or vaccines, and referrals for other care when needed. The visit is furnished at no cost when the provider accepts assignment, but additional tests or services during the same visit can trigger coinsurance, Part B deductible liability, or full liability if Medicare does not cover the added service. The distinction between a preventive visit and a routine physical exam is crucial because CMS lists routine physical exams among items that Original Medicare does not cover.

The annual wellness visit continues the preventive mapping function after the first year. CMS's 2026 handbook states that, after more than 12 months of Part B enrollment, Medicare covers a yearly Wellness visit once every 12 months. This visit is not a physical exam; it develops or updates a personalized prevention plan based on current health and risk factors, includes a health risk assessment questionnaire, and may include routine measurements, health advice, review of medical and family history, prescription review, advance care planning, and other risk-mapping components. The first yearly Wellness visit cannot occur within 12 months of Part B enrollment or within 12 months of the Welcome to Medicare preventive visit, and no prior Welcome to Medicare visit is required to qualify for later yearly Wellness visits.

The annual wellness visit also functions as a cognitive and behavioral risk-detection platform. CMS states that the provider performs a cognitive assessment to look for signs of dementia, including Alzheimer's disease, and that signs of cognitive impairment include difficulty remembering, learning new things, concentrating, managing finances, and making daily-life decisions. If cognitive impairment is suspected, Medicare covers a separate, more thorough cognitive-function review and care-plan design. CMS further states that the provider evaluates potential risk factors for substance use disorder and, where opioid medication is used, reviews the pain treatment plan, gives information about non-opioid treatment options, and may refer to a specialist as appropriate. This confirms that the wellness architecture is not a routine head-to-toe diagnostic physical. It is an actuarial risk registry translated into a clinical encounter.

Modernized screening coverage extends the same preventive-capital logic into disease-specific surveillance. CMS's 2026 handbook lists colorectal cancer screening among covered preventive services and, in the 2026 new-and-important section, notes that Medicare covers a wide range of colorectal cancer screenings, including computed tomography colonography. CMS's 2026 handbook also identifies lung cancer screenings, cardiovascular behavioral therapy, cardiovascular disease screenings, abdominal aortic aneurysm screening, bone mass measurements, mammography, cervical and vaginal cancer screening, hepatitis screenings, HIV screening, diabetes screenings, depression screening, prostate cancer screening, sexually transmitted infection screening, and tobacco-use counseling as Part B preventive-service categories across the covered-services section. These inclusions are not merely beneficiary conveniences. They represent a federal attempt to shift expenditure timing from late-stage acute illness toward earlier detection, risk stratification, behavioral intervention, and lower-cost therapeutic windows.

Screening cost sharing varies by service, but the preventive pattern is clear. CMS states that abdominal aortic aneurysm screening is covered once in a lifetime for at-risk beneficiaries with a referral, at no cost when the provider accepts assignment. CMS states that prostate-specific antigen testing is covered yearly after age 50 at no cost, while the digital rectal exam component carries 20 percent coinsurance, Part B deductible exposure, and possible hospital outpatient copayment. CMS states that hepatitis B screening, hepatitis C screening, and HIV screening can be covered at no cost when ordered and assignment conditions are satisfied. These examples demonstrate that preventive coverage is not a single cost-sharing rule. It is a service-specific statutory and administrative map, with zero-cost preventive treatment for many approved screenings and residual cost sharing for diagnostic, therapeutic, or non-preventive components.

The outpatient surgical sequence illustrates the capital-exposure problem that the Household Medicare Diagnostic Matrix is designed to surface. CMS states that tests such as X-rays, MRIs, CT scans, EKGs, and other diagnostic tests are generally covered with 20 percent coinsurance and the Part B deductible, while certain hospital outpatient diagnostic tests may also require a hospital copayment that can exceed 20 percent of the Medicare-approved amount, though in most cases it cannot exceed the Part A inpatient hospital deductible. Surgical dressing services, ambulance services, telehealth services, urgently needed care, chemotherapy in office or freestanding clinic settings, and many physician services similarly invoke the Part B deductible and 20 percent cost-sharing framework when covered. The accumulation of separate outpatient claim lines can therefore produce substantial liability even without inpatient admission.

This specific interface addresses the exact multi-variable dilemma outlined in the Household Medicare Diagnostic Matrix. A household may correctly identify Medicare eligibility, enrollment status, and physician access while still misunderstanding the outpatient exposure embedded in Original Medicare. An uncovered specialized medical necessity, a supplier that does not accept assignment, an outpatient surgical sequence with facility copayments, a high-cost imaging cascade, or a prolonged physician-administered therapeutic regimen can create compounding liabilities because the federal baseline lacks a universal Part B maximum out-of-pocket limit. CMS states the controlling rule plainly: after the yearly deductible, the ordinary assigned-claim exposure is typically 20 percent of the Medicare-approved amount, and Original Medicare has no yearly out-of-pocket limit absent supplemental coverage. The actuarial result is that Part B is simultaneously the preventive engine of modern Medicare and the principal source of open-ended outpatient coinsurance risk under the original federal benefit structure.

2.3 The Statutory Exclusions Matrix

Original Medicare is not a universal health-services entitlement. Its federal design covers defined categories of medically necessary institutional care, professional medical treatment, outpatient services, durable medical equipment, preventive interventions, and limited post-acute recovery, but it does not absorb every cost associated with aging, bodily maintenance, sensory decline, oral health deterioration, residential support, or ordinary personal assistance. Under CMS Part A and Part B exclusion specifications in the 2026 Medicare handbook, Medicare expressly states that it "doesn't cover everything," and that services outside Part A or Part B coverage must be financed by the beneficiary unless another coverage source applies; CMS then identifies several excluded categories, including long-term care, eye exams for prescription eyeglasses and corrected contact lenses, routine physical exams, hearing aids and fitting exams, and most dental care. The exclusion matrix is therefore not an accidental gap in administrative drafting. It is a deliberate statutory boundary between medical insurance and ordinary life-maintenance expenditure.

The conceptual error most likely to distort household planning is the assumption that Medicare entitlement equals comprehensive gerontological finance. That assumption collapses multiple legal categories into one misleading conclusion. Part A and Part B are federal health-insurance entitlements, not a universal elder-support annuity. Part A addresses institutional hospital risk, skilled nursing facility recovery, hospice, and home health under specified conditions. Part B addresses medically necessary physician services, outpatient care, durable medical equipment, mental health services, limited outpatient prescription drugs, and many preventive services. Yet the same federal source architecture excludes broad maintenance categories that may be predictable, expensive, and clinically meaningful. The statutory distinction is not whether a service affects health in a broad biological sense. The distinction is whether Congress and CMS have placed the service inside a defined Medicare benefit category.

This negative space performs an actuarial function. By excluding routine dental care, ordinary refractive vision correction, hearing aids, fitting examinations, routine physical examinations, and non-medical custodial long-term care, the Original Medicare baseline transfers substantial predictable and semi-predictable costs back to households. Under the 2026 CMS framework, Original Medicare may leave such costs to personal assets, Medicaid where eligibility exists, separate private coverage, employer or retiree arrangements, or federally regulated private delivery models that may offer supplemental benefits; however, those alternative arrangements do not alter the Original Medicare statutory baseline. The exclusion matrix therefore functions as a capital-risk transfer mechanism. It identifies the precise point at which federal medical insurance stops and household balance-sheet exposure begins.

Routine outpatient dental care is the clearest structural blind spot. Oral disease is not medically trivial; periodontal infection, mastication failure, denture instability, nutritional compromise, diabetes interaction, cardiovascular comorbidity, cancer-treatment preparation, and medication-related oral complications can all shape health outcomes. Nevertheless, the federal Medicare entitlement historically segregates routine oral maintenance from the core medical-insurance package. Under CMS Original Medicare exclusions in the 2026 handbook, most dental care is outside the Part A and Part B benefit design; CMS gives routine cleanings, fillings, tooth extractions, and dentures as examples of services and items that Original Medicare generally does not cover. This language is broad enough to expose the central policy choice: oral health maintenance is not treated as a general federally insured medical category under Original Medicare.

The exclusion of routine dental services is especially consequential because dental expenditure often follows an aging curve. Tooth loss, bone resorption, dry mouth, periodontal disease, prosthetic instability, crown failure, bridge failure, and extraction sequences frequently arise after retirement income has stabilized or declined. Under the CMS exclusion framework, routine cleanings, fillings, tooth removals, dentures, and most dental care remain outside Original Medicare's ordinary coverage liability, even though such services can influence nutrition, speech, infection risk, medication adherence, and social functioning. The actuarial consequence is a bifurcation between clinical importance and federal reimbursement status. A service may be highly important to physical health and still remain outside the Medicare benefit if it is classified as routine dental care rather than as a medically necessary component of a covered medical service.

Comprehensive prosthodontics illustrates the same logic. Dentures are expressly named by CMS as an example of an item Original Medicare generally does not cover in the dental category. Crowns, bridges, periodontal procedures, implant-supported restorations, and other comprehensive dental reconstructions are not converted into Original Medicare benefits merely because they are expensive or because oral function affects general health. The federal benefit boundary does not operate through household financial severity alone. It operates through statutory benefit classification. The absence of a general dental entitlement means that high-cost oral reconstruction may remain a private household liability unless another legally separate coverage source exists.

CMS recognizes narrow derivative medical-necessity exceptions, but those exceptions must not be misread as a general dental benefit. Under the 2026 Medicare handbook, Original Medicare may pay for some dental services closely related to certain covered medical services, including a heart valve repair or replacement, an organ transplant, cancer-related treatments, or dialysis services for End-Stage Renal Disease. The controlling analytical word is "closely." The dental service is not covered because routine dentistry has become a federal benefit. It is potentially covered because the dental service is operationally connected to a covered medical intervention. The exception is derivative, medical, and procedural; it is not comprehensive, preventive, prosthodontic, or routine.

This derivative structure is essential in oncology, transplant, cardiac, and renal contexts. A dental clearance or medically required dental service may be necessary to reduce infection risk, permit surgical sequencing, manage cancer-related treatment, or support ESRD-related dialysis services. Under CMS's stated exception categories, the dental service becomes intelligible to Medicare only through its relationship to the covered medical service. The same beneficiary may therefore encounter two very different legal outcomes: a dental extraction performed as ordinary dental treatment may fall outside Original Medicare, while a dental intervention closely related to a covered organ transplant, heart valve procedure, cancer treatment, or ESRD dialysis service may receive Medicare consideration. The clinical anatomy may look similar; the statutory classification may differ completely.

Refractive vision correction occupies a parallel exclusion category. Original Medicare distinguishes medical eye disease from ordinary refractive maintenance. Under CMS Part B outpatient specifications, Medicare does not usually cover eyeglasses or contact lenses; CMS separately identifies eye exams for prescription eyeglasses and corrected contact lenses among items and services Original Medicare does not cover. This framework treats ordinary refraction, eyeglass prescription maintenance, and standard corrective lenses as outside the federal medical-insurance entitlement. The policy boundary is not drawn at the eye as an organ. It is drawn between medical disease, surgical restoration, and routine optical correction.

The post-cataract exception demonstrates the exactness of the boundary. CMS states that Medicare covers one pair of eyeglasses with standard frames, or one set of contact lenses, after each cataract surgery that implants an intraocular lens. The contact lenses or eyeglasses must come from a Medicare-enrolled supplier, whether the beneficiary or provider submits the claim, and after the Part B deductible is met, the beneficiary pays 20 percent of the Medicare-approved amount for corrective lenses after cataract surgery with an intraocular lens. This rule is restorative and surgical. It does not create a general federal eyewear benefit. It compensates for a defined post-operative optical need after a covered cataract procedure involving intraocular lens implantation.

The narrowness of the post-cataract exception is critical for capital-risk analysis. A household may assume that vision decline after age sixty-five is a Medicare-covered sensory need. The CMS rule supplies a different result. Ordinary eyeglasses and contact lenses are generally excluded, while one set of corrective lenses after qualifying cataract surgery with an intraocular lens is covered under specified supplier and cost-sharing conditions. The financial baseline remains Part B rather than full federal absorption: the Part B deductible applies, and 20 percent coinsurance applies to the Medicare-approved amount. Thus, even the exception carries ordinary outpatient cost-sharing logic.

Glaucoma screening reflects the medical-disease side of the ophthalmic boundary. CMS states that Medicare covers glaucoma screening once every 12 months for persons at high risk for glaucoma, and it defines high-risk status to include diabetes, family history of glaucoma, African American status at age 50 or older, or Hispanic status at age 65 or older. The screening must be performed or supervised by an eye doctor legally allowed to do glaucoma screenings, and the beneficiary pays 20 percent of the Medicare-approved amount, with the Part B deductible and hospital outpatient copayment applying where relevant. This is not routine refractive care. It is medically targeted disease screening.

The glaucoma rule demonstrates how the Medicare system permits narrow preventive intervention while maintaining broad exclusion of ordinary optical maintenance. Under the CMS source structure, an eye-related service may be covered when it functions as disease detection for a high-risk beneficiary, while a routine eye examination for prescription eyeglasses remains outside Original Medicare. The policy logic is preventive medical surveillance rather than visual convenience. The ophthalmic exclusion matrix therefore requires classification by purpose: disease screening, post-surgical restoration, medical diagnosis, refractive correction, or consumer eyewear.

Hearing-related exclusions follow the same statutory pattern, but their household consequences are often more socially disruptive. CMS states in the 2026 handbook that Original Medicare does not cover hearing aids or exams for fitting hearing aids. The exclusion is categorical at the federal baseline. Hearing-aid acquisition, routine hearing-aid fitting, and ordinary sensory assistance are not transformed into Part B benefits merely because hearing impairment affects communication, fall risk, caregiver burden, cognitive load, social isolation, or employment continuity. The Medicare entitlement distinguishes diagnostic medical evaluation from the purchase and fitting of hearing-assistance devices.

The diagnostic exception must be kept separate from the device exclusion. CMS states that Medicare covers diagnostic hearing and balance, including fall-risk exams, when a physician or other health care provider orders them to determine whether medical treatment is needed. This coverage pathway is medical-diagnostic, not retail-sensory. A hearing or balance examination ordered to investigate an acute pathology, neurologic problem, vestibular disorder, trauma-related condition, or other medically evaluable issue can fall within Part B's diagnostic infrastructure. A routine hearing test designed to fit hearing aids falls outside Original Medicare's baseline, according to the same CMS source.

Modernized audiologist access adds nuance but not a general hearing-aid entitlement. CMS states that an audiologist visit may occur once every 12 months without an order from a physician or other health care provider, but only for non-acute hearing conditions, such as hearing loss that occurs over many years, and for diagnostic services related to hearing loss treated with surgically implanted hearing devices. CMS further states that the beneficiary pays 20 percent of the Medicare-approved amount, that the Part B deductible applies, and that a hospital outpatient copayment may also apply. The rule creates a limited diagnostic access channel. It does not finance hearing aids, fitting examinations for hearing aids, or ordinary device procurement.

The capital-preservation implications are substantial. Hearing devices can be recurring capital purchases, and their absence can reshape family communication, appointment adherence, cognitive engagement, safety monitoring, and caregiver labor. Yet under the federal baseline, CMS preserves a distinction between medically ordered diagnostic hearing or balance evaluation and excluded sensory-device acquisition. This produces a common household paradox: Medicare may participate in diagnosing the hearing problem while leaving the principal adaptive technology outside Original Medicare. The statutory matrix therefore separates knowledge of impairment from financing of the instrument used to compensate for impairment.

The custodial long-term care boundary is the largest unhedged structural risk in the Medicare exclusion architecture. CMS states that Medicare and most health insurance, including Medicare Supplement Insurance, do not pay for non-medical long-term care services, including care in a nursing home or in the community. CMS defines such non-medical long-term care to include personal care assistance with everyday activities, including dressing, bathing, and using the bathroom, and it further identifies adult day health care, personal care, transportation, home-delivered meals, and other home- and community-based services. The exclusion applies because the dominant service is custodial or personal-supportive rather than skilled medical treatment.

Custodial assistance should be understood as functional dependency rather than acute medical intervention. Activities of daily living, including bathing, dressing, eating, toileting, transferring, and continence management, are central to human survival and dignity, but they do not become Medicare-covered services simply because they are necessary. The CMS long-term care language identifies dressing, bathing, bathroom use, adult day health care, personal care, transportation, meals, and home- and community-based services as examples of non-medical long-term care services outside Medicare's ordinary payment structure. The statutory distinction is severe: necessity for daily living is not identical to Medicare-covered medical necessity.

The skilled-care boundary confirms this distinction. CMS states that skilled nursing facility care requires physician certification that daily skilled care, such as intravenous fluids, medications, or physical therapy, is needed and, as a practical matter, can be received only as a skilled nursing facility inpatient. CMS also states that Medicare does not cover non-medical long-term care. In Section 2.1, the skilled nursing facility benefit was analyzed as a short-term, medically necessary, benefit-period-limited recovery structure. That SNF benefit is not a federal long-term residence benefit. It is a skilled-care benefit bounded by eligibility criteria, daily care requirements, benefit-period accounting, and absolute exhaustion after the covered day limit.

Home health coverage likewise does not dissolve the custodial boundary. CMS's home health framework covers medically necessary part-time or intermittent skilled nursing care, physical therapy, speech-language pathology, continued occupational therapy, and related covered services when homebound status and practitioner certification requirements are satisfied. That structure differs from non-medical personal care. A homebound beneficiary needing intermittent skilled nursing after hospitalization may fall within a covered home health pathway. A chronically impaired beneficiary needing long-term assistance with bathing, dressing, toileting, meals, transportation, supervision, or ordinary household functioning may fall outside Original Medicare when the service is custodial rather than skilled medical care.

Chronic functional decline therefore does not itself convert custodial support into Medicare-covered care. Dementia, frailty, mobility loss, sensory impairment, incontinence, and progressive neurologic decline may create profound household burden, yet Medicare coverage still turns on the statutory category of the service. CMS recognizes that non-medical long-term care may occur at home, in the community, in an assisted living facility, or in a nursing home, and it identifies Medicaid eligibility, private long-term care insurance, or self-payment as possible non-Medicare financing pathways. The federal medical-insurance entitlement does not become a general custodial-income support program merely because the household's care burden becomes financially catastrophic.

The capital-preservation problem is consequently acute. Extended custodial care can consume savings, alter residence arrangements, force liquidation of assets, shift labor onto spouses or adult children, accelerate Medicaid eligibility analysis, and create conflict between medical planning and inheritance preservation. Under CMS's long-term care exclusion, the household cannot assume that a nursing home stay, assisted living support, adult day health program, home-delivered meals, personal transportation, or assistance with activities of daily living will be paid by Medicare merely because the beneficiary has Part A and Part B. The exclusion matrix therefore identifies one of the principal threats to retirement capital: the risk that the most time-intensive care need in late life is classified as personal maintenance rather than skilled medical treatment.

The relationship between Original Medicare exclusions and federally regulated private delivery models must be handled with precision. CMS states that Medicare Advantage Plans and Medicare Cost Plans may cover some extra benefits, such as fitness programs and vision, hearing, and dental services; CMS also states that this possibility exists as an alternative to the rule that certain services are not covered by Part A or Part B. This statement does not change the Original Medicare baseline. It means that supplemental benefits may exist in separate regulated delivery arrangements, subject to contract design, year-to-year changes, service-area rules, benefit terms, provider arrangements, and CMS-approved structures. The legal point for this textbook is not plan selection. The legal point is classification: supplemental benefit presence in another arrangement does not rewrite the federal exclusion matrix of Original Medicare.

This distinction preserves CMS educational compliance and analytic clarity. A generic federal discussion may acknowledge that some regulated private structures may contain additional benefits while refusing to describe proprietary benefits, local networks, allowances, copayments, carrier identities, or market-specific comparisons. The 2026 CMS handbook itself draws the distinction at a high level: Original Medicare excludes certain categories, while other coverage or certain Medicare plan types may cover some of those services. The manuscript's task is therefore to identify the federal baseline, not to substitute a private benefit catalogue for statutory analysis.

The statutory exclusions matrix also interacts with preventive medicine in a way that can confuse households. Medicare may cover specific preventive services while still excluding routine physical exams. CMS states that a yearly Wellness visit may cost nothing when the provider accepts assignment, but additional tests or services outside the preventive benefit can trigger coinsurance, the Part B deductible, or full liability if Medicare does not cover the added service, such as a routine physical exam. This confirms the central rule of the matrix: coverage turns on the statutory definition of the service, not on the setting, the patient's age, or the subjective expectation that an encounter is health-related.

The same classification logic controls every major exclusion addressed in this section. Dental work closely related to heart valve repair, organ transplant, cancer-related treatment, or ESRD dialysis services may receive Medicare consideration; ordinary cleanings, fillings, extractions, dentures, and most dental care generally do not. One pair of post-cataract corrective lenses after intraocular lens implantation may be covered through a Medicare-enrolled supplier with Part B deductible and 20 percent coinsurance exposure; ordinary eyeglasses, contact lenses, and eye exams for prescription correction generally are not. Diagnostic hearing and balance examinations may be covered under specified medical or audiology pathways; hearing aids and fitting examinations remain outside Original Medicare. Skilled nursing facility care and home health may be covered when skilled medical criteria are satisfied; non-medical long-term care, personal assistance, transportation, meals, and community-based custodial supports generally are not.

This specific interface addresses the exact multi-variable dilemma outlined in the Household Medicare Diagnostic Matrix. A household may execute the Initial Enrollment Period correctly, preserve Part B continuity, avoid late-enrollment penalties, coordinate employer coverage, manage Part D drug exposure, and still face substantial wealth erosion because entitlement status has been mistaken for absolute benefit adequacy. The exclusion matrix identifies the negative space of Medicare: services that are foreseeable, common, and often essential to independent living, but not absorbed by the Original Medicare entitlement. Routine dentistry, ordinary refractive correction, hearing aids, fitting examinations, routine physical exams, and custodial long-term care can create liabilities that are not solved by the Medicare card alone.

The analytic conclusion is therefore austere but necessary. Original Medicare protects against large categories of institutional, professional, outpatient, preventive, and post-acute medical risk. It does not comprehensively insure oral maintenance, optical refraction, hearing-device acquisition, routine physical examinations, or custodial life support. The statutory exclusions matrix is a diagnostic tool for separating covered medical insurance from excluded maintenance, sensory, dental, and custodial categories. The household that treats entitlement as synonymous with benefit adequacy may discover the error only after irreversible capital has been consumed. The household file must therefore be read not only for what Medicare covers, but for what the federal architecture intentionally leaves outside the entitlement.

MODULE II: THE CHRONOLOGICAL MATRIX & REGULATORY TIMELINES

Chapter 3: Statutory Enrollment Windows and Application Mechanics

3.1 The Initial Enrollment Period

The Initial Enrollment Period is the first chronological gate in the age-based Medicare entitlement sequence. It is not a flexible consumer shopping interval, nor is it a merely informational anniversary window. It is a statutory timing mechanism that controls the first lawful opportunity to establish Part B, and in the case of premium Part A, the first ordinary opportunity to purchase Hospital Insurance where premium-free entitlement is unavailable. A citation correction is required at the threshold. Current 42 CFR § 406.13 governs entitlement to Hospital Insurance for individuals with End-Stage Renal Disease, not the age-based Initial Enrollment Period for premium Part A. The age-based premium Part A enrollment period appears in 42 CFR § 406.21(b), while the effective-date consequences of enrollment month appear in 42 CFR § 406.22; Part B's Initial Enrollment Period appears in 42 CFR § 407.14, and Part B effective-date consequences appear in 42 CFR § 407.25. (ECFR)

The federal architecture therefore separates three related legal questions. First, whether the individual is entitled to premium-free Part A without filing a voluntary premium-Hospital Insurance application. Second, whether the individual must enroll in premium Part A because premium-free status is unavailable. Third, whether the individual must affirmatively enroll in Part B because automatic entitlement has not occurred. Under the 2026 Medicare handbook, beneficiaries already receiving Social Security or Railroad Retirement Board benefits generally receive Part A and Part B automatically beginning the first day of the month of the sixty-fifth birthday, with a first-day-of-month birthday producing coverage on the first day of the prior month. Where Social Security or Railroad Retirement Board benefits are not already being paid near age sixty-five, the handbook directs Part A and Part B applications through Social Security, with Railroad Retirement Board procedures for railroad cases.

The seven-month span is the central metric. Under 42 CFR § 407.14(a)(1), the Initial Enrollment Period for Supplementary Medical Insurance is the seven-month period beginning three months before the month in which the individual first meets the Part B eligibility requirements and ending three months after that first eligibility month. (ECFR) Under the premium Part A regulation, 42 CFR § 406.21(b)(1) similarly states that the Initial Enrollment Period for an individual age sixty-five or older extends for seven months, from the third month before the month in which the individual first meets the premium Part A eligibility requirements through the third month after that first month of eligibility. (ECFR) The 2026 Medicare handbook translates this structure into birth-month language: the ordinary age-based Initial Enrollment Period begins three months before the month of the sixty-fifth birthday and ends three months after the month of the sixty-fifth birthday.

The seven-month sequence is symmetrical in appearance but asymmetrical in legal consequence. The first three months function as a proactive filing interval. The fourth month, ordinarily the birth month, is the benchmark eligibility month. The fifth, sixth, and seventh months remain inside the Initial Enrollment Period, but they no longer preserve the same effective date as an application submitted before the eligibility month. Under the post-2023 federal effective-date rules, 42 CFR § 406.22(b) provides that when an age-sixty-five premium Part A enrollee files during the first three months of the Initial Enrollment Period, entitlement begins with the first month of eligibility; when enrollment occurs during the last four months of the Initial Enrollment Period, entitlement begins with the month following the month of enrollment. (ECFR) Part B follows the same modernized structure: 42 CFR § 407.25(a)(2) provides that, for enrollment on or after January 1, 2023, entitlement begins with the first month of eligibility when enrollment occurs during the first three months of the Initial Enrollment Period, and begins with the month following enrollment when enrollment occurs during the last four months. (ECFR)

The pre-eligibility filing period is therefore the cleanest age-based filing interval. When an individual whose sixty-fifth birthday occurs on a date other than the first day of a month files during any of the three months before the birthday month, Part A and Part B ordinarily begin on the first day of the birthday month, assuming all entitlement and enrollment conditions are otherwise satisfied. The 2026 Medicare handbook states that if enrollment in Part A or Part B occurs during the first three months of the Initial Enrollment Period, coverage generally begins the first day of the birthday month. This rule makes early filing administratively important, because it aligns the legal coverage date with the first day of the month in which age-based Medicare eligibility matures.

The first-day-of-month birthday exception is the most technical birth-month adjustment in the ordinary age-based grid. Under the 2026 Medicare handbook, when the birthday falls on the first day of the month, Part A and Part B coverage start on the first day of the prior month for those automatically enrolled, and the Initial Enrollment Period begins four months before the month of the sixty-fifth birthday and ends two months after that birthday month. The handbook gives the operative example: a person turning sixty-five on June 1 has an Initial Enrollment Period running from February through August, not March through September. The legal effect is that the preceding calendar month becomes the effective eligibility anchor, advancing the coverage start date and shifting the entire seven-month filing map backward.

This exception has consequences beyond the Medicare card. The 2026 handbook's HSA guidance states that for a birthday on the first day of the month, Medicare coverage generally begins the first day of the month before the sixty-fifth birthday, and HSA contributions should stop two months before the sixty-fifth birthday to avoid tax penalty exposure. Thus, the first-day-of-month rule is not merely an enrollment convenience. It can affect tax-advantaged account eligibility, employer health plan sequencing, Marketplace termination timing, and dependent coverage planning. A household using the ordinary birthday-month rule without auditing the first-day exception may misalign health savings contributions, coverage termination dates, or premium-tax-credit periods.

The post-eligibility filing period contains the most significant modernization relative to the pre-2023 framework. Before the Beneficiary Enrollment Notification and Eligibility Simplification reforms became operative, enrollment during the birth month or later months of the Initial Enrollment Period could trigger multi-month delays. Current 42 CFR § 406.22(b) and 42 CFR § 407.25(a)(2) now provide a simpler post-2023 rule: enrollment during the last four months of the Initial Enrollment Period begins entitlement with the month following the month of enrollment. (ECFR) The 2026 Medicare handbook states the same operational rule in beneficiary-facing form: if enrollment occurs during the month of the sixty-fifth birthday or during the last three months of the Initial Enrollment Period, coverage starts the first day of the month after enrollment.

The modernization removes legacy lag but does not eliminate coverage risk. An application filed during the seventh month of the Initial Enrollment Period still begins coverage the first day of the following month, leaving the months between first eligibility and coverage effective date without the Medicare entitlement that earlier filing would have established. Under CMS Enrollment Specifications in the 2026 handbook, failure to sign up for Part B when first eligible can lead to future delay because Part B enrollment is available only at specified times, and it can also produce a late-enrollment penalty added to the monthly premium for as long as Part B remains in force. The modernized rule shortens the historical delay; it does not convert the Initial Enrollment Period into a consequence-free rolling application window.

The legal consequence of non-action is actuarial reclassification. Once the Initial Enrollment Period closes, an individual lacking an applicable Special Enrollment Period is moved into a less favorable regulatory posture. Under the 2026 Medicare handbook, the General Enrollment Period runs from January 1 through March 31 each year for individuals who missed the Initial Enrollment Period and do not qualify for a Special Enrollment Period, with coverage beginning the first day of the month after enrollment. The Part B penalty framework then attaches a continuing premium increase of 10 percent for each full twelve-month period in which Part B could have been held but was not, unless a Special Enrollment Period or other recognized relief applies. This converts a missed chronological window into a permanent or long-duration price signal.

The active-employment safe harbor is the principal protection against that reclassification, but it is narrow. The 2026 Medicare handbook states that a Special Enrollment Period may permit Part A or Part B enrollment after the Initial Enrollment Period when non-enrollment occurred because of group health plan coverage based on current employment, including the individual's, a spouse's, or a family member's current employment in disability cases. The same source states that the enrollment opportunity extends while still covered by the current-employment group health plan and during the eight-month period beginning after employment ends or coverage ends, whichever occurs first. The handbook also states that COBRA, retiree coverage, Veterans Affairs coverage, individual Marketplace coverage, and former-employer severance or layoff coverage are not coverage based on current employment for this Special Enrollment Period.

This distinction creates one of the most important intersections between the Initial Enrollment Period and the Household Medicare Diagnostic Matrix. A household may appear insured at age sixty-five because coverage exists from a Marketplace policy, COBRA continuation arrangement, retiree plan, or former-employer severance package. The federal enrollment system, however, does not treat those coverage types as the current-employment group health plan safe harbor for delayed Part B enrollment. Under the 2026 handbook, Marketplace coverage should be transitioned when Medicare eligibility begins to avoid delay and late-enrollment penalty exposure, and Marketplace financial help generally ends once premium-free Part A eligibility or premium Part A coverage exists. Therefore, the Initial Enrollment Period must be audited by legal coverage category, not merely by whether some non-Medicare card remains active.

Application mechanics begin at the Social Security intake layer. The 2026 Medicare handbook directs individuals close to age sixty-five who are not already receiving Social Security or Railroad Retirement Board benefits to apply for Part A and Part B through Social Security's Medicare sign-up portal or through Social Security appointment procedures; railroad cases are directed to the Railroad Retirement Board. Current 42 CFR Part 406 likewise distinguishes individuals who need not file a Hospital Insurance application from those who must file, including individuals who are not already captured through automatic entitlement channels; the regulation states that an application for Part A based on certain age-sixty-five eligibility provisions may be filed no earlier than the third month before the first month of eligibility. (ECFR) The operational implication is that the federal file begins with identity, age, citizenship or lawful-presence criteria, entitlement category, and insured-status or premium-buyer status before CMS-facing coverage operations can function.

The automatic-enrollment pathway has a different administrative posture. Under the 2026 Medicare handbook, a person already receiving Social Security or Railroad Retirement Board benefits receives Part A and Part B automatically at age sixty-five, with the red, white, and blue Medicare card mailed three months before the sixty-fifth birthday or the twenty-fifth month of disability benefits; if Part B is not rejected before the coverage start date, Part B is retained and premiums are deducted from Social Security or Railroad Retirement Board benefits. This automatic process does not negate the Initial Enrollment Period. It changes the action required inside the period. For the automatic enrollee, the relevant decision may concern Part B retention, premium exposure, coordination with active-employment coverage, and downstream drug or supplemental coverage timing. For the non-automatic enrollee, the relevant task is affirmative application through Social Security or the Railroad Retirement Board.

Premium mechanics reinforce the inter-agency character of the transaction. The 2026 Medicare handbook states that Part B premiums are deducted from monthly Social Security or Railroad Retirement Board benefit payments when those benefits are being paid. For persons not receiving Social Security or Railroad Retirement Board benefits, Medicare bills Part B premiums directly, generally every three months, with monthly billing possible where Part A premiums, Part D IRMAA, or Medicare Easy Pay are involved. Thus, an Initial Enrollment Period application may establish coverage before routine premium withholding exists, and direct billing may become the temporary or ordinary premium pathway. Premium billing is not a collateral clerical matter; it is the financial proof that the enrollment file, premium responsibility, and payment channel have synchronized.

The uploaded source packet does not provide a detailed, source-verifiable description of an internal CMS Third Party System labeled "TPS" for SSA-to-CMS Part A and Part B transaction transfer. The grounded administrative rule that can be stated from the official materials is narrower: Social Security or the Railroad Retirement Board operates as the Part A and Part B intake channel for non-automatic age-based enrollment, while Medicare and CMS-administered systems become the operational environment for coverage records, premium billing, plan comparison, claims administration, and beneficiary account functions. For managed-care and Part D transactions, the CMS enrollment guidance in the source packet does describe plan receipt of enrollment requests, valid election-period determination, completed enrollment requests, entitlement evidence, and transmission to CMS after completion. Those plan-level mechanics should not be misdescribed as the internal SSA-to-CMS Part A and Part B entitlement bridge, but they do confirm the broader federal principle that Medicare enrollment is ultimately an eligibility-verified data transaction, not merely a signed paper event.

Late filing inside the Initial Enrollment Period can create practical friction even when the legal effective date is clear. An application filed during the seventh month of the Initial Enrollment Period produces coverage effective the first day of the next month under current rules, not retroactive coverage to the birthday month. (ECFR) If premium bills, Medicare cards, Medicare account records, employer-plan terminations, Marketplace termination dates, drug coverage requests, or provider intake systems do not align at the same operational speed, the household can encounter a temporary mismatch between legal entitlement, proof of coverage, provider recognition, and premium payment. The source packet's plan-enrollment guidance treats completed enrollment requests as requiring entitlement evidence and transmission to CMS, and it instructs that enrollment requests occur within valid election periods. That procedural structure illustrates the central timing lesson: valid entitlement requires not only eligibility, but also correct filing, correct window selection, complete data, and system recognition.

The birth-month grid also interacts with Part D timing. The 2026 Medicare handbook states that a Medicare drug plan or Medicare Advantage plan with drug coverage may be joined when first eligible for Medicare, and that Open Enrollment and other election periods operate separately. The source packet's Part D late-enrollment framework states that a Part D penalty may apply if, after the Initial Enrollment Period, there is a period of 63 or more days without Medicare drug coverage or other creditable prescription drug coverage. Although Section 3.1 focuses on Part A and Part B, the practical IEP file cannot be confined to hospital and medical insurance alone. The month when Part A or Part B becomes effective may become the anchor for drug-coverage election rights, creditable-coverage calculations, and future Part D penalty exposure.

The Initial Enrollment Period also determines whether workplace health arrangements remain orderly or become destabilized. Under the 2026 handbook, employer or union group health coverage based on current employment may make delayed Part B enrollment advantageous in some circumstances, while the employer or union benefits administrator can clarify coordination with Medicare. The same source states that when age sixty-five or older and covered by a current-employment group health plan, the group plan generally pays first when the employer has twenty or more employees, while Medicare pays first when the employer has fewer than twenty employees. The Initial Enrollment Period therefore cannot be evaluated without payer-order analysis. Filing too early or too late may affect premium spending, HSA eligibility, employer coverage expectations, and claim coordination.

The HSA interface is especially unforgiving because it depends on the actual Part A coverage start date. The 2026 Medicare handbook states that HSA contributions are not permitted after Medicare begins and that premium-free Part A can be retroactive six months from Part A enrollment or Social Security or Railroad Retirement Board benefit application, but not earlier than the first Medicare-eligible month. The same source states that, when enrollment occurs during the Initial Enrollment Period, the last HSA contribution should occur the month before turning sixty-five, while a first-day-of-month birthday generally moves Medicare coverage to the first day of the prior month and moves the contribution stop date two months before age sixty-five. This rule links birth-month mapping to federal tax compliance. The Initial Enrollment Period is therefore both a health entitlement calendar and a tax-disqualification calendar.

The legal architecture of Section 3.1 produces a simple but severe conclusion: the Initial Enrollment Period is a birth-month centered legal grid with financial consequences that extend beyond the Medicare application itself. The first three months before ordinary age-sixty-five eligibility preserve a first-day-of-birthday-month coverage date. The birthday month and the following three months remain valid filing months, but under current rules they produce coverage on the first day of the month after enrollment rather than the original eligibility month. (ECFR) A first-day-of-month birthday moves the entire grid backward. Non-action after the window closes shifts the beneficiary toward General Enrollment Period dependency, possible late-enrollment penalties, and avoidable coverage gaps unless a valid Special Enrollment Period applies.

This specific interface addresses the exact multi-variable dilemma outlined in the Household Medicare Diagnostic Matrix. A household may treat age sixty-five as a birthday event, but the federal system treats it as a month-based entitlement event governed by filing sequence, first-day exceptions, current-employment safe harbors, premium collection mechanisms, tax-account consequences, and downstream drug-coverage deadlines. The failure to track the birth-month alignment can produce immediate coverage gaps, premature or delayed termination of non-Medicare coverage, HSA contribution errors, Marketplace subsidy repayment exposure, employer-plan coordination failures, or late-enrollment penalty exposure. The Initial Enrollment Period is therefore the first chronological audit in the Medicare system: before any Part C, Part D, Medigap, employer, HSA, or Marketplace interface is evaluated, the household file must establish the exact first eligibility month, the exact enrollment month, the exact coverage effective month, and the exact legal status of any asserted delay protection.

3.2 The General Enrollment Period and Modern Policy Revisions

The General Enrollment Period is the statutory remedial portal for individuals who failed to enroll during the Initial Enrollment Period and who lack a valid Special Enrollment Period. It is not a discretionary second Initial Enrollment Period; it is a legally confined recovery mechanism whose use often carries penalty exposure, interim coverage gaps, and downstream coordination complications. Under CMS GEP specifications in the 2026 Medicare handbook, Part B enrollment may occur during the General Enrollment Period from January 1 through March 31 each year when the Initial Enrollment Period was missed and no Special Enrollment Period applies; premium Part A may also be purchased during this same interval when premium-free Part A is unavailable and the Initial Enrollment Period was missed. The current premium-Hospital Insurance regulation confirms the same annual architecture for premium Part A: except for specified historical or special provisions, the General Enrollment Period extends from January 1 through March 31 of each calendar year, and it exists for individuals who failed to enroll during the Initial Enrollment Period, failed to enroll during an available Special Enrollment Period, or had prior entitlement terminate (42 CFR § 406.21(c)). (ECFR)

The General Enrollment Period must be understood as a corrective window with actuarial consequences. It exists because Medicare enrollment cannot be left perpetually open without distorting the risk pool. Medical insurance systems financed through public premiums, general revenues, payroll taxes, and trust-fund mechanisms require predictable participation rules. If enrollment could be delayed indefinitely until a major diagnosis, hospital referral, outpatient procedure, or drug regimen appeared, the federal program would absorb immediate high-cost risk from persons who had avoided prior premium participation. Fixed enrollment windows function as an anti-selection discipline: they force the decision to enroll into a legally scheduled calendar rather than allowing the individual to wait until clinical need has matured. This inference follows from the structure of the enrollment regulations, which restrict premium Part A enrollment to the Initial Enrollment Period, General Enrollment Period, Special Enrollment Periods, and limited transfer enrollment periods, rather than permitting unrestricted continuous entry (42 CFR § 406.21(a)). (ECFR)

The General Enrollment Period is therefore a temporal penalty architecture as much as a filing opportunity. The 2026 Medicare handbook states that higher Part A or Part B premiums may apply for late enrollment when the General Enrollment Period is used after the Initial Enrollment Period was missed. For Part B, the penalty formula is especially durable: CMS states that the monthly Part B premium may increase by 10 percent for each full 12-month period in which Part B could have been held but was not, and that the penalty generally continues for as long as Part B remains in force. The GEP is thus not a neutral administrative reset. It is a legally available entrance point that may carry a permanently altered premium profile.

The historical General Enrollment Period was far more punitive in effective-date timing. Before the modernized rules beginning in 2023, the person who enrolled during the January through March GEP generally waited until July 1 for Part B entitlement. Current 42 CFR § 407.25(b)(1) preserves that historical rule in regulatory text by stating that enrollment or reenrollment during a General Enrollment Period before January 1, 2023, generally produced entitlement beginning July 1 of that calendar year. (ECFR) Premium Part A followed the same historical structure; 42 CFR § 406.21(c)(3) states that, before January 1, 2023, enrollment or reenrollment during the General Enrollment Period produced entitlement beginning July 1 of the calendar year. (ECFR) The old July 1 rule created a prolonged unhedged interval: a January filer, a February filer, and a March filer all could be left without the relevant Medicare coverage until midyear.

The legacy July 1 delay had harsh household consequences. A person who missed the Initial Enrollment Period and lacked a Special Enrollment Period could file in January yet remain outside active Part B for February, March, April, May, and June. During that interval, physician services, outpatient care, durable medical equipment, preventive services, diagnostic testing, and other Part B-covered categories could remain financially unprotected by Medicare. CMS's educational materials warn that failure to keep or obtain Part B when no qualifying current-employment coverage exists can force the person to pay all costs for doctors' services, outpatient care, medical supplies, and preventive services, and that delayed Part B may require waiting for the General Enrollment Period with a resulting coverage gap. The old regime therefore converted a missed enrollment window into both a premium penalty and an immediate service-access hazard.

The modernized federal rule permanently deconstructed that delay for GEP enrollments occurring on or after January 1, 2023. Under 42 CFR § 407.25(b)(3), an individual who enrolls or reenrolls in Part B during a General Enrollment Period on or after January 1, 2023, begins entitlement on the first day of the month following the month of enrollment. (ECFR) The same next-month rule applies to premium Part

A under 42 CFR § 406.21(c)(3)(ii), which states that a General Enrollment Period enrollment or reenrollment on or after January 1, 2023, begins entitlement on the first day of the month after the month of enrollment. (ECFR) CMS translates this regulation into operational language in the 2026 Medicare handbook: when enrollment occurs during the General Enrollment Period, coverage starts the first day of the month after enrollment.

The practical examples are direct. A January GEP application produces a February 1 start date. A February GEP application produces a March 1 start date. A March GEP application produces an April 1 start date. The source packet's Part C and Part D enrollment guidance demonstrates the same operational consequence in a managed-care election context: a person age 67 enrolling in Part B for the first time during the 2025 General Enrollment Period has Part B coverage beginning April 1, 2025, and the Initial Coverage Election Period tied to newly having both Parts A and B runs from January 1 through May 31, 2025. This example confirms that a late-March GEP enrollment can activate Part B at the first of the following month, not at the old July 1 date.

The acceleration reduces but does not erase household risk. A March filing no longer waits until July, but it still may follow months or years of noncoverage and may still trigger a Part B late-enrollment penalty. CMS's 2026 materials state that a person delaying Part B without Special Enrollment Period eligibility can sign up only during the January 1 through March 31 GEP and may pay 10 percent more for each full 12-month period in which Part B could have been held but was not. The modern effective-date reform therefore changes the waiting period after application, not the historical penalty count preceding application. The law now mitigates the immediate post-filing gap while preserving the actuarial sanction for late participation.

The GEP also interacts with Part D timing. The 2026 Medicare handbook states that when a person must pay for Part A and signs up for Part B during the General Enrollment Period, a Medicare drug plan may also be joined when Part B is signed up for, and the person has two months after signing up for Part B to join a drug plan; drug coverage starts the month after the plan receives the request. The Part D late-enrollment penalty remains separately governed by creditable drug coverage rules. CMS states that a Part D late-enrollment penalty may apply after the Initial Enrollment Period when there is a period of 63 or more consecutive days without Medicare drug coverage or other creditable prescription drug coverage, and that the penalty is calculated as 1 percent of the national base beneficiary premium multiplied by the number of full uncovered months. Consequently, the GEP may solve Part B entry but not automatically neutralize Part D penalty exposure.

Premium billing after GEP entry is a synchronization problem between coverage effective date, premium obligation, and payment channel. CMS states that the standard Part B premium in 2026 is $202.90 per month, with higher premiums possible through IRMAA or late-enrollment penalties. Where Social Security or Railroad Retirement Board benefits are being paid, the Part B premium is deducted from the monthly benefit payment; where those benefits are not being paid, Medicare sends a premium bill, typically quarterly, and monthly billing may occur if Part A premiums, Part D IRMAA, or Medicare Easy Pay is involved. This creates a mid-year entrance structure rather than a calendar-year premium recalculation. The premium obligation attaches by month of entitlement and applicable premium class, not through an annual lump-sum premium divided retroactively across the entire year.

The term "pro-rated" must therefore be used carefully. Medicare coverage begins on the first day of a month, and Part B premiums are stated as monthly premiums. CMS's 2026 handbook gives the standard premium as a monthly amount and explains the payment channels through benefit withholding, direct billing, online payment, Medicare Easy Pay, bank payment, or mail. In an operational sense, the household does not owe Part B premiums for months before entitlement begins merely because GEP enrollment occurs mid-year, except where a special retroactive entitlement rule separately applies. The monthly premium clock begins with the month of coverage entitlement. By contrast, the late-enrollment penalty percentage, once applicable, is incorporated into the monthly premium going forward and can remain for as long as Part B is retained.

The annual Part B deductible does not receive the same mid-year fractional treatment. CMS's 2026 Part B outpatient specifications state that when the Part B deductible applies under Original Medicare, the beneficiary pays all costs up to the Medicare-approved amount until the yearly Part B deductible is met; for 2026, that deductible is $283, and after it is met Medicare pays its share while the beneficiary typically pays 20 percent of the Medicare-approved amount when the provider accepts assignment. The deductible is annual in the sense that it is the deductible for the coverage year; it is not reduced because coverage begins in February, March, or April after a GEP filing. Thus, a person entering Part B effective April 1 through a March GEP application faces the same 2026 Part B deductible for covered services during the remaining coverage months as a person whose Part B began January 1.

This deductible rule matters because GEP enrollees often enter Medicare in proximity to medical need. The adverse-selection rationale behind fixed windows is not abstract. Many late enrollees seek Part B only after employer coverage ended, COBRA proved insufficient, Marketplace coverage became unsustainable, or an outpatient diagnostic pathway emerged. The source packet warns that failure to retain Part B without current-employment coverage can create responsibility for all doctors' services, outpatient care, medical supplies, and preventive services, and can produce both a General Enrollment Period wait and a long-term penalty. When Part B begins mid-year, the full annual deductible and ordinary 20 percent coinsurance structure become active immediately for covered services, while the federal baseline still lacks a general Original Medicare maximum out-of-pocket limit for Part B services.

The SSA application channel remains the intake mechanism for Part A and Part B enrollment. CMS's 2026 handbook directs individuals seeking Part A and Part B enrollment to Social Security's Medicare sign-up portal, while railroad cases are handled through the Railroad Retirement Board. In a GEP context, this means the household file must move from missed Initial Enrollment Period status into a manual application posture. Identity, entitlement category, premium Part A status, Part B enrollment request, and premium-billing status must be established before Medicare coverage can be operationally recognized. The GEP is not completed merely by acknowledging that January 1 through March 31 exists; the application must be executed, processed, and recognized by the federal record before the next-month entitlement rule produces practical payer status.

The uploaded source packet substantiates SSA intake, CMS premium billing, and CMS plan-enrollment systems, but it does not establish a source-confirmed Part A or Part B processing label called the "CMS Third Party System." For that reason, the defensible manuscript treatment is not a claim about a named TPS mechanism. The defensible treatment is the broader inter-agency file-synchronization risk: SSA or the Railroad Retirement Board operates the Part A and Part B intake channel, Medicare administers premium billing and coverage records, and downstream CMS systems must recognize entitlement before plans, providers, claims channels, and premium-payment mechanisms operate without friction. Where the Part C and Part D source packet describes CMS data systems, it identifies Batch Eligibility Query and MARx online query as mechanisms plans use to verify Medicare entitlement and determine whether an enrollment request is complete; it also requires plans to determine election-period eligibility and deny enrollment when eligibility cannot be confirmed after review against CMS systems.

Those managed-care and drug-plan systems illustrate a general rule of Medicare administration: coverage status must be visible in federal systems before downstream entities can reliably process elections, claims, or billing. A late-March GEP filing that is legally destined for an April 1 effective date may still create a short operational interval in which documents, Medicare account display, premium invoices, provider registration systems, and plan eligibility checks do not all update at identical speed. The source packet's CMS plan-enrollment guidance recognizes that organizations verify entitlement through CMS systems and may need additional information before completing enrollment requests. The risk is not that the regulation lacks a start date; the risk is that administrative proof, provider intake, and billing infrastructure may lag behind the legal entitlement event.

Premium-billing anomalies can arise from the same timing problem. The 2026 handbook states that if Social Security or Railroad Retirement Board benefits are being received, the Part B premium is deducted from the monthly benefit payment; otherwise, Medicare sends a bill, typically quarterly, while Medicare Easy Pay and certain premium categories can produce monthly billing. It also states that online payment, automatic bank withdrawal, bank bill payment, and mail payment are available premium-payment methods, and that retroactive Social Security benefit notices may require changes in Medicare premium payment arrangements. A GEP enrollee who is not yet drawing Title II benefits may therefore enter Medicare through direct billing even if later benefit claiming shifts the premium channel into withholding.

The General Enrollment Period also affects secondary coverage coordination. CMS's 2026 materials repeatedly distinguish current-employment group health plan coverage from COBRA, retiree coverage, Veterans Affairs coverage, Marketplace individual coverage, and former-employer severance or layoff coverage. The latter categories do not function as the current-employment safe harbor for delaying Part B enrollment. This distinction matters when a late enrollee assumes that non-Medicare coverage has protected the file. A person leaving active employment may have had eight months under the worker Special Enrollment Period; a person relying on COBRA after that employment ended may discover that the COBRA period did not extend the Part B SEP clock. CMS states that after coverage based on current employment ends, there are eight months to sign up for Part B without penalty, whether or not COBRA is elected, and that COBRA may pay only a small portion of costs when Medicare eligibility exists.

Marketplace coverage creates an additional GEP trap. CMS's educational source packet warns that Marketplace or other individual coverage not based on current employment does not generally protect against Part B delay and that a person may have to wait for the General Enrollment Period, with late-enrollment penalty exposure, if Medicare enrollment is not executed when first eligible. It further warns that Marketplace financial assistance may have to be repaid when Part A eligibility begins and assistance continues. Thus, the modern next-month effective date may reduce the length of the post-GEP waiting period, but it does not cure premium tax credit reconciliation, family coverage disruption, or months of exposure that occurred before the GEP application.

The General Enrollment Period reshapes but does not eliminate reliance on temporary coverage frameworks. Under the old July 1 rule, households often faced several months between application and Medicare activation, requiring COBRA, retiree coverage, individual coverage, Medicaid, short-term arrangements, or self-payment to bridge an extended administrative void. Under the modern next-month mandate, the bridge can be much shorter: January to February, February to March, or March to April. The GEP acceleration therefore improves healthcare continuity by reducing the period during which a person has applied for federal coverage but lacks active entitlement. Nevertheless, the underlying need for precise transition modeling remains because non-Medicare coverage termination dates, premium tax credits, HSA eligibility, prescription-drug creditability, and provider billing all operate under their own rules.

Mid-year entry also changes the timing of downstream plan election rights. The Part C and Part D enrollment guidance in the source packet gives an example in which Part B first begins April 1 after a GEP filing, and the Initial Coverage Election Period tied to having both Part A and Part B runs January 1 through May 31. That example is not a recommendation to enter a private plan. It is a federal timing illustration showing that a delayed Part B effective date can create or reposition a separate Medicare Advantage Initial Coverage Election Period. The 2026 Medicare handbook separately states that a person who must pay for Part A and signs up for Part B during the GEP can also join a drug plan, with a two-month period after signing up for Part B and drug coverage starting the month after the plan receives the request.

Late-enrollment penalties remain the principal long-term actuarial cost of GEP dependency. CMS states that the Part B penalty may be 10 percent for each full 12-month period in which Part B could have been held but was not, and it provides an example in which a 27-month delay produces a 20 percent penalty because only two full 12-month periods are counted. A separate CMS source packet example calculates a 20 percent penalty on the 2026 standard monthly Part B premium of $202.90, producing a $40.58 penalty and a rounded monthly premium of $243.50 for 2026. These examples confirm that the penalty is tied to full 12-month periods, not merely to the number of calendar months absent Part B.

The penalty formula also demonstrates why the GEP must be analyzed longitudinally. A person who misses the Initial Enrollment Period by several months but signs up before a full 12-month period has passed may avoid a Part B late-enrollment penalty under CMS's stated rule. A person who waits 24 full months without SEP protection faces a 20 percent penalty. A person who waits 36 full months faces a larger penalty under the same 10 percent-per-year architecture. The household's financial exposure therefore compounds through two channels: uninsured months before GEP filing, and premium penalty percentages after GEP entry. The modern next-month effective date only addresses the first few months after filing; it does not erase the historical count of full years without Part B.

This specific interface addresses the exact multi-variable dilemma outlined in the Household Medicare Diagnostic Matrix. A household may know that the General Enrollment Period runs January 1 through March 31, but still miscalculate the consequences of filing month, premium channel, deductible exposure, drug-coverage timing, Marketplace subsidy status, COBRA reliance, and full-year penalty accrual. The modern next-month effective rule improves the transition model: a January application can become February coverage, a February application can become March coverage, and a March application can become April coverage. (ECFR) However, the household file must still be audited for every full 12-month period without Part B, because each full year can add a continuing 10 percent premium penalty unless Special Enrollment Period protection, Medicare Savings Program enrollment, or other recognized relief applies.

The General Enrollment Period is therefore a statutory salvage mechanism, not a planning default. Its modern form is more humane than the legacy July 1 structure, but it remains an adverse-selection control embedded in federal social insurance. It opens only from January 1 through March 31. It starts coverage on the first day of the month after enrollment for post-2023 enrollments. It may impose late-enrollment premiums. It requires premium-channel synchronization through Social Security, the Railroad Retirement Board, or direct CMS billing. It does not prorate the annual Part B deductible downward for mid-year entry. It can reposition drug-plan and managed-care election windows without eliminating separate Part D creditable-coverage rules. Most importantly, it converts a missed Initial Enrollment Period into a file-audit problem whose effects can remain visible for the rest of the beneficiary's Medicare life cycle

Chapter 4: Actuarial Penalties and Enforcement Frameworks

4.1 The Part B Lifetime Late Enrollment Penalty

The Part B late enrollment penalty is best understood as a continuing actuarial enforcement device rather than as a temporary administrative fine. Part B is the Supplementary Medical Insurance component of Medicare that helps finance physician services, outpatient care, home health care, durable medical equipment, preventive services, and other medical services that are not governed by the Part A institutional benefit-period model. Because Part B is premium-financed and voluntary in the sense that many beneficiaries may decline or delay enrollment under certain circumstances, the federal system imposes a delayed-entry surcharge when a beneficiary fails to enroll during the lawful enrollment window and lacks a recognized statutory safe harbor. Under CMS Part B Enrollment Specifications in the 2026 Medicare handbook, failure to enroll in Part B when first eligible may produce a late enrollment penalty for as long as Part B remains active, and the monthly premium may increase by 10 percent for each full 12-month period during which Part B could have been held but was not elected.

The policy rationale is inseparable from the Supplementary Medical Insurance trust structure. Part B is financed through beneficiary premiums and federal general revenues, and its annual premium architecture assumes broad participation across both high-utilization and low-utilization beneficiaries. Without a delayed-entry penalty, healthier individuals could rationally remain outside the premium pool until outpatient needs became imminent, known, or financially unavoidable. Such behavior would concentrate risk among those already consuming physician services, outpatient diagnostics, durable medical equipment, and chronic disease management. The late enrollment penalty therefore functions as an adverse-selection barrier: it attaches a durable cost to late participation so that the federal medical-insurance pool is not transformed into a claims-triggered enrollment mechanism. Under CMS's 2026 penalty formulation, the surcharge is not calculated by diagnosis, claim history, or income level; it is calculated by the number of full 12-month periods during which Part B eligibility existed without Part B enrollment and without recognized penalty protection.

The trigger point begins with the expiration of the Initial Enrollment Period. CMS states that the age-based Initial Enrollment Period generally runs for seven months, beginning three months before the month of the 65th birthday and ending three months after that month; when the birthday falls on the first day of the month, the seven-month grid shifts backward, beginning four months before the birthday month and ending two months after the birthday month. Once that statutory window closes, a beneficiary who has not enrolled in Part B must either fit within a Special Enrollment Period or rely on the General Enrollment Period. CMS states that the General Enrollment Period runs January 1 through March 31 each year for individuals who missed the Initial Enrollment Period and do not qualify for a Special Enrollment Period, and that coverage begins the first day of the month after enrollment. The legal transition from Initial Enrollment Period status to General Enrollment Period dependency is the point at which actuarial penalty exposure becomes a permanent file variable.

The principal safe harbor from Part B late enrollment penalty exposure is not the mere existence of health insurance. It is coverage through a group health plan based on current employment. Under CMS Part B Enrollment Specifications, delayed Part B enrollment may be protected when a beneficiary is covered by a group health plan based on current employment, including the employment of a spouse or, in disability cases, a family member. CMS states that Part A or Part B enrollment can occur during that current-employment group health plan coverage or during the eight-month period beginning after the employment ends or the coverage ends, whichever occurs first. In the separate CMS notice material contained in the source packet, the same rule is restated as a Special Enrollment Period for persons 65 or older with employer or union group health coverage from the current job of the beneficiary or spouse, and for certain disabled persons with current-employment group health coverage from a spouse or family member.

The safe harbor is therefore occupational, not merely contractual. A private insurance card, claims administrator, network, pharmacy benefit, continuation notice, or retiree plan booklet does not establish protection unless the coverage is legally tethered to active current employment in the manner recognized by CMS. The 2026 handbook expressly excludes COBRA, retiree coverage, Veterans Affairs coverage, individual health insurance coverage through the Health Insurance Marketplace, and former-employer coverage obtained through severance or layoff from the definition of coverage based on current employment. The consequence is severe: a household may remain insured in the practical sense while failing the federal test for Part B penalty insulation. The Medicare file does not ask whether some health coverage existed; it asks whether the delay was protected by the statutory current-employment group health plan standard or by another recognized federal exception.

COBRA continuation coverage is the paradigmatic filing trap. COBRA may preserve access to a former employer's group health plan after employment ends, but CMS states that COBRA coverage is not considered coverage based on current employment and does not count as current employer coverage for the Part B Special Enrollment Period. CMS further states that after coverage based on current employment ends, the eight-month Part B enrollment period runs whether or not COBRA is elected, and a beneficiary generally is not eligible for a Special Enrollment Period when COBRA later ends. This means that COBRA can create a false sense of federal compliance. The household may perceive continuous medical coverage, yet the Medicare Part B penalty clock may already be moving because current employment has ended.

Retiree coverage creates a parallel trap. CMS states that retiree health plans are not coverage based on current employment for the Part B Special Enrollment Period, and it warns that retiree coverage may not pay for health services if both Part A and Part B are not held. The same logic applies to Veterans Affairs coverage for Part B enrollment timing; CMS lists VA coverage among the coverages that do not constitute current-employment coverage for this Special Enrollment Period. These categories may have significant value in their own legal domains, but they do not automatically protect the Medicare Part B file from late-enrollment penalty exposure. The safe harbor is not a general health-benefit adequacy test. It is a Medicare enrollment-period test.

Marketplace coverage is especially complex because it can also create tax-credit consequences. CMS states that individual Marketplace coverage is not coverage based on current employment, and it advises that Medicare enrollment at first eligibility avoids the risk of delayed Medicare coverage and possible late enrollment penalties. CMS further states that once premium-free Part A eligibility or premium Part A coverage exists, Marketplace help for premiums or other medical costs generally ends, and continued receipt of that help may require repayment during federal tax filing. Thus, Marketplace coverage can fail the Part B safe-harbor test while also creating premium tax credit reconciliation exposure. For the Household Medicare Diagnostic Matrix, this is not a side issue; it is a multi-system hazard involving Medicare enrollment law, federal tax reconciliation, and household dependent coverage continuity.

The 10 percent formula is mechanical. CMS states that the monthly Part B premium may increase by 10 percent for each full 12-month period in which Part B could have been held but was not. The operative computational unit is a full 12-month period. The law does not add a new 10 percent increment for every partial year. A delay of 11 months does not create the same penalty percentage as a delay of 12 full months. A delay of 23 months produces one full 12-month block, not two. A delay of 24 months produces two full 12-month blocks. The formula is therefore linear by completed year of exposure: penalty percentage equals 10 percent multiplied by the number of full 12-month periods during which Part B eligibility existed without Part B enrollment and without penalty protection.

The CMS example captures the significance of partial-year exclusion. The 2026 handbook states that an individual whose Initial Enrollment Period ended in December 2021 and who waited until March 2024 during the General Enrollment Period to sign up for Part B had a 20 percent Part B premium penalty, even though the gap lasted 27 months, because only two full 12-month periods were included. The 27-month timeline contains 24 completed penalty months plus three additional months. The completed 24 months form two full 12-month blocks. The remaining three months do not create a third block. The penalty is therefore 20 percent, not 30 percent. This example is essential because it prevents imprecise arithmetic from overstating the surcharge while also demonstrating the severity of completed delay cycles.

A federal calculation model follows directly from the CMS formula. For a 20 percent Part B late enrollment penalty applied to the 2026 standard monthly Part B premium of $202.90, the penalty amount equals $40.58 before rounding. CMS's source packet example adds that amount to the $202.90 standard premium and identifies the resulting rounded 2026 monthly premium as $243.50. The same example confirms that the late enrollment penalty is added to the standard premium and that the final premium amount may be rounded. The mathematical model is therefore: standard Part B premium multiplied by penalty percentage equals the monthly penalty amount; standard Part B premium plus penalty amount equals the monthly premium obligation before any separate income-related premium rules or billing adjustments apply.

The penalty's lifetime character is the central actuarial hazard. CMS states that the Part B late enrollment penalty may have to be paid for as long as the beneficiary has Part B. This duration distinguishes the Part B penalty from short-term administrative surcharges or temporary commercial penalties that expire after a defined number of months. The phrase "for as long as Part B remains active" should be read functionally. A beneficiary who incurs a 20 percent Part B LEP generally carries that surcharge across subsequent Part B premium years unless a recognized correction, Special Enrollment Period protection, Medicare Savings Program interaction, or other federal relief changes the file. The penalty is therefore not merely the cost of late entry. It is a continuing modification of the Medicare premium base.

The penalty percentage is fixed by the number of full delay blocks, but the dollar amount is dynamic because the standard Part B premium changes over time. CMS states that the standard Part B premium amount in 2026 is $202.90 and that most beneficiaries pay that amount every month, with higher-income beneficiaries potentially subject to Income-Related Monthly Adjustment Amounts. The CMS notice material also states that the Part B premium amount can change each year. Therefore, a fixed 20 percent penalty does not produce a fixed dollar amount across decades. If the standard Part B premium rises, the dollar value of the 20 percent surcharge rises. If the standard premium declines, the dollar surcharge would decline. The actuarial risk is that the penalty is attached to a national premium base that is recalibrated over time rather than frozen at the premium in effect during the enrollment error year.

This design creates long-term capital erosion without compounding in the interest-on-interest sense. The Part B LEP does not accrue compound interest on unpaid penalty amounts. Instead, it operates as a recurring percentage surcharge applied to an annually changing premium base. That distinction is important. The penalty's severity lies not in exponential finance mathematics, but in its persistence and its exposure to future premium inflation. A household with a 30 percent penalty does not merely pay more in the year of late enrollment. It pays a structurally elevated monthly Part B premium across the remaining period of Part B coverage, subject to whatever annual standard-premium increases occur in the federal SMI pricing cycle. The cash-flow consequence may therefore become more severe over time even if the penalty percentage never changes.

Premium collection mechanics translate the penalty from abstract formula into household cash-flow reduction. CMS states that when Social Security or Railroad Retirement Board benefits are being paid, the Part B premium is deducted from the monthly benefit payment. For automatic enrollees, the source packet states that the Part B premium is usually deducted from the monthly Social Security or Railroad Retirement Board benefit, and if those benefits are insufficient to cover the Part B premium, a bill is sent every three months. Thus, a Part B LEP can reduce disposable household income before the benefit payment reaches the operating account. The penalty becomes embedded in the federal withholding stream, making it less visible as a separate discretionary expense while still reducing monthly liquidity.

For households not receiving Social Security or Railroad Retirement Board benefits, CMS states that Medicare sends a Part B premium bill, typically quarterly, while monthly billing may occur when Part A premiums, Part D IRMAA, or Medicare Easy Pay applies. CMS identifies online Medicare account payment, Medicare Easy Pay automatic deductions, bank payment, and mailed payment as premium-payment methods. In a direct-bill household, the penalty may be more visible because it appears in invoice obligations rather than in net benefit withholding. However, visibility does not reduce the economic burden. The late enrollment penalty becomes part of the recurring Medicare premium liability, whether extracted through federal benefit withholding or paid from household checking, savings, card, or other authorized premium channels.

The household budget impact is broader than the premium line itself. Original Medicare's Part B design normally requires the annual Part B deductible where applicable and, after the deductible, 20 percent coinsurance for many Part B-covered services under the Medicare-approved amount when assignment applies. The 2026 handbook states that Original Medicare has no yearly limit on what is paid out of pocket unless supplemental coverage such as Medigap, Medicaid, employer, retiree, or union coverage exists. A permanent Part B LEP therefore consumes cash that might otherwise absorb Part B deductible exposure, 20 percent coinsurance, outpatient diagnostic costs, durable medical equipment cost-sharing, physician-administered therapies, or hospital outpatient copayments. The penalty interacts with the uncapped outpatient liability structure described in Section 2.2.

The purchasing-power compression is also intensified by Medicare's exclusion matrix. Section 2.3 established that Original Medicare generally excludes routine outpatient dental care, ordinary refractive vision correction, hearing aids and fitting examinations, routine physical examinations, and non-medical custodial long-term care. CMS identifies many of these exclusions directly in the 2026 handbook, including most dental care, hearing aids and fitting exams, routine physical exams, and long-term care. A permanent Part B surcharge reduces liquid resources available for precisely those services that the federal benefit does not absorb. The household may therefore experience the penalty not merely as a Medicare premium increase, but as a reduction in the reserve available for excluded dental reconstruction, hearing technology, vision correction, caregiving, transportation, home modifications, or custodial support.

The penalty can also interact with Part D and income-related premium structures. CMS states that higher-income beneficiaries may owe IRMAA for Part B, and that an additional amount may also apply to Medicare drug coverage when modified adjusted gross income exceeds the applicable threshold. The Part B LEP is conceptually distinct from IRMAA. The LEP arises from delayed enrollment without protected status. IRMAA arises from income-related premium rules based on tax-return data. Yet both affect monthly Medicare premium outflow. The presence of one does not neutralize the other. A household subject to both may face a layered premium burden: standard Part B premium, Part B late enrollment penalty, and income-related adjustment where applicable.

Medicare Savings Program interaction provides a recognized penalty relief pathway, but it must be stated cautiously. CMS states that if a beneficiary is allowed to sign up for Part B during a Special Enrollment Period, or enrolls in a Medicare Savings Program, the late enrollment penalty may not have to be paid. This statement does not convert the Medicare Savings Program into a universal retroactive cure for every late enrollment problem, nor does it supply state-specific eligibility thresholds inside a generic federal manuscript. It establishes the federal principle that low-income assistance frameworks may alter Part B premium and penalty responsibility when the beneficiary qualifies under the applicable program. The manuscript's compliance posture requires this issue to remain generic rather than advisory.

Exceptional Special Enrollment Periods also qualify the penalty analysis. CMS states that Special Enrollment Periods may be available where an enrollment period was missed because of certain circumstances, including natural disaster or emergency, incarceration, employer or health plan error, loss of Medicaid coverage, or other circumstances outside the beneficiary's control that Medicare determines are exceptional. The existence of such exceptions confirms that the penalty framework is not blind to administrative or extraordinary life events. Nevertheless, these are specific federal relief categories, not general equitable forgiveness. The household file must support the claimed exception with the relevant facts and timing, and the penalty analysis remains anchored in the federal record.

The enforcement framework ultimately rests on documentation. A Part B LEP dispute or correction requires reconstruction of the first eligibility month, the close of the Initial Enrollment Period, the date of Part B enrollment, the existence or absence of current-employment group health plan coverage, the date employment ended, the date group coverage ended, and any exceptional circumstance or Medicare Savings Program status. CMS's safe-harbor language is precise: the protected worker SEP is tied to coverage under a group health plan based on current employment and to an eight-month period after the employment or the coverage ends, whichever happens first. The evidentiary question is therefore not whether a household "had insurance." It is whether the insurance satisfied the Medicare current-employment standard during the relevant months.

This specific interface addresses the exact multi-variable dilemma outlined in the Household Medicare Diagnostic Matrix. The Part B LEP is the financial enforcement counterpart to the matrix's enrollment timeline rows. A household may preserve continuous private coverage through COBRA, retiree insurance, VA benefits, Marketplace coverage, or severance-related former-employer coverage, yet still fail the federal Part B safe-harbor test because those arrangements are not coverage based on current employment for the Part B Special Enrollment Period. The matrix therefore requires four variables to be audited before any Part B delay is treated as safe: the first month of Part B eligibility, the final month of the Initial Enrollment Period, the existence of current-employment group health plan coverage, and the number of full 12-month periods elapsed without Part B after penalty exposure begins.

The actuarial conclusion is unforgiving. The Part B late enrollment penalty converts a missed statutory window into a durable premium impairment. Its numerical rule appears simple: 10 percent for each full 12-month delay block. Its household effect is more complex: recurring withholding or billing, annual dollar variability as the standard premium changes, reduced purchasing power, interaction with uncapped Original Medicare coinsurance exposure, possible coexistence with IRMAA, and diminished liquidity for services excluded from the federal benefit. Under CMS's 2026 formulation, the penalty may remain for as long as Part B remains active. A filing delay that initially appears administrative can therefore become a persistent claim on retirement capital, measurable not only in premium arithmetic, but in reduced household capacity to absorb medical, pharmaceutical, dental, sensory, custodial, and caregiving risk across the Medicare life cycle.

4.2 The Part D Lifetime LEP Calculations

The Part D late enrollment penalty is a structural enforcement device embedded inside the voluntary prescription drug benefit. It is not a minor administrative fee imposed for clerical lateness. It is an actuarial participation mechanism designed to protect the Medicare drug risk pool from selective delayed entry. Under CMS Part D Enrollment Specifications in the 2026 Medicare handbook, the late enrollment penalty is an amount permanently added to the Medicare drug coverage premium when enrollment occurs after the Initial Enrollment Period and there has been a period of 63 or more consecutive days without Medicare drug coverage or other creditable prescription drug coverage; CMS further states that the penalty generally remains part of the monthly premium for as long as Medicare drug coverage continues, while Extra Help eliminates the late enrollment penalty for qualifying beneficiaries. This duration rule gives the penalty its institutional severity: the surcharge is not a retrospective invoice for a past enrollment error, but a continuing premium modifier attached to future drug coverage.

The voluntary structure of Part D makes such a penalty system necessary. Part D is not automatically identical to premium-free Part A entitlement or standard Part B medical insurance. It is a federally regulated prescription drug framework administered through Medicare drug coverage arrangements that follow Medicare rules, while the beneficiary decision to obtain drug coverage remains tied to election periods, creditable coverage status, and plan enrollment mechanics. Without a delayed-entry surcharge, healthy beneficiaries with low medication utilization could remain outside the drug premium pool until chronic prescriptions, oncology therapies, transplant drugs, anticoagulants, diabetes agents, pulmonary therapies, or high-cost maintenance medications became clinically foreseeable. The resulting adverse selection would concentrate drug risk among those already expecting claims.

Pursuant to 42 CFR Part 423 Subpart B, and specifically the Part D late enrollment penalty architecture of 42 CFR § 423.46, the federal system converts uncovered months after eligibility into a continuing premium surcharge, thereby preserving the economic relationship between timely participation and later claims access.

Creditable prescription drug coverage is the principal safe harbor against Part D late enrollment penalty exposure. Under CMS's 2026 Medicare handbook, creditable prescription drug coverage may include coverage from a current or former employer or union, TRICARE, the Indian Health Service, the Department of Veterans Affairs, or other recognized arrangements, but the controlling test is not the mere existence of a drug card or pharmacy benefit. CMS defines creditable prescription drug coverage as coverage expected to pay, on average, at least as much as Medicare drug coverage. Under 42 CFR § 423.56(a), the legal standard is actuarial: alternative prescription drug coverage must equal or exceed the actuarial value of the defined standard Part D prescription drug benefit under CMS rules. The safe harbor is therefore objective, documentary, and actuarial, not subjective or experiential.

This distinction is essential because a household may possess broad medical coverage while still lacking creditable prescription coverage for Part D penalty purposes. Major medical insurance, a retiree health arrangement, an individual health policy, a union benefit, a federal health arrangement, or a legacy employer plan may feel adequate in ordinary household terms; however, the Part D late enrollment penalty analysis asks whether the prescription drug component was creditable under the Medicare standard. CMS states that once Part D eligibility exists, a beneficiary cannot go 63 days or more without either Medicare drug coverage or other creditable prescription drug coverage without risking penalty exposure. The existence of medical coverage alone does not answer that question. The federal audit requires proof that the prescription component satisfied the actuarial creditability threshold.

The 63-day rule supplies the chronological trigger. Under CMS Part D Enrollment Specifications, Part D late enrollment penalty exposure may arise when a beneficiary goes 63 days or more in a row without Medicare drug coverage or other creditable prescription drug coverage after the Initial Enrollment Period has ended. The statutory distinction between days and months must be preserved. The 63-day continuous break is the threshold that triggers penalty inquiry. The penalty amount itself is not calculated by multiplying 63 days by a daily rate. Instead, once penalty exposure exists, CMS calculates the surcharge by counting the number of full uncovered months during which the individual was Part D eligible, lacked Medicare drug coverage, and lacked other creditable prescription drug coverage.

The 63-day rule is also continuous, not merely cumulative in isolated fragments. A short administrative gap below the statutory threshold does not operate like a multi-year penalty block. A continuous gap reaching 63 days can activate the uncovered-month calculation. Under the federal rule reflected in 42 CFR § 423.46, the relevant period occurs after the end of the Initial Enrollment Period and while the beneficiary is eligible for Part D but not enrolled in Medicare drug coverage and not protected by creditable prescription drug coverage. The temporal architecture thereby separates ordinary short transition intervals from sustained uncovered exposure. The household file must therefore be audited by dates: the end of the Initial Enrollment Period, the first month of Part D eligibility, the start and end dates of any alternative prescription coverage, and the presence or absence of any continuous break reaching 63 days.

The disclosure regime supplies the documentary architecture for that audit. CMS states that non-Medicare drug coverage must tell Medicare-eligible individuals each year whether the coverage is creditable prescription drug coverage. Under the regulatory disclosure framework of 42 CFR § 423.56, entities offering prescription drug coverage to Part D eligible individuals must disclose whether the coverage is creditable, and notices must be supplied at defined times, including before the individual's Initial Enrollment Period, before the effective date of prescription drug coverage, upon changes affecting creditable status, before the Annual Coordinated Election Period, and upon request. Because the Annual Coordinated Election Period begins October 15, the pre-election disclosure functions as the annual compliance notice households often associate with the October Medicare planning cycle.

The notice is not a courtesy letter. It is the evidentiary bridge between alternative prescription coverage and Part D penalty protection. Under CMS's 2026 handbook, beneficiaries are instructed to keep records showing when other creditable prescription drug coverage existed and to tell the Medicare drug coverage arrangement when asked; CMS warns that failure to provide information about previous creditable prescription drug coverage may result in paying a penalty for as long as Medicare drug coverage continues. This recordkeeping requirement is the practical foundation of the national audit framework. The household cannot prove creditable coverage through memory, general insurance status, or pharmacy receipts alone. The operative proof is the notice, certificate, employer or union verification, government-program documentation, or other record establishing dates and creditable status.

The mathematical formula is more granular than the Part B late enrollment penalty formula. Part B uses a 10 percent surcharge for each full 12-month period of delayed Part B enrollment. Part D uses a 1 percent surcharge for each full uncovered month. Under CMS's 2026 Medicare handbook, the Part D late enrollment penalty is calculated by multiplying 1 percent of the national base beneficiary premium by the number of full uncovered months during which the individual was eligible for Medicare drug coverage but lacked Part D and lacked other creditable prescription drug coverage. CMS states that the final amount is rounded to the nearest ten cents and added to the monthly premium. The computational unit is therefore monthly; every full uncovered month becomes part of the penalty percentage once the penalty conditions have been triggered.

The national base beneficiary premium is the statutory multiplier. CMS states that the national base beneficiary premium is $38.99 in 2026, and that this national base beneficiary premium may increase or decrease each year, causing the dollar penalty amount to increase or decrease. The penalty is not multiplied against the premium of any particular drug coverage arrangement. It is multiplied against the national base beneficiary premium determined by CMS. This distinction is central to the actuarial character of the penalty. The household's chosen drug coverage premium may differ from the national base beneficiary premium, but the late enrollment surcharge is tied to the federal indexing base, not to the selected coverage premium.

The formula can be expressed as a statutory sequence. The penalty percentage equals 1 percent multiplied by the number of full uncovered months. The monthly penalty dollar amount equals the national base beneficiary premium multiplied by the penalty percentage, with the result rounded to the nearest ten cents. The total monthly drug coverage premium obligation equals the applicable drug coverage premium plus the federal late enrollment penalty, with any separate income-related drug premium amount treated as a distinct federal premium component where applicable. Under CMS's 2026 calculation standard, a 24-month uncovered period produces a 24 percent penalty. Applied to the 2026 national base beneficiary premium of $38.99, a 24 percent penalty equals $9.36 before rounding, which rounds to $9.40 under the nearest-ten-cent rule. This illustration demonstrates the mechanics of the federal formula; it does not project future premiums or individualized liability.

CMS's 2026 handbook provides an official example that demonstrates annual recalculation. The example states that a 29-month uncovered period produced a 29 percent penalty. In 2025, the 29 percent penalty was applied to the 2025 national base beneficiary premium of $36.78, producing $10.66, rounded to $10.70. In 2026, Medicare recalculated the same 29 percent penalty using the 2026 national base beneficiary premium of $38.99, producing $11.31, rounded to $11.30. The example proves the penalty's dynamic character. The uncovered-month percentage remains constant unless the federal record is corrected, but the dollar amount can change each year because CMS recalculates the national base beneficiary premium.

This mechanism should not be mislabeled as compound interest. The penalty does not accrue interest on unpaid penalty amounts, nor does the prior year's dollar penalty become the next year's principal. It is cumulative because each full uncovered month becomes an additional 1 percent of the national base beneficiary premium. It is variable because the national base beneficiary premium changes annually. Therefore, the penalty's economic burden is durable and indexed, but it is not compounding in the conventional finance sense. The actuarial force lies in permanent percentage attachment to a moving federal premium base.

Administrative visibility begins when a late enrollment record or potential coverage gap appears in the Part D enrollment process. Historical CMS operational guidance in the source packet states that Part D sponsors were instructed to report creditable coverage determinations through enrollment transactions, including two data elements: a creditable coverage flag and the number of uncovered months, defined as the number of calendar months after a beneficiary's Initial Enrollment Period in which the beneficiary lacked Medicare prescription drug coverage and lacked other creditable prescription drug coverage. Although the operational systems have evolved since the early Part D implementation period, the source packet confirms the federal design: uncovered-month status is converted into reportable enrollment data, and creditable coverage status is not left to informal assumption.

The phrase "National Registry Audit Framework," used in this section as an analytic label, refers to the nationwide federal compliance architecture created by CMS enrollment records, Part D sponsor reporting, creditable coverage flags, uncovered-month calculations, employer or union disclosure notices, beneficiary attestations, reconsideration forms, and independent review pathways. It should not be read as the title of a single proprietary database unless an official CMS source uses that title. The federal recordkeeping structure instead operates through interlocking administrative artifacts. CMS enrollment data identifies potential gaps. Plan sponsors collect and transmit prior coverage information. Employers, unions, and other coverage entities issue creditable coverage notices. Beneficiaries submit prior-coverage attestations when requested. CMS calculates or finalizes the penalty. Review entities evaluate disputes. Together, these components form the national audit framework that determines whether the penalty applies.

The receiving drug coverage arrangement has an administrative role when a gap is suspected. Under 42 CFR § 423.46(b), Part D sponsors must obtain information on prior creditable coverage from enrolled or enrolling beneficiaries and report that information to CMS in the form and manner CMS specifies. The source packet's historical CMS guidance confirms that sponsors report the creditable coverage flag and the number of uncovered months through enrollment transactions. This framework explains why a beneficiary who enrolls after a potential gap may receive a request for information about prior prescription drug coverage. The request is not a private underwriting inquiry. It is part of the federal penalty-determination process.

The prior-coverage attestation process is the evidentiary checkpoint inside the audit sequence. CMS's 2026 handbook instructs beneficiaries to keep records showing when other creditable prescription drug coverage existed and to provide that information when the plan asks; failure to tell the plan about previous creditable coverage may lead to a penalty for as long as Medicare drug coverage continues. The attestation must verify dates, source of coverage, and creditable status. It is not a narrative statement that coverage seemed adequate. The relevant documentation may include employer or union creditable coverage notices, retiree drug coverage certifications, recognized government-program records, or other documentation sufficient to establish that the prescription drug coverage was creditable during the asserted months.

Reconsideration is the formal administrative pipeline for contesting an assessed Part D late enrollment penalty. CMS states in the 2026 handbook that the drug coverage arrangement sends a letter stating that a late enrollment penalty must be paid, and that disagreement with the penalty may be addressed through a review request, generally within 60 days from the date on the letter. CMS further states that the reconsideration request form is provided with the letter and that proof supporting the case may include information about previous creditable prescription drug coverage. Under 42 CFR § 423.46(c), the Part D LEP reconsideration process is conducted by CMS or by an independent review entity under CMS guidance. The reconsideration pathway therefore sits inside federal administrative review, not ordinary consumer complaint handling.

The evidentiary issues in reconsideration correspond to the statutory formula. A disputed penalty may require proof that coverage existed during some or all alleged uncovered months, proof that the coverage was creditable, proof that required disclosure notices were inadequate, proof that the uncovered-month count was erroneous, or proof that Extra Help status should eliminate the penalty. CMS's handbook expressly recognizes prior creditable prescription drug coverage information as supporting proof for review. The review is documentation-driven because the penalty itself is documentation-driven. The federal record must reconcile Initial Enrollment Period end date, Part D eligibility, drug coverage enrollment date, alternative prescription coverage dates, actuarial creditability, and any 63-day continuous gap.

The disclosure-failure rules also preserve administrative equity. CMS Part D enrollment guidance in the source packet states that a Medicare-eligible individual who was not adequately informed of the creditable status of drug coverage, or of the loss of creditable prescription drug coverage, may be eligible for a Special Enrollment Period when CMS determines eligibility on a case-by-case basis; the same guidance states that the SEP begins the month CMS determines eligibility and ends two calendar months after that determination. This relief structure confirms that the federal penalty regime depends on accurate disclosure. If an entity required to provide notice failed to give accurate and timely creditable coverage information, CMS may recognize a remedial enrollment pathway. The existence of that remedy does not eliminate the need for proof; it reinforces the importance of notice records.

The Part D late enrollment penalty also interacts with premium enforcement and household liquidity. CMS states that the LEP is added to the monthly premium for Medicare drug coverage and generally remains payable for as long as that coverage continues. Because the penalty is a premium surcharge rather than a deductible, copayment, coinsurance amount, or pharmacy point-of-sale charge, it does not function as a covered-drug out-of-pocket expense. CMS states separately that 2026 yearly out-of-pocket costs for covered Part D drugs are capped at $2,100, but that cap concerns covered Part D drug cost sharing; premium obligations and penalties remain distinct from the covered-drug cost-sharing cap. The penalty therefore occupies the premium layer of the drug architecture, not the TrOOP or pharmacy-cost layer.

This premium-layer classification matters for capital preservation. A household may focus on the 2026 Part D out-of-pocket cap because it limits covered drug cost sharing, while overlooking a monthly LEP that remains outside the cap. Under CMS's 2026 rule, the penalty is added to the monthly premium and can change each year as the national base beneficiary premium changes. The surcharge consumes recurring liquidity that might otherwise fund drug copayments, deductibles, excluded dental services, hearing aids, refractive vision correction, transportation, caregiving, home supports, or custodial long-term care. The monthly dollar amount may appear modest when isolated, but its persistence across years creates a continuing claim against retirement cash flow.

The Part D LEP's actuarial severity lies in its combination of granularity, permanency, and indexing. Granularity arises because every full uncovered month becomes 1 percent of the national base beneficiary premium. Permanency arises because CMS states that the penalty is generally owed for as long as Medicare drug coverage continues. Indexing arises because CMS recalculates the dollar amount each year using the national base beneficiary premium, which may increase or decrease annually. This architecture transforms a coverage gap into a durable premium record. The household does not merely pay for the months that were missed. The household pays an indexed premium consequence after coverage has begun.

The comparison with Part B clarifies the enforcement design. Part B imposes 10 percent for each full 12-month period of delayed enrollment. Part D imposes 1 percent for each full uncovered month. Part B therefore counts completed annual blocks, while Part D counts monthly exposure. This difference reflects the different structure of the benefits. Part B is a broad medical insurance program with a national premium architecture. Part D is a voluntary prescription drug program where creditable alternative coverage is common and where pharmacy-risk selection can change quickly as prescriptions begin or end. A monthly penalty model captures shorter drug-coverage gaps more precisely than a full-year block model.

The household planning implication is that Part D cannot be audited only at retirement. It must be audited whenever drug coverage changes. Loss of creditable employer or union drug coverage, reduction in creditable status, movement between coverage arrangements, transition from active employment to retiree benefits, entry into individual coverage, or reliance on federal non-Medicare drug sources can alter the Part D penalty file. CMS Part D guidance in the source packet recognizes a Special Enrollment Period for involuntary loss of creditable prescription drug coverage, including a reduction in the coverage level so that it is no longer creditable; the SEP begins when the individual is notified of the loss or reduction and ends two calendar months after the later of the loss or the receipt of notice. This rule confirms that loss of creditability is a distinct legal event, not merely a benefit-design inconvenience.

This specific interface addresses the exact multi-variable dilemma outlined in the Household Medicare Diagnostic Matrix. A household may hold comprehensive private medical coverage, retiree coverage, Marketplace coverage, government-related coverage, or another prescription arrangement that appears adequate from the standpoint of pharmacy access. The Part D late enrollment penalty test is narrower and more technical. The prescription component must be creditable, the coverage dates must be documented, the continuous break must remain below 63 days unless Medicare drug coverage has begun, and every full uncovered month after penalty exposure begins must be countable or defensibly excluded under federal rules.

The Household Medicare Diagnostic Matrix therefore requires a five-variable audit before delayed Part D enrollment is treated as protected. The first variable is the first month of Part D eligibility. The second is the end of the Initial Enrollment Period. The third is whether Medicare drug coverage was elected. The fourth is whether alternative prescription drug coverage was creditable under the federal actuarial standard. The fifth is whether any continuous break reached 63 days or more and how many full uncovered months resulted. These variables are not advisory preferences. They are the documentary elements from which the Part D LEP is calculated, disclosed, imposed, or contested.

The final actuarial conclusion is severe. The Part D late enrollment penalty converts a prescription coverage documentation failure into a durable premium surcharge indexed to the national base beneficiary premium. The penalty's burden is not limited to the 1 percent monthly formula. It also lies in the permanence of the uncovered-month record, the annual recalculation of the national base beneficiary premium, the evidentiary burden imposed by creditable coverage disclosures, and the liquidity drain created by a recurring surcharge layered onto drug premiums, medical coinsurance, excluded dental care, hearing technology, vision correction, custodial support, and family caregiving costs. Under CMS's 2026 framework, the household file that cannot prove creditable prescription coverage may face a rising penalty long after the original coverage gap has disappeared from ordinary memory.

4.3 Administrative Relief, Appeals, and Equitable Tolling

Medicare's penalty and enforcement architecture is strict, but it is not entirely mechanical. The federal system contains structured correction channels for unfavorable coverage or payment decisions, incorrect enrollment records, erroneous disenrollments, plan sponsor error, federal system error, missed appeal deadlines for good cause, Part D late-enrollment penalty reconsideration, and limited reinstatement after nonpayment when federally defined standards are satisfied. Under CMS appeals specifications in the 2026 Medicare handbook, an appeal is the action available when Medicare or a Medicare plan issues an unfavorable coverage or payment decision, including a denial of a requested service, supply, item, drug, or payment, or a decision changing the amount owed for a covered item or service. Administrative relief is therefore a procedural correction system, not casual equitable forgiveness.

The controlling analytic requirement is procedural classification. An Original Medicare claim denial, a Part D late-enrollment penalty, a Part B premium surcharge, an IRMAA billing issue, an erroneous plan disenrollment, a failure-to-pay reinstatement request, and a federal entitlement-file mismatch do not travel through a single universal appeal channel. CMS's 2026 handbook itself separates Original Medicare appeals, Medicare health plan appeals, drug plan coverage determinations, fast appeals before a Beneficiary and Family Centered Care-Quality Improvement Organization, and Part D late-enrollment penalty review. A household file may contain a substantively legitimate grievance, yet lose the available remedy if the filing is routed to the wrong review body, filed after the operative deadline without good cause, or supported by insufficient documentary proof.

The Original Medicare claims appeal track begins with the Medicare Summary Notice. Under CMS appeals specifications, the Medicare Summary Notice showing the disputed item or service is the first operational document; the disputed item is identified on the notice, an explanation of disagreement is supplied on the notice or through attached documentation, the Medicare number and contact information are included, and the package is sent to the Medicare Administrative Contractor listed on the notice, with supporting information from the provider permitted and Form CMS-20027 available as an appeal instrument. CMS states that the Medicare Administrative Contractor generally issues a decision within 60 days after receiving the appeal request, and if Medicare covers the disputed item or service, the result appears on the next Medicare Summary Notice. This first-level claim review is a coverage and payment pathway, not a premium-surcharge pathway.

The Qualified Independent Contractor belongs to the Original Medicare fee-for-service claims appeal structure as the second level after Medicare Administrative Contractor redetermination. CMS's fee-for-service appeal guidance identifies the second level of appeal as reconsideration by a Qualified Independent Contractor, and CMS's QIC guidance states that an appellant has 180 days from receipt of the redetermination decision to file the reconsideration request, with the redetermination decision communicated through a Medicare Redetermination Notice, Medicare Summary Notice, or Remittance Advice. (CMS) The QIC therefore functions as an independent reconsideration layer for Original Medicare claim coverage or payment disputes after the contractor stage. It should not be assigned jurisdiction over every Medicare surcharge or enrollment problem merely because the word "appeal" appears in a dispute.

This jurisdictional distinction is essential. The uploaded source packet establishes Medicare Administrative Contractor processing for Original Medicare claims and good-cause late filing for those appeals, while CMS's fee-for-service appeal materials place the QIC in the second-level claims appeal sequence. (CMS) The same source set does not establish QIC jurisdiction over Part B late-enrollment penalties, Part D late-enrollment penalties, IRMAA determinations, premium-billing disputes, or plan reinstatement after nonpayment. Part D LEP review follows a separate reconsideration pathway, and good-cause reinstatement after nonpayment follows CMS enrollment guidance rather than the QIC claims pipeline.

Good cause appears first in the Original Medicare claim appeal context as a limited tolling principle. CMS states that an Original Medicare appeal must be filed by the date shown in the Medicare Summary Notice, but that a late appeal may still receive a decision if good cause is shown for missing the deadline, with disability, illness, or accident supplied as examples of circumstances that delayed timely submission. This is not an unlimited right to reopen historical claims. It is a documentary exception to a filing deadline inside the correct claims appeal track. The timing defect may be excused only when the administrative record supports a federally recognizable reason for delay.

Fast appeals occupy a separate corridor. When Medicare-covered services from a hospital, skilled nursing facility, home health agency, comprehensive outpatient rehabilitation facility, or hospice are ending too soon, CMS states that a fast appeal, also called an immediate or expedited appeal, may be requested and decided by the Beneficiary and Family Centered Care-Quality Improvement Organization. CMS also states that a fast appeal generally covers the decision to end services or discharge, and that a separate claim appeal may still be needed for items or services received after the termination decision. This reinforces the procedural premise of the chapter: remedy depends on dispute type.

Part D late-enrollment penalty disputes do not belong in the Original Medicare QIC claims pipeline. Under CMS Part D penalty specifications in the 2026 handbook, the Medicare drug coverage arrangement sends a letter stating that a late-enrollment penalty must be paid; disagreement is handled through a review request, generally within 60 days from the letter date, using the reconsideration request form supplied with the notice, and supporting proof may include information about previous creditable prescription drug coverage. CMS's Part D LEP appeals page identifies the Part D LEP Reconsideration Request Form C2C as the form used to request appeal of a late-enrollment penalty decision and directs that the completed form be sent to the Independent Review Entity as instructed. (CMS)

The Independent Review Entity review of a Part D LEP is documentary and actuarial. The disputed data points ordinarily concern whether prior drug coverage was creditable, whether the uncovered-month count was correct, whether the 63-day continuous break rule was triggered, whether Extra Help status eliminates the penalty, or whether inadequate notice or administrative error distorted the penalty file. CMS's 2026 handbook states that creditable coverage records should be kept and supplied when requested, and that failure to provide previous creditable coverage information may result in a penalty for as long as Medicare drug coverage continues. The IRE pathway therefore examines coverage chronology and documentation, not medical necessity in the QIC sense.

Good-cause reinstatement after nonpayment belongs to yet another procedural track. Under CMS enrollment reinstatement guidance, an individual involuntarily disenrolled for failure to pay plan premiums or Part D-IRMAA may request reinstatement for good cause under 42 CFR §§ 422.74(d)(1)(v) and 423.44(d)(1)(vi) only if the request is received by the plan or CMS within 60 days of the disenrollment effective date, no prior good-cause reinstatement request has been made during that same 60-day period, good cause is shown for failure to pay within the initial grace period, plan premiums owed at disenrollment are paid in full within three months, a credible statement establishes circumstances outside the individual's control or not reasonably foreseeable, and Part D-IRMAA owed at disenrollment is paid in full within three months where applicable.

The good-cause standard is deliberately narrow. CMS states that reinstatement for good cause is provided only in rare circumstances where the individual or authorized representative was unable to make timely payment due to circumstances beyond control or not reasonably foreseeable, and that the request must be accompanied by a credible verbal or written statement explaining the unforeseen and uncontrollable circumstances causing the nonpayment. CMS-recognized examples include serious illness, institutionalization, hospitalization, unexpected deterioration of health, recent death of a spouse or immediate family member, severe home damage from fire or disaster, emergency weather or public-safety events, and federal government error by CMS, SSA, or RRB causing Part D-IRMAA payment error where the enrollee was unaware or unable to act before disenrollment.

CMS also identifies circumstances that generally do not constitute good cause. The source packet states that unreported address changes causing bills or warning notices to be missed, personal non-emergency travel, failure of an authorized representative to pay timely, lack of understanding of nonpayment consequences, inability to afford premiums during the grace period, and need for prescription medicines or other plan services generally do not satisfy the standard. This rule has severe capital implications. Financial hardship and clinical need may explain the household crisis, but CMS does not treat them as ordinary good-cause bases for reinstatement after nonpayment. The remedial inquiry is causation by unforeseen or uncontrollable circumstances, not general equity.

The operational mechanics of a favorable good-cause determination remain conditional. CMS guidance states that plans should determine good cause within five business days of initial contact when the required elements are met, obtain a credible statement, obtain affirmation of willingness and ability to pay overdue plan premiums within three months, and notify the individual of the amount owed, the payment deadline, payment location, and available payment options after a favorable determination. Reinstatement is not complete merely because good cause is accepted. CMS states that reinstatements for good cause are considered complete when the plan receives the enrollment reinstatement transaction from CMS, and that payment must still be made within the three-month payment period, with limited processing time for verification and submission.

Part D-IRMAA nonpayment adds CMS caseworker involvement. CMS guidance states that when disenrollment follows failure to pay Part D-IRMAA and the individual asserts good cause, the plan must direct the individual to contact 1-800-MEDICARE within 60 calendar days of the disenrollment effective date; a Complaint Tracking Module case is generated for CMS caseworker action, CMS reviews the request and makes a favorable or unfavorable good-cause determination, and the plan must provide documentation included in the request so that CMS can consider it. CMS also states that actual reinstatement does not occur until all required payments are made within three months of the disenrollment effective date. The process is therefore dual: CMS decides good cause for the IRMAA component, and payment completion remains mandatory.

Good-cause determinations after nonpayment are not ordinary coverage appeals. CMS guidance states that good-cause determinations are not organization determinations related to coverage and therefore are not appealable under 42 CFR Parts 422 and 423, Subpart M, although an individual has the right to file a grievance against the plan related to the involuntary disenrollment. This distinction prevents procedural misrouting. A grievance may address administrative handling, but it does not convert an unfavorable good-cause determination into a QIC appeal, a Part C organization determination appeal, or a Part D coverage determination appeal. The remedy classification is final in practical effect: without favorable good cause and required payment, reinstatement fails.

Administrative-error correction differs from good-cause reinstatement. CMS defines reinstatement as an action used to correct a disenrollment made in error or to reverse a disenrollment where good cause for failure to pay has been demonstrated; after reinstatement, the enrollment record shows active, unbroken coverage, and reinstatement does not require an election period because it is not a new enrollment request. CMS identifies common reinstatement bases including erroneous death indicator, erroneous loss of Medicare Part A or Part B indicator or Part D eligibility, erroneous incarceration or unlawful presence information, individual cancellation of a new enrollment, plan error, and good cause for failure to pay plan premiums or Part D-IRMAA timely.

Erroneous death, entitlement-loss, and eligibility-loss cases are corrective rather than discretionary. CMS guidance states that when a disenrolled individual asserts erroneous disenrollment and wishes to remain enrolled, the plan should send notification within 10 days acknowledging the erroneous disenrollment and instructing continued use of plan services, and erroneous disenrollments must be corrected with corresponding reinstatements when the individual remains eligible, regardless of when the error is disputed or evidence is provided. For erroneous incarceration or unlawful presence information, CMS guidance instructs plans to check CMS systems, ensure ongoing eligibility, and refer the individual to SSA where

CMS systems still reflect the erroneous status, with services resuming seamlessly once SSA correction updates CMS systems.

Plan error requires direct correction by the plan sponsor. CMS guidance states that when an erroneous disenrollment results from plan error, the plan reinstates the individual, and if the disenrollment transaction had been submitted to CMS, the plan must cancel the disenrollment action from CMS records through the disenrollment cancellation function within CMS system parameters. This rule separates plan error from good cause. CMS expressly states that where involuntary disenrollment for failure to pay plan premiums results from plan error, the plan-error reinstatement process applies, and the case should not be treated as a good-cause reinstatement request. The distinction matters because plan error repairs an invalid administrative action; good cause excuses a valid disenrollment caused by nonpayment under rare circumstances.

System error is a federal-file category. CMS defines system error as an unintended error or delay in enrollment request processing clearly attributable to a specific federal government system, including SSA or Railroad Retirement Board systems, and related to Medicare entitlement information or other information required to process an enrollment request. The source packet supports discussion of federal system error, MARx status checks, Daily Transaction Reply Reports, Transaction Reply Codes, Regional Processing Contractor correction, and retroactive enrollment or disenrollment processing, but it does not establish a formal "CMS Third Party System clearinghouse" as the named mechanism for the correction categories in this section. Therefore, the manuscript treats the requested clearinghouse concept as a broader federal data-synchronization problem rather than as an official system title.

Retroactive corrections are file-repair mechanisms, not preference changes. CMS guidance states that a reinstatement reverses a disenrollment and restores enrollment as if disenrollment had not occurred; it may be made back to a date when a plan was closed for enrollment because reinstatement is not a new election request. The guidance also states that where a valid cancellation request is not processed timely or CMS systems cannot complete the request, the new plan submits a request to the Regional Processing Contractor to cancel the enrollment, with complete documentation including evidence that cancellation was requested within required timeframes. The governing principle is documentary mismatch: the record is corrected only where the federal file failed to reflect the valid entitlement, enrollment, cancellation, disenrollment, or employer or union group transaction.

Contesting actuarial surcharges requires still another distinction. A Part B late-enrollment penalty dispute requires reconstruction of the first Part B eligibility month, the close of the Initial Enrollment Period, the presence or absence of current-employment group health plan coverage, Special Enrollment Period protection, and the number of full 12-month penalty blocks. CMS states that the Part B penalty is 10 percent for each full 12-month period in which Part B could have been held but was not, generally continuing for as long as Part B remains active, and that the penalty is avoided if enrollment occurs before the first full 12-month period has passed or if a Special Enrollment Period applies. CMS also states that COBRA, VA coverage, retiree health plans, and individual Marketplace coverage are not coverage based on current employment for the Part B Special Enrollment Period.

The uploaded source packet establishes the Part B formula and current-employment safe harbor, but it does not provide a complete SSA Medicare premium-determination appeal chapter for Part B LEP or premium surcharge disputes. The procedural limitation is therefore part of the manuscript's legal accuracy. A complete premium-determination review channel requires applicable SSA Medicare premium determination and reconsideration guidance, including SSA reconsideration processes such as Form SSA-561-U2 where SSA determination review is implicated. This limitation preserves the boundary among QIC claim reconsideration, Part D LEP reconsideration before the IRE, CMS or plan reinstatement correction, and SSA/CMS premium-file correction. CMS's 2026 handbook supports the Part B LEP arithmetic and current-employment safe harbor, while the QIC source supports fee-for-service claim reconsideration only. (CMS)

Administrative proof is the currency of relief. CMS's 2026 handbook instructs Original Medicare appellants to retain copies of appeal materials and submit supporting information, including provider documentation, to the Medicare Administrative Contractor. CMS's Part D penalty rules instruct beneficiaries to keep records of prior creditable prescription drug coverage and provide proof during reconsideration. CMS reinstatement guidance requires credible statements for good cause, payment verification, transaction confirmation, plan-system correction, CMS system updates, and documentation for cancellation or retroactive correction. The federal record therefore outranks household recollection.

The documentary file should be understood as an actuarial control instrument. Medicare's relief architecture must distinguish enforceable late enrollment, unpaid premiums, uncovered months, and valid claim denials from penalties or disenrollments caused by file corruption, plan error, inadequate notice, federal system error, or documented circumstances outside the enrollee's control. CMS's guidance reflects this distinction by permitting reinstatement after plan error, requiring correction of erroneous disenrollments where eligibility remains, limiting good-cause reinstatement to rare circumstances, and making good-cause determinations non-appealable as coverage determinations while preserving grievance rights. Relief therefore protects legitimacy without dissolving enforcement.

This specific interface completes the procedural repair function of the Household Medicare Diagnostic Matrix. The matrix does not merely identify enrollment windows and penalty formulas; it routes file disruptions to the correct regulatory channel. A denied Original Medicare claim belongs first to the Medicare Administrative Contractor and, after unfavorable redetermination, to QIC reconsideration. A premature facility discharge belongs to the BFCC-QIO fast-appeal channel. A Part D late-enrollment penalty belongs to the reconsideration process supported by creditable coverage documentation and, where applicable, the Independent Review Entity. A nonpayment disenrollment belongs to good-cause reinstatement only under CMS's rare-circumstance standard and payment deadlines. A Part B premium surcharge belongs to premium-determination and entitlement-file review rather than to the QIC claims pipeline.

The matrix's six diagnostic variables therefore operate as procedural triage. The first variable is the nature of the dispute: clinical claim, enrollment record, premium surcharge, creditable coverage record, IRMAA billing, or disenrollment. The second is the primary review body: Medicare Administrative Contractor, QIC, plan sponsor, CMS, SSA, Railroad Retirement Board, Independent Review Entity, BFCC-QIO, or another federally designated entity. The third is the active chronological filing window and whether good cause exists. The fourth is the root cause of file corruption, including plan error, federal system error, inadequate notice, missing documentation, or beneficiary non-action. The fifth is the remedy scope, meaning retroactive transaction correction, reinstatement, reconsideration, grievance, claim payment, or new enrollment only through a valid election period. The sixth is source completeness, distinguishing CMS packet parameters from additional SSA premium-determination manuals where the uploaded source packet does not supply the full premium review channel.

The final actuarial conclusion is that administrative relief does not weaken Medicare's penalty architecture. It preserves the legitimacy of the social insurance system by separating enforceable liabilities from liabilities created by federal file error, plan error, inadequate notice, erroneous eligibility data, documented good cause, or correctable administrative mismatch. A household may be legally entitled to relief and still lose the remedy by filing in the wrong channel, missing the applicable deadline, failing to preserve creditable coverage notices, lacking payment proof, or treating a non-appealable good-cause determination as an ordinary coverage appeal.

Section 4.3 therefore functions as the procedural counterpart to the penalty equations in Sections 4.1 and 4.2: actuarial charges are enforceable when the federal file is correct, but administrative correction is required when the file itself is defective.

Questions About This Book or Medicare Education Seminars?

Visit www.medicareigetitnow.com

to submit a general question, request information about an upcoming Medicare educational seminar, or inquire about hosting a seminar for your library, church, community, employer, or organization.

MODULE III: MACROECONOMIC INTERFACES: EMPLOYMENT, COBRA, AND TAXATION

Chapter 5: The Statutory Triad: Active Employment, COBRA, and Medicare Primary Payer Rules

5.1 The Active Employment Safe Harbor and EGHP Mechanics

The Medicare Secondary Payer architecture is one of the central revenue-preservation mechanisms in the modern Medicare system. Medicare began as a public entitlement framework designed to pay defined hospital and medical claims for qualified beneficiaries, but the working-aged provisions of the Medicare Secondary Payer regime changed the payer hierarchy when age-based Medicare entitlement overlaps with active employment group health coverage. In the TEFRA-era policy transformation reflected in the current Social Security Act and implemented through CMS regulations, Medicare does not automatically remain the first payer merely because age sixty-five has been reached; instead, where statutory working-aged conditions are satisfied, the employer group health plan occupies the primary payer position and Medicare becomes secondary. Under CMS Medicare Secondary Payer specifications, the working-aged provision applies to group health plans of employers with 20 or more employees and to multi-employer or multiple-employer group health plans in which at least one employer employs 20 or more employees. (CMS)

This payer sequencing doctrine is actuarial before it is clerical. The federal program does not merely reorder claim forms; it reallocates claim liability between private employment-based capital pools and the public Medicare trust and premium architecture. CMS explains the operative concept in direct coordination language: when another insurer pays first, that primary payer pays up to the limits of its coverage, and the secondary payer pays only if costs remain uncovered, while the secondary payer may not pay all residual costs. This rule is a priority matrix. It determines whether a physician service, hospital outpatient claim, diagnostic test, durable medical equipment claim, or other Medicare-relevant expense first draws against the employer group health plan or against the Medicare program. The sequence is therefore not a peripheral coordination issue; it determines the first balance sheet exposed to medical risk.

For age-based beneficiaries, the 20-employee threshold is the principal jurisdictional switch. Under the 2026 Medicare handbook, if an individual is age sixty-five or older and has group health plan coverage based on current employment, either through the individual's own current employment or a spouse's current employment, and the employer has 20 or more employees, the group health plan pays first; the same primary-employer rule applies when the employer has fewer than 20 employees but participates in a multi-employer plan that includes another employer with 20 or more employees. In the reverse condition, if an individual is age sixty-five or older and has group health plan coverage based on current employment with an employer that has fewer than 20 employees, Medicare pays first.

The threshold is not measured by plan participation alone. CMS's Medicare Secondary Payer Manual states that the 20-or-more requirement is met if the employer has 20 or more full-time and part-time employees for each working day in each of 20 or more calendar weeks in the current or preceding year. The same CMS manual further states that the count is based on employment rolls, that an employee is counted even if not working on a particular day, that separate daily rolls may not be manipulated, and that self-employed individuals participating in a group health plan are not counted as employees for this threshold. (CMS) CMS's employer-size training guidance confirms that full-time and part-time employees must be included, that the 20 weeks need not be consecutive, and that the requirement is based on the number of employees rather than the number of persons covered under the plan. (CMS)

The current-employment condition is equally controlling. The Medicare handbook treats active employer or union coverage as legally distinct from inactive or post-employment coverage. It states that when an individual or spouse is still working and health coverage is through that employer or union, the Medicare coordination rules depend on how the employer coverage works with Medicare; it also states that coverage based on current employment does not include COBRA, retiree coverage, Veterans Affairs coverage, individual Marketplace coverage, or former-employer coverage obtained through severance or layoff. The safe harbor is therefore not a generic insurance safe harbor. It is a current-employment group health plan safe harbor.

The 20-employee rule creates a large-employer alignment. When the age-sixty-five worker or covered spouse remains tied to a qualifying employer group health plan based on current employment and the employer-size standard is satisfied, the group health plan must occupy the primary payer position. CMS's handbook states the operational rule plainly: for age sixty-five or older persons covered by current-employment group health coverage where the employer has 20 or more employees, or where a smaller employer participates in a multi-employer plan with another employer of at least 20 employees, the group health plan pays first. The current eCFR working-aged provisions similarly provide that an employer meeting the 20-employee condition may not take into account Medicare entitlement for an age-sixty-five or older individual covered or seeking coverage by virtue of current employment status. (eCFR)

The large-employer rule is not merely permissive. It prevents the employer group health plan from treating Medicare entitlement as the reason to reduce the active worker's health benefits or relegate the worker to a Medicare-first structure. Under CMS employer-size guidance, Medicare is secondary to group health plans for the working aged when either a single employer of 20 or more full-time or part-time employees sponsors or contributes to the group health plan, or when multiple employers sponsor or contribute to a multi-employer or multiple-employer plan and at least one employer has 20 or more full-time or part-time employees. (CMS) This rule transfers first-dollar or first-layer liability, subject to the group plan's terms, away from Medicare and onto the employment-based coverage pool.

The small-employer rule reverses that alignment. CMS's 2026 handbook states that when an age-sixty-five or older individual has group health plan coverage based on current employment and the employer has fewer than 20 employees, Medicare pays first. CMS's employer-size guidance similarly states that if an employer with fewer than 20 full-time or part-time employees sponsors or contributes to a single-employer group health plan, the working-aged Medicare Secondary Payer rules applicable to age-based entitlement do not apply, and Medicare is the primary payer. (CMS) The practical effect is that the small employer plan may coordinate as secondary, even though it remains a workplace benefit in ordinary human resources language.

This reversal is the foundation of the small-group exposure. If Medicare is primary by law, the small group plan may be designed and administered as secondary to Medicare for the age-sixty-five worker or spouse. CMS's handbook states that the primary payer pays up to its limits first, that the secondary payer pays only if costs remain, and that the secondary payer may not pay all uncovered costs. It also adds the crucial warning that if group health plan or retiree coverage is secondary, Part B will likely be needed before that insurance will pay. Thus, a beneficiary who retains small-group employer coverage but declines or delays Part B may not possess a full substitute for Medicare. The plan may be present, premiums may be paid, and an insurance card may be active, while the primary payer expected by the coordination rules is absent from the claim.

The resulting "phantom primary payer" hazard should be modeled with caution and precision. Under Original Medicare, where the Part B deductible applies, the beneficiary pays all costs up to the Medicare-approved amount until the deductible is met; after the deductible, Medicare pays its share and the beneficiary typically pays 20 percent of the Medicare-approved amount when the provider accepts assignment, and Original Medicare has no yearly out-of-pocket limit without supplemental coverage. If a small-group plan coordinates on the assumption that Medicare is primary, the secondary plan may calculate its responsibility only after the Medicare-primary layer that should have been present. Because many Part B claims are built around an 80 percent Medicare share and a 20 percent beneficiary coinsurance after deductible, the household can face a practical exposure approaching the missing primary layer when Part B was not in force, although the exact result depends on the contract, service category, assignment status, and coordination terms.

This exposure is catastrophic because it is not bounded by the intuitive limits associated with ordinary employer coverage. CMS states that Original Medicare has no yearly limit on out-of-pocket costs unless supplemental coverage such as Medigap, Medicaid, employer, retiree, or union coverage applies. Yet a small-group secondary plan may not function as a full supplemental shield when the primary Medicare layer is missing. A physician-administered drug, durable medical equipment claim, outpatient surgery, diagnostic imaging sequence, emergency department episode, or recurring therapy course can generate repeated exposure. The 20 percent coinsurance figure in Original Medicare is often treated as the residual beneficiary layer after Medicare's primary payment; when Medicare is legally primary but Part B is absent, the household may confront the far larger unfunded primary segment rather than the ordinary coinsurance residue.

The capital destruction occurs because the household may have correctly preserved employment coverage but incorrectly classified payer order. The file appears insured in a conventional employment-benefit sense, yet it is uninsured for the primary Medicare layer that the small-group coordination structure expects. Claims can be delayed, reduced, denied, or paid only in the secondary posture. The household then must finance the missing primary obligation through cash reserves, retirement accounts, home equity, credit, family transfers, or deferred care. This is not a late-enrollment penalty in the narrow premium-surcharge sense. It is a coordination failure that converts a Medicare enrollment omission into uncapped clinical liability, while also potentially preserving exposure to the Part B late enrollment penalty if no valid Special Enrollment Period later applies. CMS states that delayed Part B without Special Enrollment Period protection can lead to General Enrollment Period dependency and late-enrollment penalty exposure.

The active-employment safe harbor is therefore narrower than many employment households assume. CMS states that the employer or group health plan Special Enrollment Period is generally available when the person is age sixty-five or older, the person or spouse is currently working, and employer or union group health coverage is from that job; it can be used any time while still working and covered by employer or union group health coverage from that job, or for up to eight months after group health plan coverage ends or employment ends, whichever occurs first. The operative elements are current work, group health coverage from that work, and timely filing within the statutory period after the first terminating event. Coverage from former employment does not carry the same legal character.

Inactive workforce pools must therefore be segregated. COBRA can continue group coverage after employment ends, but CMS states that COBRA is not coverage based on current employment and does not count as current employer coverage for the Part B Special Enrollment Period. Retiree health coverage is expressly classified as former-employment coverage, and the handbook states that Medicare pays first when retiree coverage exists. Veterans Affairs coverage and individual Marketplace coverage likewise fail the current-employment coverage test for this safe harbor. These exclusions are not semantic distinctions. They determine whether delayed Part B remains protected or becomes penalty-prone and medically hazardous.

Severance-based coverage is equally dangerous because it may preserve a payroll-adjacent appearance without preserving current-employment status. CMS's 2026 handbook states that coverage based on current employment does not include former-employer coverage obtained through severance or a layoff. A severed worker may still receive subsidized coverage, plan access, or employer-sponsored administrative support, but the worker is no longer in the current-employment category that supports the worker Special Enrollment Period. The Medicare file looks to the legal basis of coverage, not merely the premium source or the corporate logo on the coverage material.

SHOP coverage requires separate classification. The CMS source packet states that employer coverage through the Marketplace Small Business Health Options Program is included when the worker is still working and has employer coverage through work, and the same page applies the fewer-than-20 and 20-or-more employer-size rules to determine whether Medicare or the employer pays first. This is materially different from individual Marketplace coverage for persons and families, which CMS identifies as not based on current employment and as a potential source of Medicare delay and late-penalty risk. Thus, "Marketplace" is not a single coordination category. Employer-sponsored SHOP coverage must be separated from individual Marketplace coverage.

The disability and ESRD rules show that the 20-employee rule is part of a larger payer-order matrix, not a universal threshold. CMS states that for Medicare entitlement based on disability, current-employment group health plan coverage generally pays first when the employer has 100 or more employees, or when a smaller employer participates in a multi-employer plan where another employer has 100 or more employees; Medicare pays first when the employer has fewer than 100 employees in the disability category. CMS also states that in ESRD cases, group health plan coverage based on employment or former employment pays first for the first 30 months after Medicare eligibility, with Medicare paying first after that 30-month period. Section 5.1 focuses on age-based active employment, but the Matrix must not misapply the age-sixty-five 20-employee rule to disability or ESRD files.

The employer-size audit must therefore be conducted at the claim-date level. CMS's MSP Manual states that the 20-or-more requirement must be met at the time the individual receives the services for which Medicare benefits are claimed, and that during the time the employer has met the requirement in the current or preceding calendar year, the group health plan is primary. (CMS) The manual further states that an employer meeting the threshold must provide primary coverage even if fewer than 20 employees participate in the group health plan. (CMS) This prevents the household from relying on plan enrollment counts as a proxy for employer size. The relevant measure is the employer's employment-roll count under CMS rules, not the number of Medicare-eligible employees, the number of covered employees, or the number of workers enrolled in the plan.

Multi-employer and multiple-employer arrangements require additional care. CMS's employer-size guidance states that when at least one participating employer in a multi-employer or multiple-employer group health plan has 20 or more full-time or part-time employees, the working-aged MSP rules apply to all individuals entitled to Medicare on the basis of age, including those associated with an employer having fewer than 20 employees, unless a Small Employer Exception has been granted. (CMS) CMS further states that the Small Employer Exception request must be made in writing to the Benefits Coordination & Recovery Center, must be prospective rather than retroactive, and is not effective until granted. (CMS) The Matrix must therefore treat small-employer status inside a multi-employer plan as unresolved until the federal exception status is verified.

The coordination record itself must be maintained. CMS states that if group health plan coverage ends, Medicare should be contacted to update the record, and that other insurance changes can be reported to Medicare's Benefits Coordination & Recovery Center; CMS also instructs retiring individuals to ensure primary insurance information is correct. This operational instruction reveals the administrative side of payer sequencing. Correct law is not enough if the federal record reflects stale payer information. A file showing an incorrect primary payer can generate claim delays, mistaken denials, recovery activity, or provider billing confusion.

The active-employment safe harbor and the payer-order rule must finally be distinguished from the Part B enrollment decision. A large employer with 20 or more employees may make delayed Part B more administratively coherent because the employer group health plan pays first while current employment continues. A small employer with fewer than 20 employees creates the opposite condition because Medicare pays first. CMS's 2026 source packet states that if an employer has fewer than 20 employees, Medicare pays first, and if an employer has 20 or more employees, the employer pays first; it also warns that COBRA, Veterans Affairs coverage, and retiree health plans are not current-employment coverage for a Special Enrollment Period. The employment file must therefore answer two separate questions: whether Part B delay is penalty-protected, and whether the non-Medicare plan is primary or secondary for current claims.

This statutory triad links directly to the Household Medicare Diagnostic Matrix. Section 5.1 forms the analytical pillar for the Matrix rows addressing active workers, employer size, small-group exposure, COBRA confusion, retiree coverage, and secondary payer sequencing. A household that treats "still working" as a complete answer has not completed the audit. The file must identify whether the worker or spouse has current-employment group health plan coverage, whether the employer has 20 or more employees under CMS counting rules, whether a multi-employer plan changes the result, whether a Small Employer Exception exists, whether Part B is required before secondary insurance will pay, and whether the Medicare coordination record has been updated. (CMS)

The final actuarial conclusion is severe. Active employment can protect a Medicare file, but only when the legal ingredients align. A qualifying large employer group health plan can preserve private primary liability and place Medicare in a secondary position. A small employer plan can leave Medicare as the primary payer, making failure to enroll in Part B a direct pathway to uncovered outpatient liability. COBRA, retiree coverage, VA coverage, individual Marketplace coverage, severance coverage, and other inactive or non-current-employment arrangements may preserve practical insurance access while failing the federal safe-harbor test. Under the Household Medicare Diagnostic Matrix, employer coverage must therefore be audited by payer order, employer size, current-employment status, Part B enrollment status, and record accuracy. Without that audit, a workplace benefit that appears secure can become the mechanism by which household assets are exposed to uncapped medical risk.

5.2 Defining Factual "Active Employment Status"

The Medicare enrollment safe harbor for employment is not activated by employment language in a severance agreement, by continuation of a corporate health card, by a payroll-adjacent subsidy, or by the general social reality that a person remains connected to a former employer. It depends on the federal concept of current employment status and on group health plan coverage that arises from that status.

Under 42 CFR § 411.104, current employment status exists when an individual is actively working as an employee, is the employer, including a self-employed person, or is associated with the employer in a business relationship; the same regulation also recognizes certain nonworking persons who retain employment rights, but only under specified conditions. (eCFR) The Medicare handbook translates the practical enrollment consequence into direct operational language: delayed Part B enrollment can be protected when the beneficiary or spouse is still working and has employer or union group health coverage from that job, while coverage based on current employment expressly excludes COBRA, retiree coverage, Veterans Affairs coverage, individual Marketplace coverage, and former-employer coverage obtained through severance or layoff.

The policy rationale is actuarial and administrative. Medicare permits delayed Part B enrollment without late-enrollment penalty only when another legally recognized employment-based risk pool is already bearing or coordinating medical liability. The federal program therefore requires a verifiable relationship between work, employer responsibility, group health plan coverage, and the timing of the Special Enrollment Period. Under the Part B Special Enrollment Period regulation, current employment status has the meaning supplied by 42 CFR § 411.104, and for age-sixty-five or older individuals the relevant group health plan coverage must be by reason of the current employment status of the individual or spouse; the regulation further provides that the Special Enrollment Period ends after the eighth consecutive month during which the individual is at no time enrolled in a group health plan by reason of current employment status. (eCFR) This structure prevents generic insurance continuity from substituting for active employment.

The safest description of active employment is not merely "being on payroll." It is a legally supportable employment relationship in which services, employment rights, employer group health plan coverage, and tax records align. The IRS common-law employee standard states that an individual performing services is an employee when the business has the right to control what will be done and how it will be done, even when the worker retains freedom of action. (IRS) For payroll employees, the IRS states that employers generally must withhold and deposit income taxes, Social Security taxes, and Medicare taxes from employee wages, and must pay the matching employer share of Social Security and Medicare taxes. (IRS) These tax markers do not independently create Medicare current employment status, but they provide documentary evidence that the relationship is not merely retrospective compensation, severance continuation, or independent contractor payment.

Severance arrangements expose the most common filing trap because they imitate continuity while terminating the current-employment anchor. A departing employee may receive subsidized health coverage for a negotiated number of months, continued employer billing support, reimbursement, salary continuation, or other negotiated consideration. Yet CMS treats former-employer severance or layoff coverage as outside coverage based on current employment for the Part B Special Enrollment Period. The distinction is severe but coherent: severance is compensation or benefit continuation flowing from past labor, not ongoing labor or retained current employment status sufficient to preserve the worker Special Enrollment Period. The presence of a corporate subsidy does not transform a former worker into an active worker for Medicare enrollment purposes.

The federal regulation confirms this principle through its treatment of delayed compensation. Under 42 CFR § 411.104(f), an individual who is not working is not considered an employee solely because delayed compensation payments for earlier work are being received, even if those payments are subject to FICA taxes or would be subject to FICA taxes if the employer were not exempt. (eCFR) This rule is the statutory antidote to the severance illusion. A payment stream connected to prior service does not establish current employment status by itself. Therefore, a severance package that continues compensation, premium support, or administrative access can coexist with Medicare penalty exposure if the individual fails to enroll in Part B during the applicable post-employment window.

The timing consequence is direct. CMS states that the worker Special Enrollment Period permits Part A or Part B enrollment at any time while the individual remains covered by the group health plan based on current employment, or during the eight-month period beginning after employment ends or the coverage ends, whichever occurs first. Once actual employment ends, the eight-month clock can begin even if COBRA is elected, retiree coverage is activated, severance coverage continues, or another former-employer mechanism remains in force. CMS states that COBRA is not considered coverage based on current employment, does not count as current employer coverage for the Special Enrollment Period, and generally does not create a new Special Enrollment Period when COBRA later ends. The severance beneficiary therefore faces a hidden mismatch: a health card may remain active while the Medicare enrollment protection clock is already running.

Disability leave requires more careful analysis because federal rules do not treat every nonworking period alike. The regulation recognizes current employment status for a person who is not actively working and receives disability benefits from an employer for up to six months, with the first six months of employer disability benefits subject to FICA taxes. (eCFR) It also recognizes certain nonworking persons who retain employment rights, have not had employment terminated, are not receiving employer disability benefits for more than six months, are not receiving Social Security disability benefits, and have group health plan coverage that is not COBRA continuation coverage. (eCFR) Thus, disability leave is not automatically disqualifying, but its protective effect depends on duration, employment rights, benefit source, Social Security disability status, and whether the health coverage remains non-COBRA group health plan coverage.

The regulation's retained-rights category is broader than active labor but narrower than indefinite inactive coverage. Persons who retain employment rights include furloughed persons, temporarily laid-off persons, persons on sick leave, teachers and seasonal workers who normally do not work throughout the year, and persons with health coverage extending beyond or between active employment periods, such as hours-bank arrangements. (eCFR) This language prevents a simplistic rule that only same-day work performance counts. It also prevents the opposite error, which would treat every leave, disability period, or benefit continuation as protected indefinitely. The file must identify whether the employment relationship remains legally alive, whether coverage is based on that relationship, and whether the specific regulatory conditions remain satisfied.

Family and Medical Leave Act leave sits inside this same cautionary architecture. The Department of Labor states that FMLA provides eligible employees of covered employers with unpaid, job-protected leave and requires continuation of group health benefits under the same terms and conditions as if the employee had not taken leave. (DOL) The Department further states that employees using FMLA leave generally have the right to return to the same or an equivalent job, and that employer group health insurance coverage continues during FMLA leave on the same terms as if work had continued. (DOL) For Medicare purposes, however, FMLA terminology does not replace the 42 CFR § 411.104 analysis. The relevant Medicare question remains whether the individual retains employment rights, whether employment has not been terminated, whether group health plan coverage is based on that employment relationship, and whether COBRA continuation has not become the coverage basis. (eCFR)

Short-term and long-term disability statuses should therefore be separated. During the early employer disability phase, current employment status may survive under the six-month employer disability benefit rule. (eCFR) After that point, the file becomes more fragile. If employer disability benefits continue beyond the regulatory boundary, if Social Security disability benefits begin, if employment rights terminate, if coverage converts to COBRA, or if the employer plan reclassifies the individual into a retiree or inactive population, the Medicare safe harbor may fail. The uploaded CMS packet does not provide a complete taxonomy of every employer disability arrangement or state-mandated disability program; the controlling official Medicare source for that granular classification is 42 CFR § 411.104 and the CMS Medicare Secondary Payer Manual chapter on current employment status. (eCFR)

The independent contractor boundary is equally technical. An individual paid through an IRS Form 1099 structure is not an employee merely because services are performed for a business. The IRS states that independent contractors are self-employed, that earnings from independent contractor work are subject to self-employment tax, and that payments are generally reported on Form 1099-NEC as nonemployee compensation. (IRS) The IRS also states that a written contract calling the worker an independent contractor is not controlling by itself; the actual relationship determines whether worker status is employee or independent contractor. (IRS) For Medicare safe-harbor purposes, this means that a 1099 relationship cannot simply be relabeled as active employment to preserve delayed Part B protection.

A 1099 contractor normally does not derive coverage from an employer-employee group health plan sponsored by the contracting entity. The IRS states that employers generally do not withhold or pay employment taxes on payments to independent contractors, in contrast to the withholding and employer tax obligations tied to employee wages. (IRS) The Medicare regulation, however, does not ignore all self-employment. It contains a special rule for self-employed persons: a self-employed individual is considered to have group health plan or large group health plan coverage by virtue of current employment status during a particular tax year only if, during the preceding tax year, the individual's net earnings from work related to the employer offering the group health coverage equal or exceed the self-employment income amount specified in section 211(b)(2) of the Social Security Act. (eCFR) The boundary is therefore not "employee only." It is verifiable current employment status, including narrowly defined self-employment where the federal rule is satisfied.

This distinction prevents both over-inclusion and under-inclusion. A common-law employee with employer group health coverage may possess the safe-harbor structure if the other Medicare conditions are satisfied. A self-employed proprietor, partner, business owner, or business-associated individual may qualify only if the 42 CFR § 411.104 self-employment rule is satisfied through qualifying net earnings connected to the employer offering the group health coverage. (eCFR) A mere independent contractor relationship with a client, without employee status or a qualifying self-employed group health plan relationship, should not be treated as current employment coverage from that client. The file must be supported by employment classification, tax reporting, group health plan eligibility documents, and coverage basis.

Corporate auditing becomes unavoidable because Medicare coordination rules rely on objective records. Employer group health plan coordination turns on whether coverage is based on current employment and, for age-based Medicare Secondary Payer rules, whether the employer-size threshold produces employer-primary or Medicare-primary payer status. CMS states that if group health plan coverage ends, Medicare should be contacted to update the coordination record, and that changes in other insurance can be reported to the Benefits Coordination & Recovery Center. The same handbook states that if an individual is still working and has employer coverage through work, the employer should be contacted to determine how that coverage works with Medicare and whether Part B is needed. These instructions show that the federal record is not self-correcting.

The payroll and tax file therefore becomes an evidentiary substrate. W-2 wages, FICA withholding, employer benefit eligibility records, group health plan enrollment documents, employment-status certifications, approved leave records, disability benefit dates, COBRA election documents, severance agreements, and 1099-NEC records may each clarify whether the Medicare file is protected or exposed. The IRS employee standard depends on control over the manner and means of work, while the Medicare current-employment regulation depends on active work, employer status, business association, retained employment rights, or qualifying self-employment under the regulatory rule. (IRS) (eCFR) A contract label, payment label, or human resources shorthand cannot safely replace that legal classification.

The active employment safe harbor also interacts with payer order. The 2026 Medicare handbook states that, for an individual age sixty-five or older with group health plan coverage based on the current employment of the individual or spouse, a 20-or-more employee employer generally makes the group health plan pay first, while an employer with fewer than 20 employees makes Medicare pay first. Therefore, factual active employment is necessary but not always sufficient to determine the full exposure. A small employer may produce current-employment coverage but still leave Medicare in the primary payer position. In that scenario, failure to hold Part B can produce the small-group primary-payer gap analyzed in Section 5.1, because the secondary payer may not pay all uncovered costs and may require Part B before payment.

The Household Medicare Diagnostic Matrix therefore treats active employment as a legal file condition, not a biographical description. The matrix must distinguish between active labor, protected retained-rights leave, employer disability benefits within the regulatory boundary, severance, COBRA, retiree coverage, individual Marketplace coverage, VA coverage, and 1099 independent contracting. CMS states that COBRA, retiree coverage, VA coverage, individual Marketplace coverage, and former-employer severance or layoff coverage are not coverage based on current employment for the Part B Special Enrollment Period. That list is the operational warning label for retirement transition planning. A household may remain insured in the ordinary sense while becoming exposed in the Medicare enrollment sense.

Section 5.2 supplies the definitions required to complete the employment audit rows of the matrix. The first question is whether actual current employment status exists under 42 CFR § 411.104. The second is whether group health plan coverage is based on that current employment status rather than COBRA, retiree status, severance, individual coverage, or another excluded category. The third is whether the employer-size rule makes the group health plan primary or leaves Medicare primary. The fourth is whether any leave, disability, furlough, layoff, seasonal break, hours-bank arrangement, or self-employed relationship remains inside the regulatory boundaries. The fifth is whether tax records and benefit records support the classification. Failure at any point can convert a seemingly orderly corporate transition into a Part B late-enrollment penalty problem, a primary-payer gap, or a claim coordination failure.

The actuarial conclusion is exacting. Medicare privileges verifiable current employment status over contractual continuity, severance generosity, informal payroll labels, or deferred corporate compensation. The safest file is one in which labor status, tax treatment, employer group health plan eligibility, payer order, and Special Enrollment Period timing all point in the same direction. A severance package may preserve cash flow but fail the current-employment test. A disability leave may preserve current employment status temporarily, then lose protection when regulatory conditions fail. A 1099 contract may generate self-employment income but not create employee group coverage from the contracting entity. Under the Household Medicare Diagnostic Matrix, active employment is therefore not a story about attachment to work. It is a documentary legal status that determines whether private employment coverage can lawfully protect delayed Part B enrollment or whether the federal Medicare file has already become exposed.

5.3 The COBRA Continuation Crossover Trap

COBRA continuation coverage occupies a uniquely hazardous position in the Medicare transition architecture because it preserves the surface form of an employer group health plan after the legal foundation of current employment has ended. For a worker below Medicare age, COBRA can function as a vital temporary bridge after job loss, reduction in hours, divorce, death of a covered employee, or another qualifying event. Medicare.gov describes COBRA as a federal law that may allow continued employer group health plan coverage for a limited time after employment ends, or after loss of coverage as a spouse or dependent of the covered employee. (Medicare)

Yet the same continuation contract changes character when it intersects with age-based Medicare eligibility, because the federal Medicare enrollment system does not treat COBRA as coverage based on current employment for the Part B Special Enrollment Period. Under CMS signing-up specifications in the 2026 Medicare handbook, COBRA is not considered coverage based on current employment and does not count as current employer coverage for the Part B Special Enrollment Period.

This is the structural core of the COBRA crossover trap. A household may observe uninterrupted premium payment, the same group plan administrator, the same plan identification card, and the same provider network. The federal Medicare file, however, observes a different legal event: active employment has ended, and continuation coverage has replaced current-employment coverage. Under Social Security's Special Enrollment Period operating policy, enrollment in Supplementary Medical Insurance or premium Hospital Insurance can occur during any month in which the individual is enrolled in a group health plan or large group health plan based on current employment status, or during the eight consecutive months following the last month in which such current-employment-based coverage existed. (Social Security Administration) COBRA may preserve a private contract, but it does not preserve the current-employment status that protects delayed Part B enrollment.

The word "creditable" must be handled precisely in this context. For Part D, creditable prescription drug coverage is a defined actuarial term tied to whether alternative drug coverage is expected to pay at least as much as Medicare drug coverage. For Part B, the controlling safe-harbor term is not creditable prescription coverage, but coverage based on current employment. Nevertheless, COBRA is "non-creditable" in the functional Part B safe-harbor sense because it does not satisfy the employment-based condition required to avoid Part B late enrollment penalty exposure. CMS states that after coverage based on current employment ends, there are eight months to sign up for Part B without penalty whether or not COBRA is chosen, and that a beneficiary generally is not eligible for a Special Enrollment Period when COBRA later ends.

The legal distinction is harsh because COBRA can be financially expensive while still failing the Medicare safe-harbor test. The Department of Labor states that COBRA often makes the qualified beneficiary responsible for the full cost of coverage, and that the premium generally may reach 102 percent of the plan's total cost, including both the former employee share and the employer share, plus two percent. (DOL) A household may therefore spend substantial amounts maintaining continuation coverage while the federal Part B penalty clock remains unprotected. CMS states that if Part B is delayed without Special Enrollment Period eligibility, enrollment may be available only during the General Enrollment Period and the Part B premium may increase by 10 percent for each full 12-month period in which Part B could have been held but was not, generally for as long as Part B remains active.

The timeline mismatch is the operational danger. The Part B worker Special Enrollment Period is anchored to the end of employment or the end of active-employment group health plan coverage, whichever happens first. CMS states that the worker Special Enrollment Period permits Part B enrollment any time while still working and covered by employer or union group health coverage from that job, or for up to eight months after the group health plan coverage ends or employment ends, whichever happens first. Social Security's operating policy states the same structure: the eight-month period follows the last month in which the individual had group health plan coverage based on current employment status. (Social Security Administration) COBRA exhaustion does not reset that clock.

COBRA's duration rules intensify the trap because COBRA often lasts longer than the Part B Special Enrollment Period. Medicare.gov states that COBRA coverage is generally offered for 18 months, with 36 months in some cases. (Medicare) CMS's COBRA fact sheet states that the covered employee usually receives a maximum of 18 months after termination or reduction of hours, that disability can extend coverage to 29 months when conditions are met, and that certain spouse and dependent-child rules or second qualifying events can extend coverage to 36 months. (Centers for Medicare & Medicaid Services) The Department of Labor similarly identifies 18 months for termination or reduction in hours, 36 months for several dependent-related qualifying events, and possible disability extension to 29 months. (DOL) These COBRA durations are real, but they are not Medicare Part B Special Enrollment Period durations.

The month-nine trap follows from this misalignment. If active employment ends and COBRA begins, the Medicare Special Enrollment Period generally runs for eight months after the end of current-employment-based coverage. If the household treats an 18-month COBRA contract as an 18-month Medicare filing safe harbor, the Part B Special Enrollment Period can close while the COBRA contract still appears intact. CMS warns that after current-employment coverage ends, Part B enrollment must occur within eight months without penalty whether or not COBRA is chosen, and that there generally is not a Special Enrollment Period when COBRA later ends. Medicare.gov likewise states that missing the eight-month period can require waiting until January 1 through March 31 to sign up, with coverage starting the month after enrollment and possible lifetime Part B late enrollment penalty exposure. (Medicare)

The coverage-gap consequence is immediate rather than theoretical. CMS states that the General Enrollment Period runs January 1 through March 31 for individuals who missed the Initial Enrollment Period and do not qualify for a Special Enrollment

Period, with coverage beginning the first day of the month after enrollment and possible higher Part A or Part B premiums for late enrollment. Therefore, a household that reaches month nine of COBRA after failing to enroll in Part B may have neither a valid worker Special Enrollment Period nor active Part B. The result can be a period of reduced or nonfunctional primary coverage, followed by General Enrollment Period dependency, delayed effective coverage, and permanent premium surcharge exposure under the full 12-month penalty block formula.

The payer-order dimension compounds the filing hazard. The 2026 Medicare handbook states that the insurance paying first pays up to the limits of its coverage, that the secondary payer pays only if costs remain uncovered, that the secondary payer may not pay all uncovered costs, and that if a group health plan or retiree coverage is secondary, Part B will likely be needed before that insurance will pay. Medicare.gov's COBRA guidance applies this logic directly to continuation coverage: if COBRA exists and the beneficiary is eligible for Medicare but not enrolled, COBRA may pay only a small portion of health care services, and most costs may fall back onto the household. (Medicare) The continuation contract may exist, but its coordination position can leave a large primary payer layer unfunded.

The requested "automatic secondary shift" should be stated with official precision. The uploaded CMS packet and current Medicare.gov materials do not establish a universal rule that every commercial COBRA contract automatically drops into secondary position on the first day of the month the individual reaches age sixty-five, regardless of plan terms. The defensible official rule is more exact: qualified beneficiaries eligible for Medicare but not enrolled may have Medicare treated as primary, and COBRA coordination can affect how claims are paid; CMS states that COBRA may pay only a small portion and that the COBRA policy should be consulted for the percentage paid. (DOL) This distinction preserves technical accuracy while still exposing the same actuarial danger. The missing Medicare enrollment can create a phantom primary payer position, leaving the household responsible for a large uninsured claim layer.

The 80 percent liability model is therefore a practical illustration rather than a universal contract term. Under Original Medicare, after the Part B deductible is met, Medicare typically pays its share and the beneficiary usually pays 20 percent of the Medicare-approved amount for many Part B-covered services when assignment applies; the 2026 handbook also states that Original Medicare has no yearly out-of-pocket limit unless supplemental coverage applies. When a COBRA or former-employer contract coordinates on the premise that Medicare should be primary, the absent Part B layer can resemble the missing Medicare share of the claim, while the continuation plan may pay only a residual or secondary amount. CMS does not reduce this risk to a universal 80 percent rule for every COBRA contract, but its warning that COBRA may pay only a small portion and that most costs may fall to the beneficiary supports the same high-stakes conclusion.

The employer or plan administrator also may possess termination authority when Medicare entitlement occurs after COBRA election. CMS's COBRA fact sheet states that continuation coverage may end earlier than the maximum period if, after the COBRA election, a beneficiary first becomes entitled to Medicare benefits; the same source states the key exception, namely that if Medicare entitlement, either Part A or Part B, is effective on or before the date of the COBRA election, COBRA coverage may not be discontinued on account of Medicare entitlement, even if the individual enrolls in the other part of Medicare after the COBRA election. (Centers for Medicare & Medicaid Services) The Department of Labor's worker guide similarly states that a qualified beneficiary may lose COBRA before the maximum period ends if the qualified beneficiary becomes entitled to Medicare benefits after electing COBRA. (DOL)

This termination rule creates a second order trap. If the beneficiary elects COBRA first and later becomes entitled to Medicare, the continuation contract may terminate for that beneficiary once Medicare coverage becomes active, subject to the statutory and plan-specific rules. The Department of Labor's Medicare and COBRA table states that where a qualified beneficiary on COBRA enrolls in Medicare and was never covered under Part A or Part B before electing COBRA, COBRA coverage may end for that beneficiary once Medicare coverage becomes active, while coverage continues for other qualified beneficiaries. (DOL) Conversely, where Medicare Part A was already in effect before COBRA election and Part B is added while on COBRA, DOL states that adding Part B does not affect COBRA coverage for any qualified beneficiary. (DOL) The ordering of Medicare entitlement and COBRA election is therefore not clerical. It determines whether continuation coverage can persist.

The pre-existing Medicare enrollment exception must be isolated because it is often misunderstood. If Medicare entitlement exists before COBRA is elected, the COBRA continuation contract may remain available, but that does not transform COBRA into current-employment coverage for Part B safe-harbor purposes, nor does it guarantee primary payer status. CMS's COBRA fact sheet states that COBRA coverage may not be discontinued on account of Medicare entitlement if Medicare entitlement is effective on or before the COBRA election date. (Centers for Medicare & Medicaid Services) Medicare.gov separately warns that qualified beneficiaries eligible for Medicare but not enrolled may have Medicare treated as primary and may face unexpected financial obligations when COBRA starts. (Medicare) Thus, the pre-existing enrollment rule protects continuation eligibility in a narrow ordering circumstance; it does not erase payer coordination risk.

COBRA also differs from Part D creditable drug coverage. The Medicare handbook treats loss of employer or union coverage, including COBRA coverage, as a Special Enrollment Period event for Medicare Advantage or Medicare drug plan enrollment, with a two-full-month window after the month coverage ends. That Part C and Part D election opportunity is distinct from the Part B worker Special Enrollment Period. A household may therefore possess one timeline for Medicare health or drug plan changes after leaving COBRA and a different, earlier eight-month timeline for Part B after active employment or current-employment coverage ends. Confusing the two timelines can cause Part B penalty exposure even where another Medicare election window exists.

The household capital consequences are severe because COBRA is expensive, temporary, and legally incomplete for Medicare delay purposes. A COBRA enrollee may pay full continuation premiums while simultaneously losing the Part B Special Enrollment Period, accumulating possible Part B late enrollment penalty exposure, and facing claims coordination in which Medicare is expected to occupy the primary position. CMS states that if non-Medicare coverage might not pay medical costs without Part B, the beneficiary may have to wait for the General Enrollment Period and may pay a late enrollment penalty for as long as Part B coverage continues. This creates a three-layer erosion model: high continuation premiums paid during COBRA, uninsured or underinsured claims during Medicare-primary coordination, and durable premium surcharge exposure after late Part B enrollment.

The crossover trap becomes particularly destructive when a household treats COBRA as equivalent to active employment. Active employment creates the potential Part B Special Enrollment Period. COBRA begins only after the employment-based coverage was lost because of a qualifying event, commonly termination or reduction of hours. Medicare.gov states that COBRA may allow employer group health plan coverage for a limited time after employment ends, while CMS states that COBRA is not current-employment coverage for Part B SEP purposes. (Medicare) These two rules, read together, explain the trap. COBRA's very existence usually signals that current employment has ended, which is the event that begins the eight-month Medicare clock.

The continuation timeline must also be tested against dependent coverage. DOL and CMS state that a worker's termination or reduction in hours generally produces up to 18 months of COBRA for the employee, spouse, and dependent child, while certain dependent events and second qualifying events may extend coverage to 36 months. (DOL) (Centers for Medicare & Medicaid Services) When the employee becomes entitled to Medicare while still working and later experiences a qualifying event, DOL states that COBRA can be available after the qualifying event, with the employee receiving up to 18 months and dependents receiving up to 36 months from Medicare entitlement or 18 months from loss of coverage, whichever is later. (DOL) These dependent rules are important, but they should not be imported into the Part B filing analysis for the Medicare-eligible worker. Dependent COBRA duration does not extend the worker's Part B current-employment safe harbor.

The Matrix must therefore record three dates separately: the date active employment ended, the date current-employment group health plan coverage ended, and the date COBRA coverage ends. CMS states that the Part B Special Enrollment Period runs for up to eight months after the group health plan coverage ends or the employment ends, whichever happens first. DOL and CMS state that COBRA may run 18, 29, or 36 months depending on the qualifying event and extension rules. (DOL) (Centers for Medicare & Medicaid Services) The longest or most visible date, the COBRA exhaustion date, is not the controlling date for the Part B worker SEP. The controlling date is the earlier loss of current employment or active-employment-based group health plan coverage.

This section therefore performs the continuation and separation tracking function inside the Household Medicare Diagnostic Matrix. The Matrix cannot mark "covered" as a safe status merely because COBRA is active. It must classify COBRA as continuation coverage, test whether Part B has already been elected, determine whether Medicare entitlement preceded or followed COBRA election, identify whether the COBRA contract may terminate after Medicare entitlement, and confirm how the continuation plan coordinates claims with Medicare. CMS instructs beneficiaries with COBRA and Medicare questions to contact the Benefits Coordination & Recovery Center, and DOL directs private-sector COBRA questions to the Employee Benefits Security Administration, confirming that the crossover is a dual-jurisdiction administrative problem. (Medicare)

The final actuarial conclusion is uncompromising. COBRA can preserve access to a former employer's group health plan for a limited period, but it does not preserve the Part B current-employment safe harbor. Its continuation duration can exceed the eight-month Part B Special Enrollment Period. Its claim coordination can leave Medicare as the expected primary payer. Its contract can terminate when Medicare entitlement arises after COBRA election, while pre-existing Medicare entitlement before COBRA election creates only a narrow protection against termination, not a guarantee of primary private payment. Under the Household Medicare Diagnostic Matrix, COBRA must therefore be treated as a separation-risk instrument rather than as an active-workplace shield. A household that cross-references COBRA exhaustion against the wrong Medicare clock can transform a costly private bridge into a direct pathway for late penalties, claim denials, liquidity depletion, and long-term asset erosion.

Chapter 6: The High-Income Surcharge: IRMAA Mechanics

6.1 The Income-Related Monthly Adjustment Amount (IRMAA)

The Income-Related Monthly Adjustment Amount is a federal premium-pricing mechanism, not a late-enrollment penalty, underwriting surcharge, private-plan fee, or discretionary administrative assessment. It arises from the statutory financing structure of Supplementary Medical Insurance and applies when a Medicare beneficiary's income exceeds defined federal thresholds. Pursuant to the Social Security Act § 1839(i) framework, SSA's Part B IRMAA regulation states that beneficiaries enrolled in Medicare Part B with modified adjusted gross income above the statutory threshold pay an income-related monthly adjustment amount in addition to the standard monthly Part B premium and any applicable premium increases. (Social Security) Under CMS IRMAA specifications in the 2026 Medicare handbook, the standard Part B premium amount in 2026 is $202.90, and Medicare uses modified adjusted gross income reported on the IRS tax return from two years earlier to determine whether an additional Income-Related Monthly Adjustment Amount applies.

IRMAA therefore operates as a progressive premium-recovery instrument inside Medicare financing. It does not change the beneficiary's entitlement to covered services, does not expand or restrict the statutory benefit package, does not alter the Original Medicare exclusions matrix, and does not substitute for deductibles or coinsurance. It changes the monthly premium obligation. The macroeconomic premise is that higher-income beneficiaries finance a larger portion of Part B and Part D premium responsibility while retaining access to the same federally defined Medicare benefit categories. SSA's regulatory introduction confirms that the income-related adjustment is layered onto the Part B premium system, while CMS's 2026 cost materials express the same principle administratively: if modified adjusted gross income from the tax return two years earlier is above a specified amount, the beneficiary pays the standard Part B premium plus an income-related monthly adjustment amount. (Social Security)

The two-year MAGI lookback rule is the central timing mechanism. Under CMS's 2026 Medicare handbook, Medicare uses modified adjusted gross income from the IRS tax return from two years earlier to determine whether IRMAA applies; for the 2026 premium cycle, the relevant federal tax file is generally the 2024 return. SSA Form SSA-44 reflects the same administrative data structure by explaining that SSA asks the IRS for adjusted gross income plus certain tax-exempt income, called modified adjusted gross income, from the 2024 federal income tax return for a 2026 IRMAA determination, with 2023 data used if the 2024 return is unavailable. (Social Security)

This lookback is institutionally necessary because current-year income cannot be fully known when Medicare premiums are set, while completed IRS tax-return data provides a standardized national measurement file.

The two-year lookback creates predictable friction between prior taxable income and present retirement cash flow. A household may have recognized income in 2024 through wages, pension commencement, required minimum distributions, business-sale proceeds, capital gains, Roth conversion income, or other taxable events, yet enter 2026 with lower recurring liquidity. The federal premium file still begins with the completed tax return, not with informal current-year expectations. SSA's Form SSA-44 confirms that the review mechanism depends on MAGI and tax filing status, and defines MAGI for the form as adjusted gross income from line 11 of IRS Form 1040 plus tax-exempt interest income from line 2a of IRS Form 1040. (Social Security) This creates a tax-to-premium conversion channel: federal taxable-income reporting becomes the input for future Medicare premium classification.

The 2026 Part B bracket structure is filing-status specific. Under the 2026 Medicare Costs fact sheet contained in the CMS source packet, beneficiaries with 2024 income of $109,000 or less on an individual tax return, $218,000 or less on a joint tax return, or $109,000 or less on a married filing separately return pay the standard 2026 Part B monthly amount of $202.90. When 2024 income is above $109,000 up to $137,000 for an individual filer, or above $218,000 up to $274,000 for a joint filer, the 2026 monthly Part B amount is $284.10. When 2024 income is above $137,000 up to $171,000 for an individual filer, or above $274,000 up to $342,000 for a joint filer, the 2026 monthly Part B amount is $405.80.

The higher Part B tiers continue the same filing-status architecture. Under the CMS 2026 cost table, 2024 income above $171,000 up to $205,000 for an individual filer, or above $342,000 up to $410,000 for a joint filer, corresponds to a 2026 monthly Part B amount of $527.50. The next tier applies to 2024 income above $205,000 and less than $500,000 for an individual filer, above $410,000 and less than $750,000 for a joint filer, and above $109,000 and less than $391,000 for married filing separately; that tier corresponds to a 2026 monthly Part B amount of $649.20. The terminal tier applies to 2024 income of $500,000 or above for an individual filer, $750,000 or above for a joint filer, and $391,000 or above for married filing separately; that tier corresponds to a 2026 monthly Part B amount of $689.90.

This bracket system is not a smooth marginal tax schedule. It operates as a premium classification ladder. Ordinary federal income tax rates generally apply higher marginal rates only to income inside a higher taxable bracket. IRMAA, by contrast, places the beneficiary into a higher monthly Medicare premium category once the applicable MAGI threshold is crossed. The CMS table does not calculate a surcharge only on the incremental dollar above $109,000 for an individual filer or $218,000 for a joint filer; it assigns a higher monthly Part B premium category for the premium year once the threshold is exceeded. This produces a cliff effect. A small amount of MAGI above a threshold can produce a full-year change in monthly premium classification, even though the underlying Medicare benefits remain unchanged.

The Part B IRMAA structure must be separated from the Part D IRMAA structure. Part B IRMAA is incorporated into the monthly Part B premium amount shown in the CMS Part B table. Part D IRMAA is an additional federal amount owed in addition to the applicable Medicare drug coverage premium. CMS states in the 2026 handbook that higher-income beneficiaries may pay an extra amount for Medicare drug coverage, that this amount is paid in addition to the plan premium, and that it is required even when the drug coverage is included in another Medicare coverage arrangement. The Part D-IRMAA definition in CMS enrollment guidance further states that Part D-IRMAA is a premium amount separate from the Part D plan's monthly premium, assessed annually by SSA based on available tax information.

The 2026 Part D IRMAA brackets use the same income categories as the 2026 Part B IRMAA table, but the amounts are separate drug-coverage surcharges. Under the 2026 CMS Part D cost table, the lowest income category pays only the applicable drug plan premium, while 2024 income above $109,000 up to $137,000 for an individual filer and above $218,000 up to $274,000 for a joint filer corresponds to $14.50 plus the plan premium. Income above $137,000 up to $171,000 for an individual filer and above $274,000 up to $342,000 for a joint filer corresponds to $37.50 plus the plan premium. Income above $171,000 up to $205,000 for an individual filer and above $342,000 up to $410,000 for a joint filer corresponds to $60.40 plus the plan premium.

The upper Part D IRMAA tiers preserve the same married filing separately compression found in the Part B table. Under the 2026 CMS cost table, 2024 income above $205,000 and less than $500,000 for an individual filer, above $410,000 and less than $750,000 for a joint filer, and above $109,000 and less than $391,000 for married filing separately corresponds to $83.30 plus the plan premium. The terminal Part D IRMAA tier applies at $500,000 or above for individual filers, $750,000 or above for joint filers, and $391,000 or above for married filing separately, and corresponds to $91.00 plus the plan premium. The same CMS source states that the 2026 Part D national base premium is $38.99 and that Medicare uses that national base premium to estimate both the Part D late-enrollment penalty and the income-related monthly adjustment amounts listed in the table, with the national base amount subject to annual change.

Part D IRMAA's billing design creates a distinct administrative risk. CMS states that Medicare or the Railroad Retirement Board usually deducts the Part D IRMAA from Social Security or Railroad Retirement Board payments, but if Medicare or the Railroad Retirement Board bills the beneficiary instead, the extra amount must be paid to Medicare or the Railroad Retirement Board, not to the drug plan. CMS further states that Part D IRMAA payments must be paid separately even when an employer or another third party, such as a retirement system, pays the plan premium. This rule prevents a third-party premium payment from satisfying the separate federal Part D IRMAA obligation. A household may therefore have a drug plan premium paid externally while still owing a separate federal surcharge.

Nonpayment of Part D IRMAA can destabilize drug coverage. CMS's 2026 handbook warns that failure to pay the extra Part D IRMAA amount can result in loss of Medicare drug coverage, inability to join another plan right away, and possible Part D late-enrollment penalty exposure for as long as drug coverage continues. CMS enrollment guidance supplies the operational enforcement details: individuals with Part D IRMAA must pay the additional premium directly to the government, CMS establishes a three-month initial grace period for failure to pay Part D IRMAA, and after the grace period CMS disenrolls individuals who fail to pay from the Medicare drug coverage arrangement, with the disenrollment effective the first day of the month after the initial grace period. Thus, Part D IRMAA is not a passive accounting notation. It is a federal premium obligation whose nonpayment can terminate drug coverage.

IRMAA review is a data-alignment process, not a generalized equitable relief system. CMS's 2026 handbook states that when a beneficiary owes IRMAA and disagrees because income is lower due to a life event, the review channel runs through Social Security. SSA's public IRMAA page states that a life-changing event reducing household income can support a request to lower the additional amount paid for Medicare Part B and Part D, and identifies examples including marriage, divorce, death of a spouse, loss of income, and employer settlement payment. (Social Security) Form SSA-44 lists the specific life-changing-event categories as marriage, divorce or annulment, death of a spouse, work stoppage, work reduction, loss of income-producing property, loss of pension income, and employer settlement payment. (Social Security)

The SSA-44 instructions define the evidentiary boundaries. The form states that a life-changing-event date must be in the same year or an earlier year than the tax year requested for the income-related premium adjustment, and it explains that where 2024 tax information was used for a 2026 IRMAA determination, a beneficiary may request use of 2025 tax information instead when income was reduced in 2025 due to a life-changing event occurring in 2025 or an earlier year. (Social Security) The form also states that required evidence of MAGI and the life-changing event must be supplied, including a signed tax return or IRS transcript if the return has been filed, or a later tax return when an estimate was used. (Social Security) Therefore, the relief mechanism is documentary and chronological. It does not exist merely because a prior income spike was inconvenient.

Certain income events must be described with caution. SSA-44 recognizes work stoppage or reduction, loss of income-producing property not at the beneficiary's direction, loss of pension income through scheduled cessation, termination, or reorganization of an employer pension plan, and employer settlement payments arising from employer bankruptcy or reorganization. (Social Security) Standard capital gains, voluntary business-sale gain recognition, and planned Roth conversion income are not listed among those SSA-44 life-changing-event categories. The official source does not convert every taxable spike into a reviewable life-changing event. It permits use of more recent tax-year information only when the federal life-changing-event framework and evidentiary requirements are satisfied. (Social Security)

IRMAA's household cash-flow effect is immediate because it reduces premium-period liquidity. Part B premiums are deducted from Social Security or Railroad Retirement Board benefits when those benefits are being paid, and the 2026 handbook states that the Part B premium will be deducted from the monthly benefit payment. Part D IRMAA is likewise usually deducted from Social Security or Railroad Retirement Board payments, with separate billing by Medicare or the Railroad Retirement Board where withholding does not occur. The cash-flow consequence is that IRMAA may reduce the net amount reaching household operating accounts before discretionary medical allocation begins. It becomes a recurring claim against income rather than a claim paid only when services are used.

The recurring nature of IRMAA matters because Medicare liabilities are layered. Original Medicare generally requires payment of deductibles before Medicare pays its share, and Part B-covered services usually involve 20 percent coinsurance after the deductible under assignment rules. CMS also states that 2026 covered Part D drug out-of-pocket costs are capped at $2,100, but premium obligations and IRMAA remain separate from that covered-drug cost-sharing cap. IRMAA therefore reduces liquidity available for Part B deductibles, Part B coinsurance, Part D premiums, covered-drug cost sharing, dental care excluded from Original Medicare, ordinary refractive vision correction, hearing aids, and non-medical custodial long-term care. The surcharge is paid whether or not the beneficiary uses additional services during the month.

IRMAA must also be separated from late-enrollment penalties. A beneficiary may owe IRMAA because the two-year MAGI file exceeds the applicable threshold. A beneficiary may owe a late-enrollment penalty because Part B or Part D enrollment was delayed without recognized protection. A beneficiary may owe both, or neither, because the systems have different statutory triggers. CMS's 2026 handbook states that the Part B late-enrollment penalty may increase the monthly premium by 10 percent for each full 12-month period during which Part B could have been held but was not, while the same handbook separately states that the standard premium increases through IRMAA when MAGI exceeds threshold amounts. Part D follows the same separation: Part D IRMAA is an income-related federal amount, while the Part D late-enrollment penalty arises from uncovered months without Medicare drug coverage or other creditable prescription coverage.

This distinction is actuarially important because the household file may contain multiple premium modifiers. The 2026 Medicare Costs fact sheet states that Part B premium amounts may be higher when a late-enrollment penalty applies, and it separately provides the IRMAA-based Part B premium categories. The Part D table similarly states that the national base premium is used to estimate the Part D late-enrollment penalty and the income-related monthly adjustment amounts, and that the total premium amount may be higher if a late-enrollment penalty is paid. Therefore, IRMAA analysis cannot be performed in isolation from enrollment compliance. One premium increase may arise from income, another from delayed enrollment, and a third from the ordinary plan or coverage premium.

The Household Medicare Diagnostic Matrix must therefore include IRMAA as a tax-interface audit rather than as a coverage-selection issue. Section 6.1 supplies the matrix's high-income, business-sale, Roth conversion, capital-gain, pension, required minimum distribution, retirement, widowhood, and filing-status logic. A household file cannot be declared Medicare-stable merely because Part A entitlement, Part B enrollment, Part D coverage, and employer coordination have been executed correctly. The file must also identify tax filing status, the MAGI year used for the premium year, the applicable bracket, the Part B monthly amount, the Part D IRMAA amount, the federal billing channel, and any recognized SSA life-changing-event pathway supported by documentation. (Social Security)

The final actuarial conclusion is that IRMAA converts prior taxable income into a current Medicare premium compression. Its severity lies not in denial of care, but in bracket cliffs, two-year lookback mismatch, recurring withholding or federal billing, and liquidity reduction during years when other health-related liabilities often rise. The household that recognizes a business gain, pension distribution, Roth conversion, capital gain, or other taxable event in the lookback year may experience a Medicare premium effect two years later, even when current cash flow has changed. Under the Household Medicare Diagnostic Matrix, IRMAA is therefore the premium-pricing bridge between the tax return and the Medicare file: prior MAGI becomes present federal premium obligation, and present premium obligation reduces the capital reserve available for coinsurance, prescription costs, excluded dental and sensory services, and custodial care exposure.

6.2 The Two-Year Lookback Architecture

The two-year lookback architecture is the temporal engine that converts prior taxable income into current Medicare premium liability. It is not an accidental administrative lag. It is a federal risk-management structure built around the fact that Medicare premium determinations must be made before current-year taxable income can be finally known, verified, and processed through the federal income tax system. Under CMS lookback specifications in the 2026 Medicare handbook, Medicare uses modified adjusted gross income reported on the IRS tax return from two years earlier to determine whether an Income-Related Monthly Adjustment Amount applies; for the 2026 premium year, CMS identifies 2024 modified adjusted gross income as the income file used to determine whether a beneficiary may owe IRMAA. SSA's Program Operations Manual System states the same operational rule: MAGI used for IRMAA is generally the most recent tax information that IRS can provide, ordinarily from two years before the premium year, with 2026 premiums generally based on 2024 tax return information. (Social Security Administration)

The retrospective model protects the Supplementary Medical Insurance financing system by giving the federal government a completed, standardized, national income file rather than an estimate of current household income. Part B premiums are set annually, and the federal premium subsidy is tied to the portion of the full Part B cost paid through transfers into the Supplementary Medical Insurance Trust Fund. SSA regulations define IRMAA as an additional Part B premium amount owed when income exceeds the statutory threshold, and define the standard Part B premium as the monthly amount set annually by CMS under the Part B premium regulations. (Social Security) The lookback system therefore mediates between two incompatible timelines: the immediate premium-setting calendar for Medicare and the delayed verification calendar for federal tax administration. Current-year income cannot be conclusively audited at the moment Medicare must bill premiums, so the federal system reaches backward to a completed IRS record.

The IRS-to-SSA data exchange is the institutional bridge between federal revenue administration and federal social insurance administration. SSA's handbook states that SSA uses federal income tax return information from the IRS about beneficiaries' modified adjusted gross income to make IRMAA determinations. (Social Security) The statutory confidentiality framework in Internal Revenue Code § 6103 generally protects return information from disclosure, but it also contains specific statutory disclosure channels. Section 6103 authorizes the Secretary of the Treasury, upon written request from the Commissioner of Social Security, to disclose return information of a taxpayer whose premium may be subject to adjustment under Social Security Act § 1839(i) or increase under Social Security Act § 1860D-13(a)(7). (Legal Information Institute) The IRMAA file is therefore not built through voluntary premium reporting. It is built through a legally authorized federal data exchange.

The MAGI value used in this exchange is not ordinary household cash flow. SSA's POMS states that MAGI for IRMAA is the beneficiary's adjusted gross income from line 11 of IRS Form 1040 plus tax-exempt interest income from line 2a of IRS Form 1040. (Social Security Administration) Form SSA-44 uses the same construction, requiring adjusted gross income and tax-exempt interest income, and its instructions state that MAGI is adjusted gross income from line 11 of Form 1040 plus tax-exempt interest income from line 2a of Form 1040. (Social Security) This reconstitution matters because IRMAA does not examine spendable retirement income alone. It reassembles the federal tax return into a premium classification measure that can include taxable income and tax-exempt interest.

For the 2026 premium cycle, the mechanical result is direct. CMS's 2026 Medicare cost table classifies 2026 Part B premiums by 2024 income, beginning with the standard $202.90 monthly Part B premium when 2024 income is $109,000 or less for an individual return, $218,000 or less for a joint return, or $109,000 or less for married filing separately, and then rising through higher monthly amounts as 2024 income crosses the listed thresholds. The same CMS cost table applies 2024 income to 2026 Part D IRMAA, with the Part D national base premium identified as $38.99 and with additional Part D IRMAA amounts tied to the same income categories. Thus, the 2024 tax return becomes a 2026 healthcare premium determinant.

This architecture produces the retirement caught-in-the-middle trap. A beneficiary may earn peak wages in the final working year, receive a corporate exit payment, recognize deferred compensation, sell a business interest, realize a capital gain, or begin required distributions before the premium year in which retirement cash flow has already declined. The federal premium system nevertheless classifies the later Medicare year through the earlier tax return because the IRS record is the verified data source. CMS states that Medicare uses the modified adjusted gross income from the IRS return two years earlier, and SSA states that the most recent tax information IRS can provide is generally from two years before the premium year. (Social Security Administration) The mismatch is structural: historical taxable capacity can be converted into current premium obligation after the household's recurring income has already changed.

Real estate and portfolio events illustrate the same timing problem. A taxable sale of non-residential real property, a major capital-gain distribution from a taxable portfolio, a concentrated stock liquidation, or an unusually large required minimum distribution may create a one-year MAGI spike. The Medicare premium consequence does not necessarily appear in the same calendar year as the transaction. It appears when that tax return becomes the lookback record for a later premium year. Under the 2026 structure, 2024 MAGI controls 2026 premium classification, and the CMS table applies higher Part B and Part D IRMAA amounts once the applicable 2024 income thresholds are crossed. The result is a delayed premium shock: an income event that may have been fully spent, reinvested, taxed, or absorbed in the transaction year can still generate Medicare premium compression two years later.

Corporate exit packages create a particularly opaque version of this problem. Severance payments, accumulated vacation payouts, deferred compensation releases, retention bonuses, executive transition payments, and pension commencements may produce temporary liquidity during the employment exit year. In the later Medicare premium year, those payments may no longer exist as recurring income, but the tax return they produced remains the federal income file for IRMAA. SSA's SSA-44 instructions recognize that the agency used MAGI and tax filing status to determine the income-related monthly adjustment amount, and they require the claimant seeking adjustment to supply more recent MAGI only through the form's defined life-changing event process. (Social Security) The household may experience the payment as a one-time transition cushion; the federal system experiences it as a verified MAGI input.

The primacy of the IRS record is central to the initial assessment. SSA's handbook states that SSA uses IRS tax return information about MAGI to make IRMAA determinations. (Social Security) CMS's 2026 handbook states that Medicare uses modified adjusted gross income reported on the IRS return from two years earlier. SSA's POMS states that the MAGI used for IRMAA is the most recent tax information IRS is able to provide, generally two years before the premium year and not more than three years before. (Social Security Administration) These statements define the initial administrative baseline. SSA does not begin with a household budget, current bank balance, or retirement projection. It begins with the IRS transmission.

That baseline can be revisited only through recognized federal channels. CMS states that if a beneficiary must pay an extra amount and disagrees, for example because income is lower due to a life event, the review channel is through Social Security. SSA's public IRMAA page states that a life-changing event reducing household income can support a request to lower the additional amount paid for Medicare Part B and Part D, and identifies life-changing events including marriage, divorce, death of a spouse, loss of income, and employer settlement payment. (Social Security) Form SSA-44 provides the documentary structure for that review and requires evidence of both

MAGI and the life-changing event. (Social Security) The relief mechanism is therefore a data-alignment process, not a discretionary waiver.

The SSA-44 framework is narrow. The form's instructions state that the more recent tax year selected must reflect a reduction in income due to the life-changing event listed, and that the year must be more recent than the year of tax return information used in the IRMAA notice. (Social Security) The instructions also state that evidence must be supplied: a signed federal tax return or IRS transcript if the return has already been filed, or later proof when an estimate is used, together with original documents or certified copies of evidence of the life-changing event. (Social Security) This converts the review process into a documentary record test. A current income decline must match a recognized life event and be supported by federal evidence.

Non-qualifying financial spikes remain inside the ordinary lookback architecture. Standard portfolio gains, voluntary Roth conversion income, discretionary sale proceeds, ordinary taxable liquidation of assets, and non-pension contract settlements are not listed in the SSA-44 life-changing event categories shown in the official form and SSA summary. (Social Security) (Social Security) The source framework therefore does not create a general remedy for every one-year MAGI spike. If the event is taxable, appears on the IRS return, and does not fall within the recognized life-changing-event correction channel or amended-return procedure, it remains part of the initial IRMAA determination for the applicable premium year. This is not a moral judgment about the financial event. It is an administrative boundary.

The amended-return pathway is also distinct from the life-changing-event pathway. SSA's IRMAA page states that a person with an amended income tax return may contact Social Security to request review of the Medicare Income-Related Monthly Adjustment Amount. (Social Security) That pathway corrects or updates the IRS income file itself; it does not ask SSA to disregard a valid IRS figure because the household later dislikes its premium consequence. The structure preserves institutional hierarchy: the IRS record determines the initial MAGI baseline, an amended IRS record can alter the income data, and a recognized life-changing event can permit SSA to use more recent income information under SSA-44.

The two-year lookback also affects Part D beyond ordinary premium billing. CMS states that Part D-IRMAA is a monthly amount added to the individual's Part D premium and is based on modified adjusted gross income; individuals with Part D-IRMAA must pay this additional premium directly to the government, not to the plan. CMS enrollment guidance further states that failure to pay Part D-IRMAA triggers a three-month initial grace period, after which CMS disenrolls the individual from the Part D or MA-PD arrangement, with disenrollment effective the first day of the month after the grace period. A prior tax return can therefore mandate not only a current surcharge, but also a federal billing obligation whose nonpayment can cause drug coverage disruption.

This is why the phrase "out-of-pocket healthcare costs" must be read broadly. IRMAA is a premium obligation, not a claim cost, deductible, copayment, or coinsurance amount. Yet it functions economically as a mandatory outflow tied to the Medicare file. Part B IRMAA increases the monthly Part B premium obligation, and Part D IRMAA adds a federal amount to drug coverage premium responsibility. CMS's 2026 table states that the Part D national base premium is used to estimate the income-related monthly adjustment amounts and that the national base amount can change each year. The household therefore faces a recurring healthcare-related cash-flow charge derived from a historical tax record rather than from present medical utilization.

The cash-flow compression is magnified by the fact that Medicare liabilities are layered. Original Medicare Part B services commonly involve deductible and 20 percent coinsurance exposure after deductible, and Original Medicare has no annual out-of-pocket limit unless supplemental coverage applies, as CMS explains in the 2026 handbook's comparison of Original Medicare and Medicare Advantage. The premium layer created by IRMAA reduces liquidity before those service-use liabilities are encountered. It also reduces the cash reserve available for items excluded from Original Medicare, including routine dental care, ordinary refractive vision correction, hearing aids, and non-medical custodial long-term care, as discussed in the statutory exclusions matrix. The lookback system therefore links a prior tax return to present healthcare affordability even when no new claim has been filed.

The lookback system should not be described as compounding in the investment sense. The IRMAA surcharge does not earn interest on itself, and a prior premium obligation does not become principal for a later premium year. The escalation risk lies elsewhere: a single income event can place the household into a higher bracket for a full premium year, and multiple income events across successive tax years can produce repeated premium-year consequences. CMS's 2026 table shows bracketed Part B and Part D premium effects tied to 2024 income, while SSA's POMS states that the tax information used is generally the most recent IRS information available for the premium year. (Social Security Administration) The actuarial issue is not interest-on-interest. It is year-to-year premium classification through trailing tax files.

The Household Medicare Diagnostic Matrix therefore must treat tax timing as a Medicare variable. A current-year retirement budget cannot be evaluated without identifying the tax year that will become the Medicare premium-year lookback file. For the 2026 cycle, the matrix must identify 2024 MAGI, filing status, tax-exempt interest, Part B bracket, Part D IRMAA category, federal billing channel, and whether a recognized SSA-44 life-changing event or amended-return pathway exists. CMS's source packet gives the 2026 income brackets and premium amounts; SSA's POMS supplies the MAGI definition and two-year lookback rule; SSA-44 supplies the evidence and more-recent-income framework. (Social Security Administration) (Social Security)

The concluding principle is exacting. The Medicare premium file is not driven solely by current income, current medical need, current liquidity, or current retirement status. It is driven first by a verified federal tax record transmitted through authorized inter-agency channels. A liquidation, Roth conversion, business sale, capital gain, pension event, required distribution, or corporate exit package may appear as a short-term financial decision in the tax year, but it can reappear as a Medicare premium consequence two years later. Section 6.2 therefore supplies the chronological data interface for the Household Medicare Diagnostic Matrix: prior MAGI must be mapped against future Medicare premium years, because the failure to track the 24-month federal reporting pipeline can convert a standard financial transition into recurring premium compression precisely when the household's out-of-pocket healthcare liabilities are expanding.

6.3 Statutory Life-Changing Events (LCE)

Statutory Life-Changing Event relief is the narrow corrective counterweight to the two-year IRMAA lookback architecture. The ordinary IRMAA determination begins with historical tax data: Medicare uses modified adjusted gross income reported on the IRS tax return from two years earlier to determine whether an Income-Related Monthly Adjustment Amount applies, and the 2026 premium year generally uses 2024 MAGI. SSA's IRMAA operating policy states the same premise, namely that MAGI used for IRMAA is generally the most recent tax information IRS can provide, ordinarily from two years before the premium year, with 2026 premiums generally based on 2024 tax return information. (Social Security Administration) Life-Changing Event relief exists because that retrospective tax file can overstate current household income after a federally recognized disruption. The relief mechanism is therefore not equitable forgiveness, tax-planning relief, investment-loss relief, or a general hardship waiver. It is a bounded federal data-alignment doctrine that permits SSA to substitute a more recent tax year only when a qualifying event causes a significant MAGI reduction.

The actuarial purpose of the Life-Changing Event framework is to preserve the legitimacy of income-related premium recovery without converting a stale tax return into an excessive premium charge after a recognized disruption. SSA Handbook § 2507 states that a beneficiary or spouse may experience events causing a significant reduction in MAGI, and that a significant reduction is one that decreases or eliminates

IRMAA for a specific year; the same provision allows a request for a new initial determination using a more recent tax year when a life-changing event caused the reduction. (Social Security) This framing is exact. A reduction in income is not enough by itself. A qualifying event is not enough by itself. Relief depends on both: an enumerated event and a resulting MAGI reduction that changes or removes the surcharge.

Form SSA-44, Medicare Income-Related Monthly Adjustment Amount, Life-Changing Event, is the principal administrative instrument for this correction. The current SSA-44 form states that when a major life-changing event occurs and income has gone down, the form may be used to request a reduction in the income-related monthly adjustment amount. (Social Security) The form explains that SSA asked IRS for adjusted gross income plus certain tax-exempt income, called MAGI, from the federal income tax return used for the IRMAA determination, and it then requires the applicant to identify the life-changing event, the event date, the more recent tax year, adjusted gross income, tax-exempt interest income, and filing status. (Social Security) The administrative significance is substantial: SSA-44 is not an automatic surcharge cancellation device. It is a documentary request for SSA to make a new premium determination.

The form's own threshold logic prevents unnecessary or unsupported filings. SSA-44 states that if the most recent filed tax return shows MAGI below the IRMAA trigger amount, no income-related monthly adjustment amount is owed and the form should not be completed even if a life-changing event occurred. (Social Security) Conversely, when MAGI remains above the applicable threshold after the event, the surcharge may continue at the recalculated level. The 2026 CMS materials identify the standard Part B premium as $202.90 and state that IRMAA may apply when 2024 MAGI exceeds $109,000 for individual filers or $218,000 for joint filers; CMS also states that Part D IRMAA may apply when MAGI exceeds the applicable threshold. Therefore, the relief analysis is bracket-sensitive. The question is not merely whether income declined. The question is whether the accepted evidence moves the file into a lower IRMAA classification for Part B, Part D, or both.

SSA recognizes eight life-changing events for IRMAA adjustment purposes. SSA Handbook § 2507 identifies death of spouse, marriage, divorce or annulment, work reduction, work stoppage, loss of income-producing property, loss or reduction of pension income, and receipt of employer settlement payment as the eight events. (Social Security) The regulation at 20 CFR § 418.1205 likewise identifies spouse death, marriage, divorce or annulment, work stoppage or reduction in work hours, loss of income-producing property, loss or reduction of pension income, and employer settlement payment as major life-changing events. (Social Security) These categories are administrative gateways, not open-ended examples. The federal system does not authorize a general appeal whenever a tax return produced an inconvenient premium result.

Marriage, divorce or annulment, and death of a spouse can alter the income composition and filing-status architecture of the IRMAA file. A marriage can combine income streams and change filing status; a divorce or annulment can sever a joint tax unit; a spouse's death can move a surviving spouse from joint-filing thresholds into individual-filing thresholds while income-producing assets, survivor benefits, distributions, capital transactions, or pension streams may remain elevated. SSA-44 requires the life-changing event date and more recent income data, while 20 CFR § 418.1265 requires evidence that one or more major life-changing events caused a significant MAGI reduction for the tax year SSA is asked to use. (Social Security) The family-status event therefore must be documented, and the income reduction must be demonstrated. A marital-status change without a lower bracket does not by itself eliminate IRMAA.

Work stoppage and work reduction are the most common retirement-transition categories because the two-year lookback often captures peak wages from a final employment year while the current premium year reflects lower post-employment income. SSA-44 lists work stoppage and work reduction as distinct life-changing events, and its instructions require the more recent tax year to reflect a reduction in income due to the listed event. (Social Security) A work stoppage represents complete cessation of compensated labor, including retirement or other termination of work activity, while work reduction represents a decrease in work hours or income-producing labor activity. The administrative file must show the event date, the changed work status, and the resulting reduced MAGI. Retirement terminology alone is insufficient; the federal record must tie the employment event to a lower income year.

The evidence architecture for work stoppage and work reduction is necessarily documentary. SSA-44 instructs that the selected tax year must be more recent than the tax year used in the IRMAA notice, and it permits use of the premium year estimate when income is lower in that year or the prior year's tax information when that year reflects the reduction. (Social Security) The same instructions define MAGI for the form as adjusted gross income from line 11 of IRS Form 1040 plus tax-exempt interest income from line 2a, and require actual or estimated amounts and filing status. (Social Security) Generic evidence may include employer separation letters, retirement notices, payroll records, pension statements, tax returns, or other SSA-accepted proof. The institutional question is whether the evidence demonstrates a recognized work event and a MAGI reduction that changes the IRMAA result.

Loss of income-producing property is one of the most misunderstood Life-Changing Event categories. SSA-44 includes "Loss of Income-Producing Property" as a selectable event, and SSA Handbook § 2507 includes the same category among the eight recognized events. (Social Security) The category should not be expanded into ordinary investment disappointment. It does not mean a voluntary sale at a gain, a tactical portfolio liquidation, a planned reallocation, a Roth conversion, or the ordinary decline of a marketable-security portfolio. It concerns the loss of property that produced income, where the loss is consistent with the SSA life-changing-event framework and produces a significant MAGI reduction. The distinction is actuarially essential because IRMAA relief is designed to correct income disruption, not to neutralize chosen taxable income recognition.

The qualifying and nonqualifying boundaries can be expressed without turning the text into advice. An income-producing property destroyed by disaster may fit the conceptual frame if the documentary record establishes the loss and the resulting income reduction. A voluntary sale of rental real estate producing a capital gain generally does not become a "loss of income-producing property" merely because the gain produced IRMAA two years later. A portfolio decline generally does not become a Life-Changing Event merely because market value fell. A Roth conversion generally does not become a Life-Changing Event because it was a voluntary taxable income event, even where it was undertaken for long-term asset positioning. SSA's recognized categories and evidence rule require an enumerated event and a significant MAGI reduction, not merely a high-income year followed by displeasure with premium consequences. (Social Security)

Loss or reduction of pension income is a separate category because pension income may stop or decrease for reasons outside ordinary household choice. SSA Handbook § 2507 lists loss or reduction of pension income as one of the eight recognized Life-Changing Events, and SSA's POMS table of contents identifies a specific operating section for reduction or loss of pension income. (Social Security) In this category, the administrative issue is whether the pension income stopped or decreased because of a qualifying pension event, such as scheduled cessation, termination, or employer plan reorganization, rather than because the household elected a different income strategy. Documentation may include pension notices, plan termination materials, income statements, employer or plan communications, and tax filings. The LCE framework recognizes structural income reduction, not broad preference for a lower premium.

Employer settlement payment is also limited. SSA Handbook § 2507 lists receipt of employer settlement payment as a Life-Changing Event, and SSA's POMS table of contents identifies a dedicated operating section for that category. (Social Security)

The category is tied to employer-related disruptions such as closure, bankruptcy, or reorganization as reflected in SSA materials, not to any ordinary private settlement, consulting buyout, non-pension contract settlement, or elective income acceleration. The evidentiary distinction is the same one that controls the entire LCE framework: the federal record must show a recognized event, a relevant date, and a resulting income change capable of producing a new IRMAA determination.

The evidentiary burden is rigorous because SSA is being asked to override the presumptive force of IRS lookback data. Under 20 CFR § 418.1265, the claimant must provide evidence that one or more major life-changing events resulted in a significant MAGI reduction for the tax year SSA is asked to use, and preferred evidence includes a retained copy of the filed federal income tax return, an amended return with IRS receipt, proof of IRS correction, or comparable IRS-derived documentation for the more recent tax year. (Social Security) Where a filed return is not available, the regulation permits equivalent evidence together with a signed statement under penalty of perjury that the information provided is true and correct. (Social Security) The file must therefore prove both sides of the case: the event and the income.

SSA-44's instructions reinforce this evidentiary architecture. The form instructs the claimant to provide required evidence of MAGI and the life-changing event, and it explains that if income is estimated, SSA may later use the filed tax return or IRS information to adjust Medicare premiums if necessary. (Social Security) The regulation similarly provides that SSA may later verify the information when IRS data for the relevant tax year becomes available. (Social Security) This later verification rule protects the integrity of the premium system. SSA can act on beneficiary-provided information when IRS data is not yet available, but the file remains subject to reconciliation when the tax record matures.

Nonqualifying financial spikes must be separated from recognized Life-Changing Events. Ordinary capital gains, voluntary Roth conversions, ordinary required minimum distributions, discretionary business-sale gain recognition, speculative investment losses, non-pension contract settlements, and general cash-flow discomfort do not automatically qualify under SSA's enumerated LCE categories. SSA-44 lists the recognized events directly, and the CFR evidence rule ties relief to those events and to a significant MAGI reduction. (Social Security) If a taxable event appears on the IRS return and does not fall within a recognized LCE category or another official correction channel, the IRMAA surcharge may remain for the premium year. The administrative file is not permitted to disregard valid taxable income merely because the event was unusual, one-time, or financially inconvenient.

Amended tax returns occupy a different channel from Life-Changing Events. SSA's public IRMAA page states that amended income tax returns can support a request to lower IRMAA, and 20 CFR § 418.1265 identifies a retained copy of an amended return with IRS receipt, or proof of corrected IRS information, as preferred evidence where applicable. (Social Security) That pathway corrects the income record itself. It is different from asking SSA to use a more recent income year because a recognized Life-Changing Event reduced income. The distinction matters because an amended IRS record changes the data baseline, while SSA-44 LCE relief changes the tax year used for the determination only when the statutory event and income-reduction conditions are satisfied.

Life-Changing Event relief can affect both Part B IRMAA and Part D IRMAA because both are driven by MAGI classification. CMS states that Medicare uses the modified adjusted gross income from the IRS return two years earlier to determine whether Part B IRMAA applies, and that an extra amount may also apply to Medicare drug coverage when MAGI exceeds the applicable amount. CMS's Part D materials state that a higher-income beneficiary may pay an extra Part D IRMAA amount in addition to the drug coverage premium, that the amount is usually deducted from Social Security or Railroad Retirement Board payments or billed by Medicare or the Railroad Retirement Board, and that payment must go to the government rather than to the plan. Thus, a successful SSA-44 adjustment may reduce premium pressure across both premium systems where the recalculated MAGI moves the file into a lower bracket.

Part D IRMAA also carries its own enforcement consequence. CMS states that failure to pay the extra Part D IRMAA amount can result in loss of Medicare drug coverage, inability to join another plan right away, and possible Part D late-enrollment penalty exposure for as long as drug coverage continues. CMS enrollment guidance states that Part D-IRMAA is a monthly amount added to the Part D premium, based on MAGI, paid directly to the government, and subject to a three-month initial grace period before CMS disenrolls an individual from drug coverage for nonpayment. Life-Changing Event relief therefore has cash-flow and coverage-stability implications, but it does not erase billing duties before SSA changes the file. The federal premium obligation remains operative unless and until a new determination changes it.

Timing is a central feature of the relief mechanism. SSA-44 explains that the life-changing event date must be in the same year or an earlier year than the tax year requested for the new determination; for example, if 2024 tax information was used for a 2026 IRMAA determination, 2025 tax information can be requested if income was reduced in 2025 due to a life-changing event that occurred in 2025 or earlier. (Social Security) The form also allows use of the premium year estimate when the income reduction occurs in the premium year or when the premium year is expected to be lower than the prior year. (Social Security) SSA regulations provide that when

MAGI for the more recent tax year is significantly reduced as a result of a major life-changing event, the new initial determination is generally effective January 1 of the year in which the request is made, subject to limited prior-year circumstances. (Social Security)

The premium correction itself should not be overstated beyond the source record. An accepted SSA adjustment may lower prospective billing and may support correction of over-collected amounts where the federal record supports a new determination, but exact refund timing is not established by the uploaded CMS materials. SSA's regulation provides the effective-date rule for new determinations, while SSA-44 and 20 CFR § 418.1265 explain the evidence and verification architecture. (Social Security) The manuscript's safe conclusion is therefore procedural: when SSA accepts a qualifying LCE and revised income evidence, the premium file can be recalibrated to the applicable income category. The outcome depends on the recalculated MAGI, filing status, premium year, and official determination.

The Household Medicare Diagnostic Matrix treats Section 6.3 as the IRMAA correction interface. The matrix must distinguish a valid IRS lookback result from an amended-return correction, a recognized Life-Changing Event, a nonqualifying taxable spike, and a billing or withholding issue. Under CMS specifications, IRMAA begins with the two-year MAGI lookback and may affect both Part B and Part D premium obligations; under SSA procedures, LCE relief requires a recognized event and a significant MAGI reduction supported by evidence. (Social Security) The diagnostic file must therefore record the tax year used, the MAGI and filing status in that year, the alleged LCE category, the event date, the reduced income year, the documentary support, and whether the adjustment affects Part B IRMAA, Part D IRMAA, or both.

The final actuarial conclusion is that Life-Changing Event relief is the narrow statutory safety valve inside the IRMAA system. It prevents the two-year lookback from overpricing current premiums after recognized income-disrupting events such as spouse death, marriage, divorce or annulment, work stoppage, work reduction, loss of income-producing property, loss or reduction of pension income, or employer settlement payment. It does not erase ordinary taxable spikes, voluntary income recognition, generalized financial discomfort, or investment outcomes that fall outside the federal categories. The Household Medicare Diagnostic Matrix therefore treats SSA-44 not as a universal appeal form, but as a document-driven premium recalibration instrument for specific federal life-changing events that materially reduce MAGI and alter the income-related premium classification.

Chapter 7: The Health Savings Account (HSA) and IRS Tax Coordination

7.1 The Statutory Contribution Disqualification

The statutory disqualification of Health Savings Account contributions after Medicare enrollment is a structural feature of federal revenue policy, not an administrative inconvenience or a discretionary Medicare enrollment side effect. The HSA is a tax-exempt trust or custodial account designed to pay or reimburse qualified medical expenses, and the tax preference exists only for an "eligible individual" under the Internal Revenue Code and IRS Publication 969. IRS Publication 969 states that an eligible individual must be covered under a high deductible health plan on the first day of the month, must have no other health coverage except permitted coverage, must not be enrolled in Medicare, and must not be claimed as a dependent on another taxpayer's return. Internal Revenue Code § 223 states the same architecture in statutory form by permitting an HSA deduction only for an eligible individual and defining eligible individual status through high deductible health plan coverage, absence of disqualifying non-HDHP coverage, and absence of Medicare entitlement. (U.S. Code)

The Medicare-HSA collision therefore arises from a conflict between two federal subsidies. The HSA allows pre-tax or tax-deductible contributions, tax-deferred accumulation, and tax-free qualified medical distributions; IRS Publication 969 describes deductible non-employer contributions, exclusion of employer contributions from gross income, tax-free account earnings, tax-free qualified medical distributions, and portability across employers or workforce exit. Medicare, by contrast, is a federal health insurance entitlement that supplies hospital, medical, private-plan, or drug coverage depending on the enrollment configuration. Once Medicare enrollment exists, the exclusive HDHP alignment required for HSA contribution eligibility is broken. Under IRS Publication 969, beginning with the first month of Medicare enrollment, the HSA contribution limit becomes zero, and this zero-limit rule also applies to periods of retroactive Medicare coverage.

This distinction must be framed as contribution disqualification, not account invalidation. Medicare enrollment does not destroy the HSA account itself, erase prior lawful contributions, or prevent later tax-free distributions for qualified medical expenses. The statutory wall applies to new contributions. IRS Publication 969 states that contributions remain in the account until used, that the interest or earnings on account assets are tax free, and that distributions may be tax free when used for qualified medical expenses. The prohibited act after Medicare enrollment is the ongoing capital infusion into the HSA, whether from salary reduction, direct individual contribution, employer contribution, cafeteria-plan contribution, family contribution, or other contribution source. The account may remain a tax-favored reservoir; the contribution valve closes when Medicare enrollment makes the individual no longer HSA-eligible.

The month-by-month nature of eligibility is the operational engine. IRS Publication 969 states that HSA eligibility is tested on the first day of the month, requiring HDHP coverage on that day, no disqualifying other coverage, no Medicare enrollment, and no dependent status. Consequently, HSA contribution capacity is not determined by a vague annual impression that a household was "mostly" covered by an HDHP. It is calculated through monthly legal status. If the individual satisfies the eligible-individual test on the first day of a month, that month can enter the contribution-limit computation. If Medicare enrollment exists on the first day of a month, that month contributes zero HSA contribution capacity under IRS Publication 969's Medicare rule.

The proration formula follows directly from this monthly architecture. IRS Publication 969 states that the amount that can be contributed depends on the type of HDHP coverage, age, the date eligible individual status begins, and the date eligible individual status ends, and it identifies the Form 8889 Line 3 limitation chart and worksheet for individuals who are not eligible for the entire year or who change coverage during the year. The IRS examples show the mathematical operation: monthly limits are totaled and divided by 12, and where an individual turns 65 in July, enrolls in Medicare, has self-only HDHP coverage, and is eligible for the $1,000 additional contribution, the contribution limit is calculated as $5,300 multiplied by 6 and divided by 12, producing $2,650 for the six eligible months before Medicare enrollment.

The 2026 annual dollar limits demonstrate the same structure. IRS Publication 969 states that for 2026, self-only HDHP coverage permits contributions up to $4,400, while family HDHP coverage permits contributions up to $8,750, before any applicable age-related additional contribution is considered. Those figures represent full-year limits only when full-year eligible-individual status exists or when a special last-month rule validly applies. Where Medicare begins during the year, the annual limit must be reduced to the eligible months before Medicare enrollment unless a rule separately applies and remains satisfied. The mechanical formula is therefore annual HSA contribution limit multiplied by eligible months divided by 12, adjusted for coverage category, age, employer contributions, and any other statutory reductions.

The last-month rule is especially dangerous in a Medicare transition because it can create an artificial full-year contribution assumption that later collapses. IRS Publication 969 states that an individual who is an eligible individual on the first day of the last month of the tax year is treated as an eligible individual for the entire year under the last-month rule, but the individual must remain eligible during the testing period beginning with the last month of the tax year and ending on the last day of the twelfth month following that month. If eligible status fails during the testing period for reasons other than death or disability, the amount contributed solely because of the last-month rule is included in income and is subject to a 10 percent additional tax, calculated on Form 8889. This rule is distinct from the 6 percent excess contribution excise tax, but it illustrates the same federal principle: accelerated HSA funding must remain aligned with verified eligible-individual status.

The legal difference between Medicare eligibility and Medicare entitlement is the first analytic hinge. Reaching age 65 creates Medicare eligibility, but HSA contribution disqualification is triggered by Medicare enrollment or entitlement, not by birthday status alone. Internal Revenue Code § 223 frames the statutory disqualification through entitlement to Medicare benefits, while IRS Publication 969 uses the administrable phrase "enrolled in Medicare" for the eligible-individual test. (U.S. Code) The 2026 Medicare handbook states that an individual is not eligible to make HSA contributions after having Medicare and advises that the last HSA contribution occur the month before Part A coverage begins to avoid a tax penalty. Thus, a household that merely reaches age 65 while delaying Medicare may still require a separate HSA eligibility analysis, but the execution of Medicare enrollment or automatic Medicare activation through benefit receipt closes contribution eligibility.

Automatic Part A activation creates the most common invisible trap. The 2026 Medicare handbook states that beneficiaries already receiving Social Security or Railroad Retirement Board benefits automatically receive Part A and Part B starting the first day of the month of the 65th birthday, or the first day of the prior month when the birthday falls on the first day of the month. The same handbook states that premium-free Part A coverage can go back retroactively 6 months from the date of Part A sign-up or application for Social Security or Railroad Retirement Board benefits, but not earlier than the first Medicare-eligible month. That retroactive Part A rule can disqualify months that the household had already treated as HSA-eligible, converting post-dated or payroll-driven HSA contributions into excess contributions after the fact.

The Medicare handbook converts that retroactive rule into concrete stop-contribution timing. For Medicare sign-up during the Initial Enrollment Period, CMS states that a tax penalty can be avoided by making the last HSA contribution the month before turning 65; when the birthday falls on the first day of the month, Medicare coverage generally begins the first day of the prior month, and the last HSA contribution should occur two months before turning 65. For delayed Medicare sign-up less than 6 months after age 65, CMS states that HSA contributions should stop the month before turning 65; for Medicare sign-up 6 or more months after age 65, CMS states that HSA contributions should stop 6 months before the month of Medicare application. These timing rules convert Medicare filing strategy into federal tax-accounting exposure.

The prohibition applies equally to employee salary-reduction contributions and employer contributions. IRS Publication 969 states that an employee, an employer, or both may contribute to an employee's HSA in the same year, and that employer contributions, including cafeteria-plan contributions, reduce the amount that the individual or any other person can contribute. Once Medicare enrollment makes the contribution limit zero, both employee and employer deposits collide with that zero limit. IRS Publication 969 states that beginning with the first month of Medicare enrollment, the contribution limit is zero, and that if enrollment is later backdated, contributions made during retroactive Medicare coverage are excess. A payroll system that continues salary reductions or employer matching deposits after Medicare entitlement therefore converts a routine fringe benefit into an employee-side tax compliance problem.

Employer contributions require special accounting clarity. IRS Publication 969 states that employer contributions may be excluded from gross income when made for an eligible employee, but it also states that excess contributions made by an employer are included in the employee's gross income; if the excess is not included in Form W-2, box 1, the excess must be reported as other income on the tax return. The uploaded source materials establish employee-side income inclusion and HSA contribution reporting through Form 8889, Form 5498-SA, and Form W-2 code W, but they do not establish a categorical rule that every employer deduction is permanently forfeited in every excess-contribution case. The manuscript's accurate conclusion is therefore narrower and stronger: the employee file bears excess-contribution income and excise exposure, while employer-side deduction treatment requires separate employer tax-accounting authority beyond the HSA contribution-limit materials in the source packet.

The excise tax framework supplies the enforcement penalty. IRS Publication 969 states that excess contributions exist when HSA contributions for the year exceed the applicable limits, that excess contributions are not deductible, that excess employer contributions are included in gross income, and that a 6 percent excise tax generally applies to excess contributions. Internal Revenue Code § 4973 imposes a 6 percent tax for each taxable year on excess contributions to specified tax-favored accounts, including health savings accounts, subject to the statutory definition of excess HSA contributions. (U.S. Code) IRS Publication 969 further states that the excise tax applies for each tax year the excess contribution remains in the account. (IRS)

The annual persistence of the 6 percent excise tax creates a compounding-like asset erosion vector, although the tax is not interest-on-interest in the conventional finance sense. The repeated annual tax arises because the excess remains in the HSA at year end, not because the prior year's excise tax becomes a new account principal. Internal Revenue Code § 4973 applies a 6 percent tax for each taxable year to the excess-contribution amount, while IRS Publication 969 states that the excise tax applies each tax year the excess contribution remains in the account. (U.S. Code) The economic effect is persistent erosion: the same uncorrected excess can repeatedly generate excise exposure, while the original deposit also loses its intended tax-advantaged character.

Corrective withdrawal is the primary mitigation pathway. IRS Publication 969 states that some or all excess contributions may be withdrawn to avoid the excise tax on the withdrawn amount when the required conditions are satisfied, and the IRS source explains that the correction must occur by the due date of the tax return, including extensions, with net income attributable to the excess contribution also addressed under the correction rules. (IRS) The operative point is procedural: an excess contribution is not neutralized by leaving it in the account and describing it as a harmless payroll error. The contribution must be identified, attributed to the correct year, adjusted for related earnings where required, reported on the appropriate tax forms, and removed within the federal filing-deadline framework if the excise trajectory is to be avoided.

The Medicare retroactivity rule intensifies the corrective burden because excess contributions may not be visible when made. IRS Publication 969 states that if Medicare enrollment is backdated, contributions made during the retroactive coverage period are excess. CMS states that premium-free Part A may go back 6 months from Part A sign-up or Social Security or Railroad Retirement Board benefit application, subject to the limit that coverage cannot begin before the first month of Medicare eligibility. This creates a backward-looking tax trap: a payroll deposit that appeared permissible in March can become excess after a later Part A application retroactively establishes Medicare coverage for March. The HSA audit therefore must examine the actual Part A effective date, not merely the application date or payroll contribution date.

A mid-year transition example demonstrates the operational arithmetic. For 2026, a self-only HDHP limit of $4,400 would produce a monthly base fraction of $366.67 before any applicable catch-up contribution, calculated by dividing the annual limit by 12. If Medicare enrollment begins in July and no retroactive period changes that

date, only January through June remain eligible months, producing a six-month base limit of $2,200 for self-only coverage before any applicable age-55 additional amount. IRS Publication 969's own Medicare example uses the same method, applying a six-month fraction to a self-only limit plus the age-55 additional contribution and producing a $2,650 limit when the relevant annual number is $5,300. For family HDHP coverage, the 2026 annual base limit of $8,750 would likewise require monthly proration when Medicare entitlement ends eligibility before year end.

The first-day-of-the-month rule makes the precise Medicare effective date decisive. An individual who becomes enrolled in Medicare effective July 1 has a zero contribution limit beginning in July, while the months before July remain subject to the ordinary eligible-individual test. IRS Publication 969 states that eligibility to qualify for an HSA contribution requires HDHP coverage on the first day of the month and no Medicare enrollment. Medicare's first-day birthday rule and retroactive Part A rule can therefore move the disqualification date earlier than a household expects. The 2026 handbook states that when the birthday falls on the first day of a month, Medicare coverage generally starts the first day of the prior month, and HSA contributions should stop two months before the 65th birthday to avoid penalty exposure.

The distinction between using existing HSA assets and funding new HSA assets should remain explicit. IRS Publication 969 states that an HSA is portable and that account funds remain until used, while distributions for qualified medical expenses may be tax free. Medicare enrollment blocks additional contributions, but it does not require immediate liquidation of the account. This distinction matters for household capital allocation. Existing HSA balances can remain a medical-liability reserve, while new salary reductions, employer matching deposits, personal cash contributions, or family contributions after Medicare entitlement create excess-contribution risk. The wealth-building function changes from accumulation to controlled deployment.

The Household Medicare Diagnostic Matrix treats Section 7.1 as the primary tax-coordination pillar for HSA, payroll, employer benefit, and Medicare Part A timing rows. The matrix must capture the HDHP coverage category, first eligible month, first Medicare entitlement month, Part A retroactive effective date, Social Security or Railroad Retirement Board application date, employer payroll contribution schedule, employer contribution amount, employee salary-reduction election, catch-up contribution status, Form 8889 reporting position, and any excess-contribution correction. CMS states that HSA contributions are not permitted after Medicare begins and that retroactive premium-free Part A may require stopping contributions 6 months before the month of Medicare application when Medicare is delayed 6 or more months after age 65. IRS Publication 969 states that retroactive Medicare coverage converts contributions during that period into excess contributions.

The final actuarial conclusion is severe but precise. The HSA is one of the most powerful tax-favored medical savings instruments in the federal tax system, but its contribution privilege depends on uninterrupted eligible-individual status. Medicare enrollment, especially retroactive premium-free Part A, can convert ordinary payroll deposits into excess contributions, taxable income, and recurring excise exposure. Under Internal Revenue Code § 223 and IRS Publication 969, the contribution limit drops to zero beginning with the first month of Medicare enrollment, and under Internal Revenue Code § 4973 and IRS Publication 969, uncorrected excess contributions can generate a 6 percent annual excise tax for each year the excess remains. (U.S. Code) The Household Medicare Diagnostic Matrix therefore treats Medicare-HSA coordination not as an optional payroll footnote, but as a statutory risk-isolation system separating lawful pre-tax accumulation from post-entitlement tax exposure.

7.2 The Six-Month Retroactivity Lookback Trap

The six-month retroactivity lookback trap arises from the collision between two federal systems that were not designed around the same timing objective. Medicare's retroactive premium-free Part A rule is a coverage-preservation mechanism. The Health Savings Account contribution system is a tax-expenditure control mechanism. The first can move health-insurance entitlement backward; the second tests eligibility for tax-favored contributions by month. Under CMS Part A retroactivity specifications in the 2026 Medicare handbook, premium-free Part A coverage can go back retroactively 6 months from the date of Part A sign-up or the date of application for Social Security or Railroad Retirement Board benefits, but not earlier than the first month of Medicare eligibility. Under IRS Publication 969, beginning with the first month of Medicare enrollment, the HSA contribution limit is zero, and this zero-limit rule applies to periods of retroactive Medicare coverage, so contributions made during a backdated Medicare period are excess contributions. The trap is therefore not conceptual. It is calendar-based, statutory, and arithmetically enforceable.

The retroactive Part A rule is protective in the Medicare system because it can prevent an older worker or delayed retiree from losing hospital-insurance entitlement for a period immediately preceding application. That policy premise is intelligible inside Medicare's insurance architecture. A late retiree who deferred monthly Social Security benefits, remained covered under an employer group health plan, and later applied for Social Security or Medicare may receive premium-free Part A back to a prior month, subject to the six-month cap and the rule that coverage cannot precede the first Medicare-eligible month. Yet the same protective backdating becomes destructive inside the HSA tax architecture because HSA contribution eligibility requires that the individual not be enrolled in Medicare. IRS Publication 969 states that an eligible individual must have high deductible health plan coverage on the first day of the month, must have no disqualifying other health coverage, must not be enrolled in Medicare, and must not be claimed as a dependent on another person's return. A Medicare rule designed to avoid coverage gaps can therefore retroactively erase HSA contribution eligibility for months in which payroll deposits had already occurred.

The key operational event is the Medicare effective date, not the date the household remembers stopping work, the date the employer plan ended, the date payroll contributions were made, or the date a human resources department adjusted benefit elections. CMS states that a beneficiary is not eligible to make HSA contributions after having Medicare and that the last HSA contribution should generally occur the month before Part A coverage begins to avoid a tax penalty. IRS Publication 969 supplies the corresponding revenue rule: when Medicare enrollment is backdated, HSA contributions made during the retroactive coverage period are considered excess contributions. The retroactive date therefore becomes the true HSA termination date. The filing date is merely the event that reveals it.

The disqualification operates through eligible-individual status. Before Medicare entitlement, a late-career worker may maintain self-only or family high deductible health plan coverage, receive employer HSA funding, execute employee salary-reduction contributions through a cafeteria plan, and satisfy the HSA rules month by month. After backdated Part A attaches, the same months are reclassified. The individual is deemed to have had Medicare enrollment during those months, and IRS Publication 969 states that the contribution limit is zero beginning with the first month of Medicare enrollment, including retroactive months. This is the involuntary conversion problem. Contributions that were mechanically valid in payroll practice become unlawful for tax-account purposes because a later federal entitlement transaction rewrites the coverage calendar.

Late-retirement households are the highest-risk population because the ordinary workplace record can mask the tax exposure. A beneficiary working beyond age 65 for a large employer may be enrolled in an employer group health plan that pays first under Medicare Secondary Payer rules, while Part B is delayed under the current-employment Special Enrollment Period. CMS states that when an individual age 65 or older has group health plan coverage based on current employment and the employer has 20 or more employees, the group health plan pays first. That payer-order rule may make delayed Medicare medical enrollment operationally rational in the health-claims system, but it does not preserve HSA contribution capacity after Part A begins.

The HSA exposure often appears only when the same worker later applies for Social Security retirement benefits or executes delayed Medicare enrollment and discovers that Part A has been backdated.

The Medicare handbook's stop-contribution chart converts the abstract rule into a strict planning timeline. When Medicare sign-up occurs during the Initial Enrollment Period, CMS states that a tax penalty can be avoided by making the last HSA contribution the month before turning 65. When the birthday falls on the first day of the month, CMS states that Medicare coverage generally starts the first day of the prior month, and the last HSA contribution should occur two months before turning 65. When Medicare sign-up is delayed less than 6 months after age 65, CMS states that HSA contributions should stop the month before turning 65; when Medicare sign-up is delayed 6 or more months after age 65, CMS states that HSA contributions should stop 6 months before the month of Medicare application. These rules are not advisory preferences. They are risk-isolation dates designed to prevent a retroactive Part A period from swallowing HSA eligibility.

The mathematical subtraction is straightforward but unforgiving. If the Medicare application month is December and the beneficiary is more than 6 months beyond age 65, the retroactive Part A period ordinarily reaches back 6 months, subject to the first-eligibility limit. A December application can therefore produce a Part A effective date of June 1. Under IRS Publication 969, the HSA contribution limit is zero beginning with the first month of Medicare enrollment, including retroactive Medicare coverage. Therefore, May is the last potentially HSA-eligible contribution month under the Medicare backdating rule, assuming the individual otherwise satisfied the eligible-individual test through that month. A payroll deposit made for June, July, August, September, October, November, or December would need to be measured against a zero-limit period.

The pro-rata HSA formula follows the first-day-of-the-month rule. IRS Publication 969 states that eligibility for HSA contributions depends on high deductible health plan coverage on the first day of the month, absence of disqualifying other coverage, absence of Medicare enrollment, and absence of dependent status. It also states that the contribution limit depends on coverage type, age, the date eligible-individual status begins, and the date eligible-individual status ends, and that the Line 3 Limitation Chart and Worksheet in the Instructions for Form 8889 governs cases where eligible-individual status does not last for the entire year or coverage changes. The algebraic expression is therefore annual limit multiplied by eligible months divided by 12, with additional contribution rules, employer contributions, and coverage category applied according to the Form 8889 framework.

For 2026, IRS Publication 969 states that self-only high deductible health plan coverage permits HSA contributions up to $4,400, while family high deductible health plan coverage permits contributions up to $8,750, before any applicable age-55 additional contribution is considered. A self-only late retiree whose retroactive Part A date is June 1 therefore has five eligible months, January through May, if all other HSA criteria were satisfied during those months. The base contribution ceiling would be five-twelfths of $4,400, or $1,833.33 before any applicable additional contribution computation and before accounting for employer deposits. A family-coverage file with the same retroactive Medicare date would begin with five-twelfths of $8,750, or $3,645.83 before applicable additional contribution considerations. These examples illustrate the statutory fraction; the actual return file must reconcile all employer, employee, family, and qualified HSA funding contributions through Form 8889.

The age-55 additional contribution must be prorated with equal care when Medicare interrupts eligibility. IRS Publication 969's Medicare example states that an individual who turned 65 in July, enrolled in Medicare, had self-only HDHP coverage, and was eligible for an additional $1,000 contribution had a contribution limit of $2,650, calculated as $5,300 multiplied by 6 and divided by 12. This example is the model for the transition-year computation. The total annual amount for which the individual would otherwise have been eligible, including the age-55 additional contribution, is multiplied by the eligible-month fraction. Medicare enrollment in July leaves six eligible months, January through June. Retroactive Medicare enrollment can move that endpoint backward, reducing the numerator.

The most dangerous error is annual front-loading without retroactive adjustment. IRS Publication 969 states that HSA contributions may be made for the tax year through the due date for filing the return, and that employer contributions may be made after year end when allocated to the prior year under specified reporting rules. This timing flexibility can encourage early or accelerated funding. Yet if Medicare later backdates Part A, the contribution ceiling shrinks. A January lump-sum contribution made when the individual appeared HSA-eligible for the year may become excessive after a later Medicare application establishes a June 1 Part A effective date. The contribution's original timing does not protect it. The final contribution limit is determined by eligible months under IRS Publication 969 and Form 8889 mechanics.

Form 8889 is the reporting platform for the boundary line between permissible HSA funding and excess contributions. IRS Publication 969 states that all HSA contributions must be reported on Form 8889 and filed with Form 1040, 1040-SR, or 1040-NR; it also states that employer contributions and qualified HSA funding distributions are shown on the form, that Form 5498-SA should show HSA contributions reported by the trustee, and that employer contributions appear on

Form W-2, box 12, code W. IRS Publication 969 further states that Form 8889 must be filed when there is HSA activity during the year, even if only an employer or spouse's employer made contributions. Thus, the retroactive Medicare date must be reflected not merely in payroll discussion, but in the federal tax return architecture.

The calculation requires identification of the excess asset bubble. The first step is to determine the actual Medicare Part A effective date, including any six-month retroactive period. The second step is to count the months before that effective date in which the individual satisfied all HSA eligible-individual criteria on the first day of the month. The third step is to apply the annual contribution limit for the applicable coverage category and age status to that eligible-month fraction. The fourth step is to aggregate actual HSA funding, including employee salary-reduction contributions, employer contributions, family or other-person contributions, and qualified HSA funding distributions. IRS Publication 969 states that excess contributions exist when HSA contributions for the year are greater than the applicable limits, and that amounts contributed for the year include contributions by the individual, employer, any other person, and any qualified HSA funding distribution. The difference between actual aggregate funding and the computed limit is the excess contribution.

Excess contributions carry both income and excise consequences. IRS Publication 969 states that excess HSA contributions are not deductible, that excess employer contributions are included in gross income, and that if the excess employer contribution is not included in Form W-2, box 1, the excess must be reported as other income on the tax return. The same IRS source states that a 6 percent excise tax generally applies to excess contributions and that the excise tax applies for each tax year the excess contribution remains in the account. This is the compounding-like penalty vector. The same uncorrected excess can trigger repeated annual excise charges, even though the legal mechanism is a recurring annual excise tax rather than interest on a prior penalty.

Corrective distribution is the principal excise-tax mitigation mechanism. IRS Publication 969 states that some or all excess contributions may be withdrawn to avoid paying the excise tax on the withdrawn amount if the excess contributions are withdrawn by the due date, including extensions, of the tax return for the year the contributions were made, and if any income earned on the withdrawn contributions is also withdrawn and included as other income on the tax return for the year of withdrawal. This corrective channel is strict. The HSA custodian must distribute the excess principal and attributable earnings within the tax-filing deadline architecture. A household cannot erase the excise exposure merely by internally labeling the funds as mistaken or by intending to reduce future payroll deposits.

The earnings component is not incidental. IRS Publication 969 requires withdrawal of any income earned on the withdrawn contributions and inclusion of those earnings in other income for the year in which the contributions and earnings are withdrawn. The rule prevents the account from retaining tax-favored earnings on funds that should never have entered the HSA. If the corrective distribution occurs properly by the filing deadline, the withdrawn excess principal can avoid the 6 percent excise tax on that amount. If the correction is late, Publication 969 states that a distribution of an excess contribution taken out after the due date, including extensions, is subject to tax even if used for qualified medical expenses. The filing deadline therefore marks the boundary between manageable correction and persistent tax exposure.

Later-year absorption is a narrower residual mechanism, not the preferred cure for a Medicare retroactivity mistake. IRS Publication 969 states that excess contributions from previous years still in the HSA may be deductible in a later year only to the extent of the lesser of the current-year maximum HSA contribution limit reduced by amounts contributed for the year, or the total excess contributions in the HSA at the beginning of the year; any excess remaining at the end of a tax year remains subject to the excise tax. For a beneficiary enrolled in Medicare, however, the current-year HSA contribution limit is generally zero beginning with Medicare enrollment, including retroactive coverage. That zero-limit environment can make later-year absorption unavailable or severely constrained. The corrective withdrawal deadline becomes correspondingly more important.

The late-retirement exposure can be modeled as a sequence. A corporate employee works beyond age 65, remains covered by a large employer high deductible health plan, delays Medicare because the employer plan pays first, and continues salary-reduction HSA contributions plus employer HSA deposits. In November, monthly Social Security retirement benefits are claimed, or delayed Medicare enrollment is executed. CMS states that premium-free Part A can be retroactive 6 months from Part A sign-up or Social Security or Railroad Retirement Board benefit application, but no earlier than the first Medicare-eligible month. If Part A becomes effective May 1, IRS Publication 969 reclassifies HSA contributions from May forward as excess because the contribution limit is zero beginning with the first month of Medicare enrollment, including retroactive Medicare coverage. The payroll ledger and Medicare ledger have become misaligned.

The same sequence explains why the formal filing month cannot be used as the tax cutoff. The Medicare application may occur in November, but the HSA disqualification date may be May 1. CMS's HSA chart states that when Medicare sign-up is delayed 6 or more months after age 65, HSA contributions should stop 6 months before the month of Medicare application to avoid tax penalty exposure. The phrase "before the month" is operationally critical. A November application generally means HSA contributions should have stopped before May when the six-month retroactive period reaches May 1. The November payroll contribution is not merely too late by one month. It may be too late by an entire retroactive coverage period.

This rule also interacts with the first-day-of-month birthday exception. CMS states that when the birthday falls on the first day of a month, Medicare coverage generally starts the first day of the prior month, and the last HSA contribution should occur two months before turning 65 to avoid tax penalty exposure. The HSA rule tests eligible status on the first day of each month, so a Medicare effective date shifted to the prior month can remove an entire month from the contribution numerator. This is not a rounding error. A single month can represent one-twelfth of the annual contribution ceiling, plus a share of the age-55 additional contribution if applicable.

The account itself remains valuable after the contribution window closes. IRS Publication 969 states that an HSA is generally exempt from tax, that amounts remaining at the end of the year carry over, that earnings on amounts in the HSA are not included in income while held, and that tax-free distributions may be received for qualified medical expenses. The retroactivity trap therefore should not be misread as a command to close the account. The risk lies in ongoing contributions after the true Medicare effective date. Existing account balances may continue to function as a medical expense reserve, while new deposits after Medicare enrollment create excess contribution exposure.

The Household Medicare Diagnostic Matrix treats Section 7.2 as the chronological bridge between Medicare enrollment, employer payroll, HSA contribution limits, Form 8889 reporting, and excise-tax prevention. The matrix must identify the month of age-65 eligibility, the month of Part A application, the Social Security or Railroad Retirement Board benefit application date, the Part A effective date, the six-month retroactive span if applicable, the final permissible HSA contribution month, the actual employer and employee contribution months, the annual self-only or family HDHP limit, the age-55 additional contribution amount where applicable, and the Form 8889 contribution limit. CMS supplies the retroactive Part A stop-contribution rule, and IRS Publication 969 supplies the retroactive Medicare excess-contribution rule and Form 8889 reporting architecture.

The final actuarial conclusion is absolute. The six-month Part A retroactivity rule transforms late-career HSA planning from an annual contribution decision into a backward-looking Medicare effective-date audit. A household can preserve valid employer coverage, delay Medicare enrollment under employment coordination rules, and continue contributing to an HSA in apparent good faith, yet still create excess contributions when Part A later reaches back six months. The permissible funding ceiling is not determined by payroll intent. It is determined by the number of months in which the individual was an eligible individual under IRS Publication 969, reduced to zero beginning with the first retroactive month of Medicare enrollment. Failure to coordinate that rule with Form 8889, Form 5498-SA, Form W-2 code W, and the excess-contribution correction deadline converts a valid retirement transition into a structural tax penalty vector, precisely the kind of asset erosion the Household Medicare Diagnostic Matrix is designed to isolate before it becomes irreversible.

7.3 Post-Medicare HSA Capital Deployment

Medicare entitlement closes the Health Savings Account contribution gate, but it does not extinguish the account, confiscate accumulated balances, or disqualify reserves that were lawfully accumulated before Medicare enrollment. Under IRS Publication 969 distribution specifications, contributions remain in the HSA until used, earnings on HSA assets are tax free while held in the account, distributions may be tax free when used for qualified medical expenses, and the HSA remains portable after a change in employment or departure from the workforce. The post-Medicare HSA therefore changes legal function. It is no longer an accumulation vehicle for new pre-tax contributions once Medicare enrollment destroys eligible-individual contribution status; it becomes a decumulation reservoir for healthcare liabilities, subject to the qualified medical expense rules and insurance-premium limitations imposed by Internal Revenue Code § 223 as operationalized through IRS Publication 969.

The distinction between contribution disqualification and distribution utility is central to Medicare tax coordination. IRS Publication 969 states that an eligible individual for contribution purposes must have high deductible health plan coverage on the first day of the month, must have no disqualifying other coverage, must not be enrolled in Medicare, and must not be claimable as another taxpayer's dependent. Those contribution rules do not state that Medicare enrollment makes prior HSA assets unusable. Instead, the distribution rules state that an HSA is generally exempt from tax, that amounts remaining at year end generally carry over, that earnings remain untaxed while held, and that distributions used exclusively for qualified medical expenses are tax free. The account's actuarial character therefore changes from tax-favored capital formation to tax-favored medical liability liquidation.

Qualified medical expense classification supplies the distribution boundary. IRS Publication 969 defines qualified medical expenses for HSA purposes as amounts paid by the HSA beneficiary for medical care, as defined in Code § 213(d), for the individual, spouse, and dependents, but only to the extent those amounts are not compensated by insurance or otherwise. The same IRS source states that qualified expenses include expenses incurred by the account beneficiary and spouse, all dependents claimed on the tax return, and persons who could have been claimed as dependents except for specified tax-return or gross-income limitations. HSA tax-free status is therefore not determined merely by Medicare status, age, or the presence of a medical invoice. It depends on whether the expense is a qualified medical expense, who incurred it, whether it was reimbursed elsewhere, and whether the HSA was established before the expense was incurred.

The anti-duplication rule prevents a second federal tax benefit from attaching to the same expense. IRS Publication 969 states that qualified medical expenses equal to the tax-free distribution from an HSA cannot also be deducted as itemized medical expenses on Schedule A. This rule preserves the integrity of the HSA structure. A tax-free HSA reimbursement already removes the expense from taxable income; a Schedule A medical deduction for the same reimbursed amount would create an impermissible duplication. Recordkeeping therefore becomes part of the account's legal architecture. IRS Publication 969 states that records must be kept sufficient to show that distributions were exclusively used to pay or reimburse qualified medical expenses, that the expenses had not previously been paid or reimbursed from another source, and that the expenses had not been taken as an itemized deduction in any year.

The documentary file should be understood as the evidence layer beneath the tax-free distribution. Medicare Summary Notices, explanation-of-benefits records, plan statements, provider invoices, pharmacy receipts, premium bills, HSA custodian records, Form 1099-SA distribution reports, Form 8889 reporting, and bank or payment confirmations each perform a different evidentiary function. IRS Publication 969 states that the HSA trustee reports distributions to the account holder and IRS on Form 1099-SA, and that qualified medical distributions must still be reported on Form 8889 even though they are not taxed. The tax-free result therefore depends on later substantiation, not merely on the mechanics of swiping an HSA debit card or transferring money from the account.

Insurance premiums occupy a more restrictive category than ordinary medical expenses. IRS Publication 969 states that HSA funds generally may not be used to pay insurance premiums, except for specified categories: long-term care insurance, health care continuation coverage such as COBRA, health care coverage while receiving unemployment compensation under federal or state law, and Medicare and other health care coverage if the account beneficiary is age 65 or older, other than premiums for a Medicare supplemental policy such as Medigap. This framework is the controlling post-Medicare premium rule. The general prohibition remains, but age 65 creates a Medicare and other health coverage premium exception, while the Medigap premium exclusion remains expressly preserved.

The Medicare premium exception must be applied with precision. Medicare Part B premiums, Medicare drug coverage premiums, and other Medicare coverage premiums may fall within the IRS age-65 exception when the account beneficiary is age 65 or older and the payment is for Medicare or other health care coverage rather than an excluded supplemental policy. Medicare & You 2026 states that Medicare Advantage is another way to receive Part A and Part B coverage, that most Medicare Advantage Plans include Part D, and that beneficiaries generally continue paying the Part B premium and may also pay a plan premium. The IRS premium rule therefore must be tested by coverage category, age, and exclusion status. It does not convert every private premium, convenience charge, ancillary membership, or nonmedical service fee into a qualified HSA distribution.

The Medigap exclusion is categorical in the IRS text. IRS Publication 969's insurance-premium exception expressly excludes premiums for a Medicare supplemental policy, such as Medigap, from the age-65 Medicare premium exception. Medicare & You describes Medigap as supplemental coverage that may help pay some out-of-pocket costs that Original Medicare does not cover, such as the 20 percent coinsurance, and states that a beneficiary pays a private insurance company a separate monthly premium for a Medigap policy in addition to the Part B premium paid to Medicare. The tax classification is therefore not controlled by the fact that Medigap relates to Medicare. Medigap premium payments are excluded from the IRS Medicare-premium exception, even though eligible medical cost sharing that Medigap might otherwise cover can be a qualified medical expense when paid directly by the HSA beneficiary and otherwise satisfies IRS rules.

The word "Supplement" in the section subtitle therefore requires careful interpretation. Accumulated HSA reserves may be deployed against eligible supplemental liabilities in the economic sense of paying qualified medical expenses that supplement Medicare's payment, but that does not mean the premium for Medicare Supplement Insurance is HSA-qualified. IRS Publication 969 excludes Medicare supplemental policy premiums such as Medigap from the premium exception. The distinction is between cost sharing and premium funding. A deductible, coinsurance amount, copayment, or qualified out-of-pocket medical expense may be eligible for HSA reimbursement when it satisfies the qualified medical expense rule; the Medigap policy premium itself generally falls outside the HSA premium exception.

Original Medicare cost sharing illustrates the decumulation function most clearly. Medicare & You 2026 states that under Original Medicare, beneficiaries generally pay a deductible before Medicare begins paying its share, then pay coinsurance or copayments for covered services and supplies, and that there is no yearly limit on out-of-pocket spending unless other insurance such as Medigap, Medicaid, or employer, retiree, or union coverage applies. The same handbook states that for Part B-covered services under Original Medicare, the beneficiary usually pays 20 percent of the Medicare-approved amount after the deductible. IRS Publication 969 permits tax-free HSA distributions for qualified medical expenses not compensated by insurance or otherwise. Accordingly, accumulated HSA balances may function as a tax-free reserve for eligible Original Medicare deductibles, coinsurance, and copayments when those liabilities are qualified medical expenses and are properly substantiated.

The cost-sharing categories are broad because Medicare-covered medical care creates multiple qualified-expense candidates. Medicare & You identifies Part A hospital insurance as covering inpatient hospital care, skilled nursing facility care, hospice care, and some home health care; it identifies Part B medical insurance as covering physician and other provider services, outpatient care, home health care, durable medical equipment, and many preventive services. Medicare & You's service chapters repeatedly assign 20 percent coinsurance and Part B deductible exposure to covered services such as prosthetic and orthotic items, pulmonary rehabilitation, rural health clinic services, and second surgical opinions. When those amounts are paid by the HSA beneficiary, spouse, or qualifying dependent and are not reimbursed elsewhere, the HSA tax-free distribution rule can apply under IRS Publication 969.

Medicare Summary Notices become particularly important in this environment. Medicare & You states that an MSN lists services billed to Medicare, shows what Medicare paid and what the beneficiary may owe, and can be used to review whether services, supplies, or equipment were actually received. For HSA purposes, that document can help link a distribution to a covered medical service, an amount owed, and a date of service. IRS Publication 969 states that records sufficient to show exclusive use for qualified medical expenses, absence of prior reimbursement, and absence of Schedule A deduction must be retained with tax records. The MSN is therefore not merely a Medicare audit document. It becomes part of the HSA substantiation file.

Part D drug coverage creates both premium and cost-sharing deployment opportunities. Medicare & You 2026 states that Medicare drug coverage costs may include a premium, deductible, copayments, or coinsurance, and that out-of-pocket costs for covered Part D drugs are capped at $2,100 in 2026. IRS Publication 969's qualified medical expense rule covers medical care expenses not compensated by insurance or otherwise, and its insurance-premium exception permits Medicare and other health care coverage premiums after age 65, other than Medicare supplemental policy premiums such as Medigap. Accumulated HSA reserves may therefore be used for eligible prescription drug costs and, where the IRS premium exception is satisfied, for Medicare drug coverage premiums. The Part D out-of-pocket cap reduces covered-drug cost-sharing exposure after the cap is reached, but it does not eliminate premium obligations or noncovered expense categories.

The Medicare Prescription Payment Plan should not be confused with an HSA tax benefit. Medicare & You 2026 states that the Medicare Prescription Payment Plan allows Part D enrollees to spread out-of-pocket costs for covered prescription drugs across the calendar year, and that the payment option may help manage expenses but does not save money or lower drug costs. A tax-free HSA distribution has a different legal effect. It may reimburse a qualified medical expense with tax-favored HSA assets when IRS requirements are met. The Prescription Payment Plan changes timing of payment; it does not change the amount owed. HSA reimbursement changes the tax character of the funding source; it does not change Medicare's cost-sharing formula or the drug plan's underlying covered-drug liability.

Managed care cost sharing requires a separate but parallel analysis. Medicare & You states that Medicare Advantage Plans are Medicare-approved plans that offer another way to receive Part A and Part B coverage, that they must follow Medicare rules, that they may charge different out-of-pocket costs and impose different service-access rules, and that they set annual limits on what beneficiaries pay out of pocket each year for services covered under Part A and Part B. IRS Publication 969 does not create a separate HSA rule for managed care labels. It asks whether the distribution is for a qualified medical expense, whether the expense was incurred by a permitted person, and whether the expense was uncompensated by insurance or otherwise. Copayments, coinsurance, and other medical cost-sharing amounts under a Medicare Advantage arrangement may therefore be HSA-qualified when they satisfy the IRS qualified medical expense standard.

The managed care analysis must not be expanded beyond the medical expense rule. Medicare & You states that Medicare Advantage Plans may offer extra benefits that Original Medicare does not cover, including vision, hearing, dental, and more, but it does not convert every plan-related charge into medical care under Code § 213(d). IRS Publication 969 requires qualified medical expense classification and excludes insurance premiums except for enumerated categories. Therefore, supplemental benefits, nonmedical convenience items, fitness programs, transportation, allowance-style benefits, over-the-counter items, or other extras must be tested under the IRS medical expense standard rather than assumed qualified. Some expenses may qualify, some may not, and the determinant is federal tax classification, not Medicare marketing terminology or plan benefit design.

The other premium exceptions remain distinct from the Medicare premium exception. IRS Publication 969 permits HSA funds to pay long-term care insurance, health care continuation coverage such as COBRA, health care coverage while receiving unemployment compensation under federal or state law, and Medicare and other health care coverage after age 65, other than Medicare supplemental policies such as Medigap. This means that COBRA premiums can occupy an unusual dual status. For Medicare enrollment coordination, COBRA can be a dangerous non-current-employment continuation trap; for HSA distribution purposes, COBRA can still be an enumerated premium category under IRS Publication 969. The two systems answer different questions. Medicare enrollment rules determine coverage timing and payer coordination; IRS distribution rules determine whether a premium payment can be reimbursed tax free from an HSA.

Qualified long-term care insurance also requires classification discipline. IRS Publication 969 lists long-term care insurance among the premium categories that may be paid with HSA funds, while separately identifying long-term care as a permitted coverage category in the broader HSA health coverage framework. Medicare & You states that Original Medicare generally does not cover long-term care, also called custodial care, when that is the only care needed, and lists long-term care among excluded or limited categories. The HSA distribution rule for qualified long-term care insurance premiums should not be conflated with unlimited tax-free payment for all custodial care charges. Premium qualification, medical expense qualification, and Medicare coverage are separate classifications requiring separate documentation and federal rule support.

Nonqualified distributions remain taxable even after Medicare age. IRS Publication 969 states that if an HSA distribution is not used for qualified medical expenses, the amount must be reported on Form 8889 and included in income, and an additional 20 percent tax may apply. The same IRS source states that there is no additional tax on distributions made after the account beneficiary reaches age 65, becomes disabled, or dies. Therefore, after age 65, a nonqualified HSA distribution generally remains taxable as income, but the additional 20 percent tax is removed by the statutory age exception. The age-65 exception does not transform nonmedical spending into a tax-free distribution. It removes the additional penalty layer while preserving ordinary income inclusion for nonqualified distributions.

Prohibited transactions and pledging HSA assets create a more severe failure mode. IRS Publication 969 states that if an account holder engages in a prohibited transaction under section 4975 with respect to an HSA, the account ceases to be an HSA as of the first day of the tax year and the fair market value of all account assets must be included on Form 8889. The same publication states that using any portion of an HSA as security for a loan requires inclusion of the fair market value of the assets used as security as income, and that deemed distributions are not treated as used to pay qualified medical expenses and are included in income and subject to the additional 20 percent tax unless an exception applies. Post-Medicare HSA deployment therefore requires not only expense classification, but also account-integrity control.

Reimbursement timing is another documentary principle. IRS Publication 969 states that expenses incurred before the HSA is established are not qualified medical expenses, and that an HSA funded by rollover from an Archer MSA or another HSA is considered established on the date the prior account was established. The publication also states that amounts paid for medical care qualify only to the extent not compensated by insurance or otherwise. This permits accumulated reserves to reimburse current or previously unreimbursed qualified medical expenses only when the HSA existed before the expense was incurred and the expense was not otherwise reimbursed or deducted. Poor recordkeeping can convert a distribution that might have been tax-free in substance into a taxable distribution in examination because the taxpayer cannot prove the expense, date, amount, payee, qualified status, and non-reimbursement position.

The post-Medicare cash-flow value of HSA reserves is actuarial rather than promotional. Existing HSA capital can reduce pressure on Social Security income, pension income, taxable brokerage sales, retirement-account withdrawals, or emergency cash reserves by funding eligible medical expenses on a tax-free basis. IRS Publication 969 states that distributions used exclusively to pay qualified medical expenses are tax free and that earnings on HSA amounts are not included in income while held in the account. Medicare & You identifies recurring liability categories that can consume household liquidity: Part B premiums, deductibles, coinsurance, copayments, no yearly out-of-pocket limit under Original Medicare without supplemental coverage, Medicare drug coverage costs, and excluded services such as routine dental care, ordinary eyeglasses, hearing aids, and long-term custodial care.

The presence of IRMAA intensifies this cash-flow function without changing the HSA rules. CMS materials state that higher-income beneficiaries may pay extra amounts for Part B and Part D through income-related monthly adjustment amounts, while IRS Publication 969 separately governs whether a distribution is tax-free. A beneficiary with IRMAA may use existing HSA reserves for eligible Medicare premiums where the IRS premium exception applies, but the income-related surcharge itself must still be tested under the Medicare and other health coverage premium category and documentation requirements. The HSA does not reduce the IRMAA assessment; it may change the tax character of the funds used to satisfy eligible premium obligations.

The Household Medicare Diagnostic Matrix treats Section 7.3 as the decumulation-side counterpart to Sections 7.1 and 7.2. The earlier sections identify when HSA contributions must stop, how retroactive Part A can create excess contributions, and why Form 8889 becomes the reporting boundary for contribution eligibility. This section identifies how lawful accumulated balances may still be deployed after Medicare entitlement. IRS Publication 969 states that the HSA remains exempt from tax, distributions may be taken at any time, and only those amounts used exclusively for qualified medical expenses are tax free. The matrix must therefore separate contribution eligibility from distribution eligibility. A closed contribution gate does not imply a closed distribution gate.

Every post-Medicare HSA distribution file should therefore be audited through six variables. The first is whether the HSA was established before the expense was incurred, because IRS Publication 969 excludes expenses incurred before HSA establishment from qualified medical expense status. The second is whether the expense qualifies as medical care under the HSA rule. The third is whether the expense was incurred by the account beneficiary, spouse, or qualifying dependent. The fourth is whether the expense was already reimbursed or deducted elsewhere. The fifth is whether a premium payment falls within an IRS premium exception or within an excluded category such as Medigap premiums. The sixth is whether records support the date, amount, provider, payee, coverage category, distribution, and non-reimbursement status.

The final actuarial conclusion is that Medicare entitlement closes the HSA contribution gate, but it does not erase the value of accumulated HSA reserves. The post-Medicare HSA becomes a statutory medical-liability liquidation account, capable of absorbing eligible premiums, deductibles, coinsurance, copayments, prescription drug costs, and other qualified medical expenses while preserving taxable household liquidity. Its value depends on disciplined classification, documentary control, and strict separation between qualified medical deployment and nonqualified premium or lifestyle spending. Under the Household Medicare Diagnostic Matrix, the HSA after Medicare is no longer a payroll savings channel. It is a controlled federal tax reservoir whose utility survives only when each distribution can be traced to an eligible person, an eligible expense, an eligible date, and an unreimbursed qualified medical liability under IRS Publication 969.

Chapter 8: The Affordable Care Act (ACA) and Individual Marketplace Crossover

8.1 The Anti-Duplication Statute and 45 CFR Restrictions

The Affordable Care Act individual Marketplace and Medicare are not parallel consumer options after Medicare entitlement has attached. They are separate statutory systems with different eligibility rules, financing mechanisms, enrollment safeguards, and risk-pool purposes. The federal anti-duplication rule is the legal firewall at their point of contact. Pursuant to Social Security Act § 1882(d), codified at 42 U.S.C. § 1395ss(d)(3)(A), it is unlawful to sell or issue to an individual entitled to Medicare Part A or enrolled in Medicare Part B a health insurance policy with knowledge that the policy duplicates health benefits to which the individual is already entitled under Medicare or Medicaid, and the statute attaches criminal exposure, imprisonment of up to five years, and civil money penalties of up to $25,000 for an issuer or $15,000 for a non-issuer seller for each prohibited act. (U.S. Code) The anti-duplication statute therefore operates as a consumer protection mandate and a public-finance control. It prevents a Medicare beneficiary from being steered into redundant individual commercial coverage that cannot properly function as a Medicare supplement and that may impose premiums without providing an integrated Medicare coordination structure.

The statutory prohibition is not merely a technical Medigap rule. The CMS Medicare and Marketplace FAQ applies Social Security Act § 1882(d) directly to individual Marketplace Qualified Health Plans and individual market coverage outside the Marketplace, stating that it is illegal to knowingly sell or issue an Individual Marketplace QHP, or other individual market policy, to a Medicare beneficiary. Medicare.gov states the same public-facing rule in current operational language: it is against the law for someone who knows that an individual has Medicare to sell that individual a Marketplace plan, even when the individual has only Medicare Part A or only Medicare Part B. (Medicare) The policy reason is not that individual Marketplace coverage is inherently defective for the pre-Medicare population. It is that, after Medicare entitlement or enrollment exists, the individual market product becomes legally incompatible with the federal entitlement system when sold or issued with knowledge of duplicative benefits.

This anti-duplication rule must be separated from the period before Medicare coverage begins. CMS states that a person who is over age 65, eligible for premium-free Part A, not collecting Social Security benefits, and not covered by either Medicare Part A or Part B may purchase a QHP or other individual market coverage because the anti-duplication statute would not prohibit issuance where the individual has neither

Part A nor Part B. That pre-entitlement interval is narrow and hazardous. The same CMS source warns that failure to enroll in Part B when first eligible may lead to late enrollment penalties for as long as Part B remains in force. Thus, the legal boundary is not age 65 in isolation. It is Medicare coverage status: actual Part A entitlement or Part B enrollment activates the anti-duplication wall, while mere eligibility without enrollment does not by itself trigger the sale-or-issuance prohibition.

Title 45 of the Code of Federal Regulations supplies the Marketplace architecture that interacts with this anti-duplication statute. Under 45 CFR § 155.305(a), an Exchange determines eligibility for enrollment in a QHP through the Exchange by testing citizenship or lawful presence, incarceration status, and residency, rather than by treating Medicare eligibility itself as the ordinary QHP enrollment screen. (eCFR) Under 45 CFR § 155.305(f), however, eligibility for advance payments of the premium tax credit requires, among other conditions, that at least one applicant who meets QHP enrollment requirements not be eligible for minimum essential coverage for the full calendar month, except for individual market coverage. (eCFR) Medicare Part A is minimum essential coverage for these purposes, and the uploaded ACA tax materials state that premium tax credit eligibility generally requires Marketplace enrollment during a month in which the enrolled individual was not eligible for other minimum essential coverage such as Medicare.

The regulatory system therefore creates two distinct consequences. First, the anti-duplication statute blocks knowing sale or issuance of duplicative individual market coverage to an existing Medicare beneficiary. Second, the premium tax credit and cost-sharing reduction system shuts down federal subsidy eligibility once Medicare coverage, especially Part A, makes the individual eligible for government-sponsored minimum essential coverage. The uploaded CMS Marketplace materials state that once a person is eligible for premium-free Part A, or already has Part A with a premium, the person does not qualify for savings on Marketplace plan premiums or other medical costs, and continued use of premium tax credits may require repayment when federal income taxes are filed. The ACA tax materials similarly state that an individual eligible for government-sponsored coverage such as Medicare is not a member of the coverage family for months in which the individual is eligible for that government-sponsored coverage, and that no premium tax credit is allowed for that individual's coverage for those months.

The Marketplace platform cannot be described accurately as a universal automatic termination engine. CMS states that if an individual already has Individual Marketplace QHP coverage and later enrolls in Medicare, the individual can keep the Marketplace QHP, but premium tax credits and reduced cost sharing end once Part A coverage begins. CMS further states that issuers may not terminate enrollees whom they later find to be eligible for or enrolled in Medicare unless the enrollee requests termination or another legal basis for termination applies. This is a critical compliance distinction. The illegality attaches to knowing sale or issuance of duplicative individual market coverage to a Medicare beneficiary; it does not authorize an issuer to retroactively purge every issued individual-market contract merely because Medicare status is later discovered. The resulting framework is not a simple cancellation rule. It is a sale-and-issuance prohibition, subsidy termination rule, and consumer-initiated or legally authorized termination regime.

The 45 CFR termination rules reinforce this controlled separation. Under 45 CFR § 155.430, the Exchange must permit an enrollee to terminate QHP enrollment, including because the enrollee obtains other minimum essential coverage, and must provide an opportunity at plan selection for the enrollee to choose to remain enrolled in a QHP if the enrollee later becomes eligible for other minimum essential coverage and does not request termination. (eCFR) The same regulation permits retroactive termination in specified circumstances, including erroneous enrollment caused by error or misconduct, enrollment without knowledge or consent, and, where available, Medicare Part A or Part B enrollment with a retroactive effective date when the enrollee requests retroactive termination within the regulatory period. (eCFR) This regulatory structure recognizes the operational reality that Marketplace enrollment records, Medicare entitlement dates, subsidy eligibility, and consumer termination requests may not move simultaneously.

The definition of knowledge must be understood through both statutory text and administrative systems. Social Security Act § 1882(d) uses a knowledge standard: the prohibited sale or issuance occurs when a person sells or issues coverage with knowledge that the policy duplicates Medicare benefits. (U.S. Code) The Marketplace verification system creates an evidentiary environment in which knowledge may be difficult to disclaim. Under 45 CFR § 155.320, an Exchange verifying eligibility for insurance affordability programs must verify whether an applicant is eligible for minimum essential coverage other than through an eligible employer-sponsored plan, Medicaid, CHIP, or the Basic Health Program by transmitting identifying information specified by HHS to HHS for verification purposes. (eCFR) The same regulation authorizes disclosure of eligibility and enrollment information to HHS for verification of minimum essential coverage as part of advance premium tax credit and cost-sharing reduction determinations. (eCFR)

The data line continues after initial application. Under 45 CFR § 155.330, the Exchange must redetermine eligibility during the benefit year if it receives and verifies new information reported by the enrollee or identifies updated information through data matching, and it must periodically examine available data sources to identify, for enrollees receiving advance premium tax credits or cost-sharing reductions, eligibility determinations for or enrollment in Medicare, Medicaid, CHIP, or the Basic Health Program. (eCFR) The same regulatory framework requires the enrollee to report changes affecting the eligibility standards in § 155.305 within 30 days, subject to specific exceptions. (eCFR) Knowledge in this environment is therefore not limited to a face-to-face admission. It can arise through application data, verification records, data matching, enrollment transactions, and issuer communications before coverage is issued.

The federal sources support severe federal penalty exposure, but they do not create a uniform federal producer-license revocation rule. The anti-duplication statute provides criminal and civil money penalties for prohibited sale or issuance; separate producer licensing consequences are generally matters of state insurance law and Marketplace participation agreements rather than a universal federal penalty stated in the retrieved source packet. (U.S. Code) The official CMS FAQ nevertheless establishes the compliance baseline for issuers and enrollment systems: if an issuer learns before the individual market coverage effective date that the enrollment is for someone whose Medicare Part A or Part B start date precedes the individual market coverage effective date, the issuer should cancel the enrollment before the policy is issued. Conversely, if coverage has already been issued, CMS states that the issuer may not terminate merely because it later finds Medicare eligibility or enrollment, unless the enrollee requests termination or another legal basis applies.

The anti-duplication statute also distinguishes individual market coverage from employer-sponsored group health coverage. CMS states that the prohibition does not apply in the SHOP market or to employer coverage outside SHOP, because employer-sponsored coverage is explicitly exempted and SHOP coverage is sold to the employer rather than directly to the Medicare beneficiary. This distinction is essential to the Chapter 5 employment analysis. A Medicare beneficiary who is an active employee covered through employer group coverage may be inside the Medicare Secondary Payer system, while an individual purchasing an individual Marketplace QHP is not. CMS states that Medicare beneficiaries whose employers purchase SHOP coverage are treated like other persons with employer group health plan coverage, and that Medicare Secondary Payer rules govern coordination where applicable. The legal status of the risk pool, individual market versus employer group, controls the analysis.

Individual Marketplace coverage is structurally incompatible with Medicare supplementation. CMS states that if someone is enrolled in both Medicare and an Individual Marketplace QHP, Medicare is the primary payer and Medicare does not provide coordination of benefits. Medicare.gov likewise explains that Medicare is not part of the Marketplace and that the Marketplace does not offer Medigap policies,

Medicare Advantage Plans, or Medicare drug coverage. The consequence is administrative and actuarial: an individual Marketplace QHP is not a federal Medicare supplement, not a Medicare Advantage plan, not a Part D plan, and not a Medicare Secondary Payer group health plan. It is an individual commercial contract that may continue after issuance under limited circumstances, but it is not designed to wrap around Medicare claims.

The creditable-coverage illusion is most dangerous in the Part B enrollment context. Medicare & You 2026 states that coverage based on current employment does not include COBRA, retiree coverage, VA coverage, individual health insurance coverage such as Marketplace coverage, or former-employer severance or layoff coverage. The same handbook states that a Part B Special Enrollment Period is available after the Initial Enrollment Period when the individual delayed Part B because of group health plan coverage based on current employment, with enrollment allowed while still covered by that group health plan or during the eight-month period after employment or coverage ends, whichever occurs first. Individual Marketplace coverage is therefore not a Part B safe harbor. Retaining Marketplace coverage after age 65 does not protect against delayed Part B enrollment exposure.

The penalty consequence follows directly. Medicare & You 2026 warns that if Part B is not taken when first eligible, future Part B coverage may be delayed because enrollment is available only at certain times, and a late enrollment penalty may be added to the monthly premium for as long as Part B is held. CMS's Medicare and Marketplace FAQ similarly states that individuals enrolled in an Individual Marketplace QHP who delay Medicare enrollment will be able to enroll only during the General Enrollment Period if they miss the Initial Enrollment Period and may be subject to late enrollment penalties, with the Part B penalty lasting as long as Part B remains in effect. The Marketplace account therefore supplies no actuarial shield against Part B penalty accumulation. It can preserve some form of private insurance continuity, but it does not preserve the federal worker Special Enrollment Period.

Part D requires a more precise statement. A Marketplace prescription drug benefit is not automatically creditable prescription drug coverage. CMS states that although prescription drug coverage is an essential health benefit, ACA rules do not require Individual Marketplace or SHOP QHP drug coverage to be at least as good as Medicare Part D, which is the general test for creditable coverage; private insurers offering prescription drug coverage must determine annually whether the coverage is creditable and notify CMS and Medicare-eligible enrollees of that determination. Therefore, individual Marketplace coverage should not be treated as a reliable Part D late-enrollment penalty shield unless the issuer's written creditable coverage notice establishes that status for the relevant period. The illusion is not that Marketplace drug coverage can never be creditable; the illusion is assuming creditability without the required annual determination and written notice.

The premium tax credit system imposes a separate household tax exposure. The uploaded ACA materials state that advance premium tax credits are reconciled on the federal income tax return through Form 8962, and that if excess advance payments were made, the taxpayer enters the excess amount on the return and repays all or part of it when filing. The same materials state that taxpayers should notify the Marketplace about changes in circumstances, including gaining or losing eligibility for government-sponsored health care coverage, so that advance credit payments can be adjusted and large reconciliation differences reduced. When Medicare Part A eligibility or enrollment removes Marketplace subsidy eligibility, the household risk is not only duplicate premium payment. It is also repayment of federal advance subsidy amounts that should have stopped when government-sponsored coverage became controlling.

The regulatory data systems are designed to discover this problem, but they are not designed to eliminate every household consequence automatically. The ACA tax materials state that the Marketplace verifies information through data sources including prior-year tax information, Social Security Administration data, and state wage data in order to estimate advance premium tax credit eligibility. 45 CFR § 155.320 requires verification of minimum essential coverage eligibility for affordability-program determinations, and 45 CFR § 155.330 requires periodic data matching for Medicare enrollment or eligibility determinations for enrollees receiving advance premium tax credits or cost-sharing reductions. (eCFR) (eCFR) The presence of federal data matching does not eliminate the obligation to classify coverage correctly, report changes, terminate duplicate coverage when appropriate, and reconcile subsidies through the tax return.

The Household Medicare Diagnostic Matrix treats Section 8.1 as the primary anti-duplication and individual-market crossover row. The matrix must separate five statuses that are often conflated: Marketplace coverage before Medicare begins, Marketplace coverage continuing after Medicare begins, knowing sale or issuance of individual market coverage to a Medicare beneficiary, employer-sponsored SHOP or other group coverage, and premium tax credit eligibility after Part A entitlement. CMS's official Medicare and Marketplace materials state that Medicare is not part of the Marketplace, that the Marketplace does not offer Medigap, Medicare Advantage, or Part D coverage, and that Marketplace savings end once Part A coverage begins. CMS's FAQ adds that individual Marketplace QHPs are not appropriate for persons with Medicare, that knowing sale or issuance is illegal, and that Medicare is primary when individual Marketplace QHP and Medicare coexist.

The final synthesis is exacting. Individual Marketplace coverage can be a legitimate pre-Medicare bridge, but after Medicare Part A entitlement or Part B enrollment exists, the federal system changes the legal character of the transaction. The anti-duplication statute prohibits knowing sale or issuance of duplicative individual market coverage to the Medicare beneficiary; Title 45 Marketplace regulations restrict subsidy eligibility, require verification, require change reporting, and permit controlled termination; CMS guidance confirms that issued coverage is not automatically terminated merely because Medicare status is later discovered, but that pre-effective issuance should be stopped when Medicare coverage is known. (U.S. Code) (eCFR) Under the Household Medicare Diagnostic Matrix, failure to distinguish individual commercial coverage from current-employment group coverage converts a temporary bridge into a source of federal subsidy repayment, missed Part B enrollment protection, possible Part D creditability exposure, duplicate premiums, and household asset erosion. The individual Marketplace is not a Medicare supplement, not a Medicare enrollment safe harbor, and not a substitute for timely entitlement coordination.

8.2 Instantaneous Premium Tax Credit (PTC) Forfeiture

The Premium Tax Credit is not a general healthcare allowance that can be preserved by personal preference once Medicare eligibility crosses the statutory boundary. It is a refundable federal tax credit governed by Internal Revenue Code § 36B, and its availability depends on whether a month is a qualifying "coverage month" for an individual enrolled in a qualified health plan through an Exchange. Section 36B excludes from the definition of a coverage month any month in which the individual is eligible for minimum essential coverage other than individual market coverage; the statutory mechanism therefore treats access to government-sponsored Medicare coverage as a direct disqualifier for Marketplace subsidy eligibility. (U.S. Code) The uploaded IRS Affordable Care Act tax materials state the same rule in administrative form: a taxpayer is allowed a Premium Tax Credit only for months in which a family member is enrolled in a Marketplace qualified health plan and is not eligible for other minimum essential coverage, including government-sponsored coverage such as Medicare.

The disqualification vector is especially severe because premium-free Medicare Part A is treated as government-sponsored minimum essential coverage. IRS Publication 974 identifies Medicare Part A coverage and Medicare Advantage coverage as government-sponsored minimum essential coverage, and it states that, in general, a taxpayer cannot receive the Premium Tax Credit for qualified health plan coverage if the individual is eligible for government-sponsored minimum essential coverage. (IRS) Medicare & You 2026 gives the public-facing Medicare counterpart: once a person is considered eligible for premium-free Part A, or already has Part A with a premium, Marketplace help for premiums or other medical costs no longer applies; if Marketplace premium tax credit assistance continues, some or all of that assistance may have to be repaid when federal income taxes are filed. The subsidy loss is therefore not merely an Exchange billing adjustment. It is a federal tax eligibility event.

The word "eligible" must be interpreted with technical precision. IRS Publication 974 states that an individual is generally considered eligible for a government-sponsored program if the individual meets the criteria for coverage under the program, but the Premium Tax Credit is not lost until the first day of the first full month in which benefits can be received. (IRS) The same IRS rule requires completion of the steps necessary to receive the government-sponsored benefits, such as submitting an application or required information, by the last day of the third full calendar month after the event establishing eligibility; if those steps are not completed within that period, Premium Tax Credit eligibility is lost beginning with the first day of the fourth calendar month after the eligibility event. (IRS) Thus, the forfeiture is "instantaneous" only in the sense that it attaches to the first day of a full calendar month once the federal eligibility rule has matured. It is not a mid-month fractional sharing arrangement between Medicare and the Exchange.

This calendar rule becomes decisive during the age-sixty-five transition. IRS Publication 974 illustrates the rule with an individual who turns 65 on June 3, applies for Medicare by the last day of the third full calendar month after reaching Medicare eligibility, and becomes eligible to receive Medicare benefits beginning December 1; the individual may receive the Premium Tax Credit through November but not beginning December. (IRS) The same IRS example states that if the application steps are not completed by the end of the third full calendar month, the individual is considered eligible for government-sponsored coverage beginning October 1, the first day of the fourth calendar month after turning 65, and Premium Tax Credit eligibility ends as of that date. (IRS) The result is a statutory anti-overlap rule. The household cannot indefinitely delay Medicare enrollment solely to preserve individual Marketplace subsidies.

Premium-free Part A is the most important trigger because it is broadly available at age 65 for individuals with sufficient work history or derivative entitlement. Medicare & You 2026 states that if an individual close to age 65 is not already receiving Social Security or Railroad Retirement Board benefits, Medicare enrollment generally must be initiated through Social Security, while individuals already receiving those benefits are automatically enrolled in Part A and Part B when Medicare eligibility begins. When automatic Medicare activation occurs, the Marketplace subsidy analysis can become a tax reconciliation problem rather than a consumer election problem. HealthCare.gov states that Marketplace coverage does not end automatically when Medicare starts, that a Medicare start date can be reported up to three months before Medicare begins, and that Marketplace coverage can be ended the day before Medicare coverage starts. (HealthCare.gov) If the Marketplace application is not updated, advance credits can continue to flow even after the legal subsidy basis has disappeared.

This communication gap is the administrative trap at the center of Section 8.2. The Marketplace may continue transmitting advance premium tax credit amounts to the issuer because the consumer's account has not been updated, while the Internal Revenue Code has already removed the individual from the coverage family for subsidy purposes. HealthCare.gov warns that if premium tax credits are used to lower monthly premiums and Marketplace coverage is not ended, the credits used must be repaid when federal taxes are filed. (HealthCare.gov) Medicare & You 2026 similarly states that Marketplace coverage should be ended in a timely manner when Medicare eligibility begins to avoid overlap, and that continued Marketplace help after premium-free Part A eligibility may have to be repaid at tax filing. The unauthorized subsidy does not become valid merely because the Marketplace account remained open. It becomes a reconciliation liability.

The HHS enrollment data system is designed to identify this overlap, but it is not designed to protect the household from every tax consequence automatically. Under 45 CFR § 155.320, an Exchange determining eligibility for insurance affordability programs must verify whether an applicant is eligible for minimum essential coverage other than employer-sponsored coverage, Medicaid, CHIP, or the Basic Health Program by transmitting identifying information specified by HHS to HHS for verification purposes. (Legal Information Institute) Under 45 CFR § 155.330, the Exchange must redetermine eligibility during the benefit year when verified new information is received or when updated information is identified through data matching; the same provision requires enrollee reporting of changes affecting eligibility standards within the regulatory timeframe. (eCFR) These verification rules create an administrative detection system, but detection can occur after months of advance subsidy payments have already been made.

Periodic data matching confirms the same integrity function. CMS's Medicare periodic data matching materials state that Exchanges periodically examine available data sources to identify consumers enrolled in Exchange coverage with financial help at the same time they are determined eligible for or enrolled in Medicare Part A or Medicare Advantage, because those Medicare categories are minimum essential coverage; the same CMS materials state that consumers with Medicare minimum essential coverage do not qualify for APTC or cost-sharing reductions for Exchange coverage after they are considered eligible for Medicare minimum essential coverage. (Centers for Medicare & Medicaid Services) This is the federal data architecture behind the household tax event. The Exchange may identify the overlap and stop savings prospectively, but the IRS reconciliation process remains the final mathematical audit for advance payments already made.

The annual tax reconciliation machinery begins with Form 1095-A. The uploaded IRS ACA tax materials state that the Marketplace sends Form 1095-A, Health Insurance Marketplace Statement, to taxpayers who enrolled themselves or a dependent in Marketplace insurance, and that the form includes monthly enrollment premiums, the applicable second lowest cost silver plan premium used to compute the credit, the amount of advance credit payments, covered individuals' identifying information, and other required information; the Marketplace also reports this information to the IRS. The current IRS Instructions for Form 8962 state that for 2025 coverage the Marketplace was required to provide or send Form 1095-A by January 31, 2026, and that a corrected Form 1095-A must be used rather than an original form when a correction is issued. (IRS) Form 1095-A is therefore the historic ledger of monthly subsidy payments, not merely a consumer notice.

Form 8962 is the federal reconciliation platform. The IRS states that Form 8962 is used to figure the Premium Tax Credit and reconcile it with advance payments of the Premium Tax Credit. (IRS) The uploaded IRS ACA materials state that taxpayers receiving advance credit payments must file a federal income tax return even when otherwise not required to file, compute the Premium Tax Credit on Form 8962, and subtract advance credit payments from the credit calculated on the return. If the calculated credit exceeds advance payments, the difference increases the refund or lowers tax owed; if advance payments exceed the allowable credit, the excess increases tax liability and can produce a smaller refund or a balance due. The Marketplace overlap therefore moves from health insurance administration into the federal income tax account.

The reconciliation calculation is month-by-month when coverage, subsidy, household, or eligibility facts change during the year. The uploaded IRS ACA materials state that the Premium Tax Credit is the sum of the credit amount for each month, and that the monthly credit is the lesser of the enrollment premium or the applicable second lowest cost silver plan premium minus the taxpayer's monthly contribution amount. The IRS Instructions for Form 8962 state that if coverage existed for fewer than twelve months or if amounts varied during the year, lines 12 through 23 must be used for monthly reporting, with Form 1095-A monthly enrollment premium, second lowest cost silver plan premium, and APTC amounts flowing through the monthly columns.

(IRS) Where Medicare eligibility changes the coverage family for only part of the year, the annual shortcut cannot accurately capture the liability. The month of Medicare transition becomes a line-item tax calculation.

The individual must be excluded from the coverage family for the months in which government-sponsored Medicare minimum essential coverage disqualifies the Marketplace subsidy. The uploaded IRS ACA tax materials state that a person eligible for government-sponsored coverage such as Medicare is not a member of the coverage family for the months of eligibility, and that a Premium Tax Credit is not allowed for that individual's coverage for those months. The same material states that a person is considered eligible for government or employer-sponsored coverage for a month only if eligible for that coverage for every day of the month; if eligibility begins on the fifth day of a month, the person may still be treated as not eligible for that coverage for the month and may be allowed a Premium Tax Credit for that month, but not for the following month. This is the source of the first-full-month rule. The tax file turns on complete calendar-month eligibility, not on a vague sense that Medicare began "sometime during the month."

The retroactive clawback is actuarial rather than punitive in form. When APTC is paid for a month in which no Premium Tax Credit is allowable for the Medicare-eligible individual, the advance payment is no longer supported by the final tax calculation. The IRS PTC overview states that advance credit payments are reconciled against the Premium Tax Credit allowed for the year, and when advance payments exceed the allowable credit, the excess APTC is added to tax liability on Form 1040, Schedule 2, producing either a smaller refund or a larger balance due. (IRS) The uploaded IRS ACA materials state the same rule, describing excess advance credit payments as amounts that increase tax liability and are entered in the Tax and Credits section of the federal return. The subsidy was paid to reduce monthly premiums, but the year-end return reclassifies unsupported subsidy as a tax repayment obligation.

The repayment limitation system modifies that result only for certain income ranges. The uploaded IRS ACA tax materials state that if excess advance credit payments were made, the taxpayer enters the excess on the return and increases tax liability by the excess, subject to a repayment cap if household income is under 400 percent of the federal poverty line. The current IRS Instructions for Form 8962 provide the 2025 repayment limitation table: if Form 8962 line 5 is less than 200 percent of the federal poverty line, the repayment limitation is $375 for single filing status and $750 for other filing statuses; at least 200 percent but less than 300 percent produces $975 and $1,950; at least 300 percent but less than 400 percent produces $1,625 and $3,250; and at 400 percent or more there is no repayment limitation. (IRS) These caps are not subsidy forgiveness for Medicare months. They are statutory limits on the amount of excess APTC that must be repaid for certain lower-income households.

The high-income threshold removes the protective cap. The IRS Instructions for Form 8962 state that if Form 8962 line 5 is 400 or more, there is no repayment limitation and the full excess advance credit amount from line 27 must be repaid on line 29. (IRS) The IRS PTC overview, updated in 2026, states the broader current-law rule that household income above 400 percent of the federal poverty line generally prevents Premium Tax Credit eligibility, with temporary elimination of the 400 percent ceiling having applied only for tax years 2021 through 2025. (IRS) The practical consequence is severe in Medicare crossover years. A middle or higher income household that fails to terminate APTC after premium-free Part A eligibility can face full dollar-for-dollar repayment of the unauthorized subsidy, rather than a capped correction.

The expiration of the temporary 2021 through 2025 expansion makes precision even more important. IRS Publication 974 for tax year 2025 states that taxpayers with household income exceeding 400 percent of the federal poverty line may be allowed a Premium Tax Credit for 2025, while the IRS's 2026 PTC overview states that the special rule applied only for tax years 2021 through 2025 and that above-400-percent households generally are not allowed the credit under current post-expansion rules. (IRS) (IRS) The manuscript cannot treat the 400 percent threshold as a static historical footnote. It is a cliff line for repayment limitation purposes in the Form 8962 system and, under current law after the temporary expansion, a substantive eligibility ceiling as well. The household Medicare transition must therefore be synchronized with the applicable tax year's PTC statute and instructions.

The Medicare crossover also interacts with family composition. A Medicare-eligible individual may leave the Marketplace coverage family while a spouse or dependent remains eligible for Marketplace coverage and subsidies. HealthCare.gov states that when reporting a Medicare start date, the application must confirm the plan for other household members who need to keep Marketplace coverage; it also explains that if savings are stopped for a person with Medicare, other people on the application may keep Marketplace coverage and their savings are rechecked. (HealthCare.gov) This is not a household-wide automatic subsidy death in every case. It is an individual-by-individual coverage-family adjustment. The Medicare-enrolled or Medicare-eligible person may lose APTC eligibility, while non-Medicare family members may remain inside the Marketplace subsidy computation if they otherwise qualify.

The non-coordination rule is equally important. Marketplace coverage does not lower Medicare out-of-pocket costs and is not used in place of Medicare Part B, according to HealthCare.gov's Medicare and Marketplace guidance. (HealthCare.gov) Medicare & You 2026 states that individual health insurance coverage such as Marketplace coverage is not coverage based on current employment for the Part B Special Enrollment Period. Therefore, a household that attempts to preserve Marketplace subsidies by delaying Medicare creates two independent exposures: the tax exposure of APTC repayment after Medicare eligibility, and the Medicare enrollment exposure of Part B late enrollment penalty or General Enrollment Period delay if the Marketplace account is mistaken for an active-employment safe harbor.

The premium-free Part A trigger must also be distinguished from premium Part A. Medicare & You 2026 states that once an individual is considered eligible for premium-free Part A, or already has Part A with a premium, Marketplace help for premiums or other medical costs ends. IRS Publication 974 adds a narrower tax-rule exception: coverage under Medicare Part A for which the individual must pay a premium is a program for which the individual is considered eligible for government-sponsored coverage only if enrolled. (IRS) This distinction prevents an overly broad conclusion. Premium-free Part A eligibility is the dominant age-based subsidy disqualifier; premium Part A can be treated differently for PTC purposes until enrollment, subject to the exact IRS and Marketplace rules.

The administrative audit sequence is therefore predictable. First, the Marketplace estimates APTC during enrollment based on projected household income, family composition, and eligibility for other coverage, using data sources that can include prior-year tax information, Social Security Administration data, and wage data. Second, if the individual later becomes eligible for premium-free Part A or Medicare minimum essential coverage and the Marketplace account is not updated, advance subsidy payments may continue. Third, Form 1095-A records the monthly enrollment premium, applicable SLCSP, and APTC amounts and reports them to the taxpayer and IRS. Fourth, Form 8962 recomputes the allowable Premium Tax Credit month by month and reconciles it against actual APTC. (IRS) Fifth, any excess APTC becomes tax liability, subject to the repayment limitation rules only where household income and filing status allow. (IRS)

The Household Medicare Diagnostic Matrix treats Section 8.2 as the tax pillar for the individual Marketplace crossover. The matrix must identify the Medicare eligibility event, the Part A premium status, the first full month in which Medicare benefits can be received, the third-full-month completion deadline when applicable, the Marketplace termination or savings-stop date, the Form 1095-A monthly APTC record, the Form 8962 coverage-family months, the FPL percentage on line 5, and the repayment limitation category. IRS Publication 974 supplies the government-sponsored MEC rule and the first-full-month transition rule; Medicare & You supplies the Marketplace-to-Medicare warning and repayment exposure; Form 8962 supplies the reconciliation and repayment limitation machinery. (IRS) (IRS)

The final actuarial conclusion is uncompromising. Marketplace subsidies are temporary bridge financing before Medicare, not parallel financing after Medicare minimum essential coverage becomes controlling. Premium-free Part A eligibility can terminate PTC eligibility even when the Marketplace policy remains active, and Marketplace coverage does not end automatically merely because Medicare begins. (HealthCare.gov) The household that fails to synchronize the Marketplace account with the Medicare start date can convert affordable interim coverage into a year-end tax debt, because Form 1095-A records the subsidy stream and Form 8962 retroactively tests whether each month remained eligible for federal credit support. Under the Household Medicare Diagnostic Matrix, the essential rule is chronological: the Marketplace subsidy file must be closed, corrected, or recalibrated before the first full month of Medicare minimum essential coverage disqualifies the individual, because after that point the APTC is no longer financial assistance. It is a federal advance payment awaiting reconciliation, recovery, and possible dollar-for-dollar repayment.

8.3 Coordination of Health Benefits (COB) Rules

Coordination of benefits is not a clerical claims convention. It is a federal risk-allocation architecture that determines which capital pool bears medical liability first when a Medicare beneficiary is covered by more than one health arrangement. CMS describes coordination of benefits as the process by which plans providing health or prescription coverage for a person with Medicare determine their respective payment responsibilities, including which insurance plan has primary payment responsibility and the extent to which other plans contribute. (Centers for Medicare & Medicaid Services) Medicare's public coordination guidance states that the primary payer pays up to the limits of its coverage and that the secondary payer pays only if costs remain after the primary payer has acted; if the secondary payer does not cover the remaining balance, the beneficiary may be responsible for the rest. (Medicare) The Medicare handbook expresses the same structure for 2026: the insurance that pays first pays up to its limits, the insurance that pays second only pays if costs remain uncovered, and the secondary payer may not pay all uncovered costs.

The macro-fiscal premise is that Medicare should not become the primary payer when Congress has assigned primary liability to another legally responsible payer. CMS defines Medicare Secondary Payer as the circumstance in which Medicare does not have primary payment responsibility because another entity has responsibility for paying before Medicare. (Centers for Medicare & Medicaid Services) That rule is not activated by the retail generosity of a private policy, the premium volume paid by a household, or the fact that an individual commercial policy appears comprehensive. It is activated by statutory classification. A group health plan based on current employment, liability insurance, workers' compensation, no-fault insurance, or another recognized category may alter payer order. An individual Marketplace contract purchased through a retail exchange does not become an employer group health plan merely because it resembles one in benefit design.

The working-aged Medicare Secondary Payer rule is the controlling employer-based contrast. Pursuant to 42 CFR § 411.170, Medicare's age-based secondary payer rules apply to group health plans of employers that meet the twenty-employee threshold, and the regulation prohibits such a plan from taking into account the Medicare entitlement of an individual age 65 or older, or the spouse of a worker, when coverage is by virtue of current employment status. (eCFR) The related rule at 42 CFR § 411.172 specifies that Medicare benefits are secondary when an individual age 65 or older is entitled to Medicare Part A, is enrolled in Part B, meets the federal current-employment coverage conditions, and is covered under a group health plan of an employer with at least twenty employees, including applicable multi-employer arrangements. (Legal Information Institute) The safe-harbor logic is therefore not simply "other insurance." It is employer group coverage based on current employment, inside a statutory MSP category.

The 2026 Medicare handbook's payer-order table translates that regulatory architecture into household terms. For an individual age 65 or older with group health plan coverage based on the current employment of the individual or spouse, the group health plan pays first when the employer has twenty or more employees, or when a smaller employer participates in a multi-employer plan that includes an employer with twenty or more employees; Medicare pays first when the employer has fewer than twenty employees. The same CMS material states that when coverage is retiree health coverage from former employment, Medicare pays first. Payer order therefore depends on employment status, employer size, and plan classification. It does not turn on the household's subjective belief that a non-Medicare policy is "good coverage."

The Part B Special Enrollment Period uses the same current-employment foundation. Medicare & You 2026 states that after the Initial Enrollment Period, a person may have a Special Enrollment Period for Part B if Part B was delayed because of group health plan coverage based on current employment, with enrollment permitted while covered by that group health plan or during the eight-month period beginning after employment ends or coverage ends, whichever happens first. The worker safe harbor is therefore a timing rule attached to an employment-based group plan, not a general rule protecting every non-Medicare insurance arrangement. It is this current-employment status, not private premium payment, that allows the federal enrollment system to tolerate delayed Part B without immediate late-enrollment penalty exposure.

Individual Marketplace coverage fails that standard by design. Medicare & You 2026 states explicitly that coverage based on current employment does not include individual health insurance coverage, including coverage through the Health Insurance Marketplace. The same handbook states that even if Marketplace coverage or other individual health coverage not based on current employment exists, Medicare should be joined when first eligible to avoid delay in Medicare coverage and possible late-enrollment penalty exposure. This is the first fracture in the Marketplace creditable-coverage illusion. A household may possess an individual exchange policy, may pay substantial premiums, and may have broad medical benefits, yet the federal Part B safe harbor remains absent because the policy is not group health plan coverage based on current employment.

The retail character of individual exchange coverage is legally decisive. Individual Marketplace coverage is purchased by or for an individual or family through an individual commercial market structure, not through an employer's group health plan based on current employment. Medicare's Marketplace guidance states that Medicare is not part of the Marketplace and that the Marketplace does not offer Medicare Supplement Insurance policies, Medicare Advantage Plans, or Medicare drug coverage. CMS's Medicare and Marketplace materials further state that if someone is enrolled in both Medicare and an Individual Marketplace qualified health plan, Medicare is the primary payer and Medicare does not provide coordination of benefits with that individual Marketplace QHP. (Centers for Medicare & Medicaid Services) The individual exchange policy therefore cannot be repurposed as a Medicare wraparound system by private election.

The distinction between individual Marketplace coverage and employer Marketplace coverage must be preserved. The uploaded CMS materials state that employer coverage through the Small Business Health Options Program, or SHOP, is employer coverage through the Marketplace, and that if an employer has twenty or more employees the employer pays first, while Medicare pays first when the employer has fewer than twenty employees. This is not a contradiction. SHOP coverage is employer group coverage purchased by an employer in a small-business marketplace structure, while an individual Marketplace account is retail individual coverage. The Part B safe harbor depends on the employment-based group health plan relationship, not on the mere word "Marketplace." The Household Medicare Diagnostic Matrix must therefore separate individual Marketplace coverage from employer SHOP or other employer group coverage.

The requested phrase "creditable coverage" also requires technical discipline. For Part B, the controlling safe-harbor term is not creditable prescription drug coverage; it is group health plan coverage based on current employment. Medicare & You uses that exact standard for the Part B Special Enrollment Period and expressly excludes individual Marketplace coverage from it. For Part D, the controlling term is creditable prescription drug coverage, meaning drug coverage expected to pay on average at least as much as Medicare drug coverage. Medicare's penalty guidance states that a Part D late-enrollment penalty can arise after a continuous period of 63 or more days without Medicare drug coverage or other creditable prescription drug coverage. (Medicare) Thus, Marketplace coverage is categorically nonqualifying for Part B delay, but Marketplace prescription coverage requires a separate Part D creditability analysis.

The official Part D marketplace rule is not that every individual Marketplace prescription benefit is automatically noncreditable. It is that Marketplace prescription drug coverage is not required to be at least as good as Medicare drug coverage, and the issuer must notify Medicare-eligible enrollees each year in writing whether the coverage is creditable. Medicare & You 2026 similarly states that creditable prescription drug coverage may include drug coverage from a current or former employer or union, TRICARE, the Indian Health Service, or the Department of Veterans Affairs, and that the plan must tell the beneficiary each year if non-Medicare drug coverage is creditable. The Marketplace illusion is therefore evidentiary as well as legal: an individual Marketplace account does not by itself prove Part D creditability. The written annual creditable-coverage notice is the operative evidence.

The secondary-payer prohibition is most accurately stated as a non-coordination rule rather than a universal plan-contract cancellation rule. CMS training materials state that, generally, there is no coordination of benefits between Medicare and an individual Marketplace QHP purchased through the Health Insurance Marketplace. (Centers for Medicare & Medicaid Services) The CMS Medicare and Marketplace FAQ states that where both Medicare and an individual Marketplace QHP exist, Medicare is the primary payer and Medicare does not provide coordination of benefits. (Centers for Medicare & Medicaid Services) The uploaded 2026 handbook confirms that Marketplace coverage is not a Medicare plan, not Medigap, not Medicare Advantage, and not Part D. The source-controlled conclusion is therefore clear without overstatement: individual Marketplace coverage is not a recognized Medicare secondary payer vehicle and should not be treated as a formal wraparound supplement.

The claim-payment consequence is an uninsured primary-layer risk. If an individual who should have enrolled in Medicare fails to do so because a Marketplace plan appears comprehensive, the individual may confront a medical claim system in which Medicare was expected to be the federal primary payer, while the individual commercial policy is not structured to coordinate as a Medicare supplement. CMS's

Medicare and Marketplace guidance states that Medicare is primary where Medicare and individual Marketplace QHP coverage overlap, and that Medicare does not provide coordination of benefits. (Centers for Medicare & Medicaid Services) Medicare's general coordination guidance states that a secondary payer pays only if costs remain after the primary payer pays and may not cover all remaining costs. (Medicare) When the expected Medicare layer is missing because Part B was delayed, the household may face the actuarial equivalent of a phantom primary payer gap.

The chronological exposure begins with the Initial Enrollment Period. Medicare & You 2026 states that the Initial Enrollment Period generally lasts seven months, beginning three months before the month of the 65th birthday and ending three months after that month, with a first-day-of-month birthday rule that shifts the period earlier. If enrollment is completed during the first three months of the Initial Enrollment Period, coverage generally begins the first day of the birthday month, or the first day of the prior month when the birthday falls on the first day of the month; if enrollment occurs during the birthday month or the last three months of the Initial Enrollment Period, coverage starts the first day of the month after sign-up. Individual Marketplace coverage does not extend that window, does not convert it into an employer Special Enrollment Period, and does not prevent the IEP from closing.

Once the Initial Enrollment Period closes without valid Part B enrollment or a qualifying employer-based Special Enrollment Period, the file enters late-enrollment territory. The 2026 Medicare materials state that Part B delayed without a Special Enrollment Period can require waiting for the General Enrollment Period from January 1 through March 31, and coverage begins the first day of the month after enrollment. The same materials state that if Part B is taken later after a delay without a Special Enrollment Period, the late-enrollment penalty is 10 percent for each full 12-month period during which Part B could have been held but was not, and in most cases the penalty lasts as long as Part B remains in force. This is not a temporary surcharge. It is a durable premium impairment caused by a missed federal timing rule.

The Part B penalty mechanics make the Marketplace misconception financially durable. The 2026 CMS example states that a two-full-year Part B delay produces a 20 percent late-enrollment penalty, calculated as 10 percent for each full 12-month period, and applies that penalty to the 2026 standard Part B premium of $202.90, producing a rounded monthly premium of $243.50 for the year in the example. A Marketplace premium paid during the delay does not offset that penalty calculation. The penalty is keyed to months during which Part B could have been held and was not, unless a recognized Special Enrollment Period protects the delay. Individual Marketplace coverage is expressly outside the current-employment coverage category that protects the Part B delay.

The Part D exposure uses a different clock. Medicare & You 2026 states that a Part D late-enrollment penalty can apply if, after the Initial Enrollment Period ends, there is a period of 63 or more days in a row without Medicare drug coverage or other creditable prescription drug coverage, and that the penalty is generally paid as part of the monthly premium for as long as Medicare drug coverage continues. The 2026 formula is 1 percent of the national base beneficiary premium, $38.99 in 2026, multiplied by the number of full uncovered months without Medicare drug coverage or other creditable prescription drug coverage, rounded to the nearest ten cents and added to the monthly premium. Marketplace prescription coverage may protect the Part D file only if the annual written notice confirms creditable status; absent that evidence, the 63-day exposure must be treated as active.

The two penalty systems therefore do not move together. Part B requires coverage based on current employment to delay without penalty after the Initial Enrollment Period, while Part D requires Medicare drug coverage or other creditable prescription drug coverage and applies a 63-day continuous uncovered period threshold. A single individual Marketplace policy can fail the Part B safe harbor categorically while simultaneously requiring written creditability verification for Part D. This is the analytic reason the Household Medicare Diagnostic Matrix cannot contain a single row labeled "other insurance." It must split medical coverage, drug coverage, employment basis, payer order, creditability documentation, and enrollment timing.

The General Enrollment Period gap is the administrative consequence of failing that split analysis. Medicare & You 2026 states that a person who misses the Initial Enrollment Period and does not qualify for a Special Enrollment Period may sign up for Part B during the General Enrollment Period from January 1 through March 31, with coverage beginning the first day of the month after sign-up. The updated 2026 guide warns that without Part B and without employer health coverage based on current employment, a person may have to pay all costs for doctors' services, outpatient care, medical supplies, and preventive services, may have to wait for the General Enrollment Period to enroll later, and may face a gap in health coverage. That gap is not cured by the fact that a Marketplace policy existed during the months before Medicare enrollment. The federal enrollment system treats the Marketplace policy as individual coverage, not as a Part B delay credential.

The revenue-policy consequences also extend beyond claims. Medicare & You 2026 states that once a person is considered eligible for premium-free Part A, or already has Part A with a premium, the person no longer qualifies for Marketplace help paying Marketplace plan premiums or other medical costs, and continued premium tax credit assistance may have to be repaid on the federal income tax return. The ACA tax materials in the source packet state that an individual eligible for government-sponsored coverage such as Medicare is not a member of the coverage family for months of government-sponsored eligibility, so the Premium Tax Credit is not allowed for that individual's coverage for those months. The same misconception that causes delayed Medicare enrollment can therefore create subsidy repayment exposure.

The anti-duplication rule compounds the coordination analysis. Medicare's Marketplace guidance states that the Marketplace is for people who do not have health insurance, that the Marketplace does not affect Medicare choices or benefits, and that it is illegal for someone who knows an individual has Medicare to sell that person a Marketplace plan, even where only Part A or only Part B exists. That prohibition underscores the structural incompatibility. A Marketplace plan is not sold as a Medicare supplement, not issued as a Medicare Advantage substitute, and not designed as a Part D plan. Once Medicare exists, the individual-market transaction becomes legally constrained, while the already-issued individual policy does not create MSP payer status or a delayed-enrollment safe harbor.

The actuarial misclassification is often caused by the phrase "full coverage." A Marketplace policy may include hospital benefits, physician benefits, preventive benefits, prescription drug benefits, and an out-of-pocket maximum. None of those features supply current-employment status. None convert the individual policy into a group health plan under the working-aged Medicare Secondary Payer rules. None establish the twenty-employee employer threshold required for the age-based group health plan primary-payer rule. (eCFR) (Legal Information Institute) None create a Medicare Supplement Insurance policy, a Medicare Advantage plan, or a Medicare drug plan, because the Marketplace does not offer those Medicare coverage categories. The statutory classification, not the private contract's perceived adequacy, controls.

The Household Medicare Diagnostic Matrix must therefore make the Marketplace row a negative gate rather than a comfort indicator. The matrix should identify whether the coverage is individual Marketplace coverage, employer SHOP coverage, other employer group coverage, retiree coverage, COBRA, Medicaid, TRICARE, Veterans Affairs coverage, or a Medicare coverage product. CMS states that individual health insurance coverage through the Marketplace is not coverage based on current employment for Part B Special Enrollment Period purposes, while SHOP or employer coverage must be analyzed under employer-size and current-employment rules. It should then identify whether Part D creditable coverage has been documented through the required annual written notice, because Marketplace prescription drug coverage is not required to be as good as Medicare Part D.

Section 8.3 therefore supplies the coordination-of-benefits pillar for the matrix. It separates three distinct inquiries that households frequently collapse into one: which payer pays first, whether Part B can be delayed without penalty, and whether prescription drug coverage is creditable for Part D. Medicare's coordination rules decide payer order; the current-employment Special Enrollment Period decides Part B delay protection; the creditable prescription drug coverage standard decides Part D penalty exposure. (Centers for Medicare & Medicaid Services) Individual Marketplace coverage fails the Part B current-employment test, generally does not coordinate with Medicare as a secondary wraparound payer, and requires written drug-creditability documentation before it can be treated as Part D protective. (Centers for Medicare & Medicaid Services)

The final actuarial conclusion is direct. Individual commercial exchange coverage is a retail insurance contract, not an active, FICA-backed employer group health plan and not a Medicare secondary payer instrument. It can function as a pre-Medicare bridge before entitlement becomes controlling, but it does not protect a delayed Part B file after the Initial Enrollment Period, does not create an eight-month worker Special Enrollment Period, does not become Medigap, does not become Medicare Advantage, and does not become Part D by nomenclature. The household that mistakes individual Marketplace coverage for creditable secondary Medicare coverage risks a closed Initial Enrollment Period, forced General Enrollment Period dependency, a lifetime Part B penalty, possible Part D late-enrollment penalty exposure, premium tax credit repayment, and uncovered primary-payer liability. Under the Household Medicare Diagnostic Matrix, the decisive classification is not whether the commercial policy appears comprehensive; it is whether the coverage is legally tied to current employment, recognized in Medicare payer-order rules, and documented under the correct Part B and Part D standards.

MODULE IV: SECONDARY PRIVATIZED HEALTH FRAMEWORKS

Chapter 9: The Standardized Supplemental (Medigap) Architecture

9.1 The Federal Lettering Matrix

Medicare Supplement Insurance, commonly called Medigap, is the federal system's standardized private mechanism for financing portions of Original Medicare cost sharing that remain after Medicare has made its primary payment. Its modern form is the product of federal intervention into a market that had become administratively opaque, difficult to compare, and vulnerable to overlapping benefit designs. The uploaded 2026 Medicare source packet states the current operative rule plainly: Medigap policies must follow federal and state laws designed to protect beneficiaries, must be clearly identified as Medicare Supplement Insurance, and, in most states, may be sold only as standardized plans named by letters A through D, F, G, and K through N; policies with the same letter provide the same basic benefits regardless of residence or issuing company, so price is the difference between same-letter policies sold by different companies. Official CMS historical analysis of the 1990 Medigap reform legislation identifies the same regulatory objective: federal reform sought to make comparison easier, promote market stability and competition, and avoid policy designs that impeded rational consumer comparison. (Centers for Medicare & Medicaid Services)

The statutory and regulatory architecture should therefore be understood as a national simplification project rather than as ordinary private insurance cataloging. Prior to standardization, supplemental policies could be arranged through multiple overlapping and non-comparable benefit structures, making it difficult to determine whether a premium bought a materially different risk transfer or merely a differently labeled version of the same narrow protection. The Omnibus Budget Reconciliation Act of 1990 amended the federal Medicare supplement framework, and CMS's official Medigap model regulation materials define "1990 Standardized Medicare supplement benefit plan" and "1990 plan" as categories within the standardized Medicare supplement policy regime. (Centers for Medicare & Medicaid Services) The resulting federal-lettering matrix limits benefit design variation. In most states, an insurer selling Plan G is not selling a privately invented Plan G. It is selling the federally standardized Plan G benefit package, subject to state oversight and permitted pricing variation.

The standardization rule also explains why Medigap competition is structurally different from Medicare Advantage or individual commercial health insurance competition. Medigap is not a substitute pathway for receiving Medicare benefits. The 2026 Medicare source packet states that Medigap is extra insurance purchased from a private health insurance company to help pay the beneficiary's share of out-of-pocket costs in Original Medicare, such as copayments, coinsurance, and deductibles; Medicare pays its share of the Medicare-approved amount for covered care, and then the Medigap policy pays its share. The same source distinguishes Medigap from Medicare Advantage: Medicare Advantage is another way to receive Medicare coverage, while a Medigap policy only helps pay costs that Original Medicare does not cover. This distinction is the foundation of the entire chapter. Medigap is a secondary privatized cost-sharing instrument attached to Original Medicare, not a replacement entitlement platform.

The federal lettering matrix is not literally a currently sold A-through-N alphabetic run. Current standardized plans in most states are A, B, C, D, F, G, K, L, M, and N; Plans E, H, I, and J are no longer sold, although a person already holding one of those older plans can generally keep it. The phrase "Plans A through N" therefore functions as historical shorthand for the standardized letter architecture, while the operative 2026 marketplace in most states uses the ten standardized letter categories identified by CMS. The same source packet notes important state deviations: Massachusetts, Minnesota, and Wisconsin standardize Medigap differently, and Medicare SELECT may exist in some states as a standardized policy requiring use of network hospitals and, in some cases, doctors for full benefits except in emergencies. These exceptions do not undo federal standardization. They illustrate federalism inside a federally constrained supplement architecture.

The required core logic begins with Plan A. The source packet states that all insurance companies that sell Medigap policies must offer at least Plan A, while companies do not have to offer every Medigap plan and may choose which standardized plans to sell, subject to federal and state law. Plan A represents the core benefit package. In the 2026 standardized chart, every plan letter covers Part A coinsurance and hospital costs up to an additional 365 days after Medicare benefits are used, Part B coinsurance or copayment at the plan's stated level, the first three pints of blood at the plan's stated level, and Part A hospice care coinsurance or copayment at the plan's stated level. This core structure is not incidental. It is the minimum Medigap logic: the policy stands behind Original Medicare's residual cost-sharing exposure after Medicare has adjudicated the claim.

The continuum from Plan A to higher-benefit plans is a sequence of risk-transfer increments. Plan A provides the basic core package but does not cover the Part A deductible, skilled nursing facility coinsurance, the Part B deductible, Part B excess charges, or foreign travel emergency coverage. Plan B adds full Part A deductible coverage to the core package, but does not add skilled nursing facility coinsurance, Part B excess charge protection, or foreign travel emergency coverage. Plan C historically added broader coverage, including the Part B deductible, skilled nursing facility coinsurance, Part A deductible, and foreign travel emergency coverage, but, as discussed below, Plan C is closed to individuals newly eligible for Medicare on or after January 1, 2020 because it covers the Part B deductible.

Plan D and Plan G illustrate the modern post-2020 replacement logic. The source packet states that people new to Medicare on or after January 1, 2020 cannot buy Plans C and F, but have the right to buy Plans D and G instead, which provide the same benefits as C and F respectively except for coverage of the Part B deductible. Plan D therefore resembles the old Plan C structure without the Part B deductible. Plan G resembles the old Plan F structure without the Part B deductible and includes 100 percent coverage of Part B excess charges, a category not covered by Plan D. From an actuarial standpoint, Plan G occupies the highest standardized non-grandfathered protection tier in most states for a newly eligible Medicare beneficiary because it absorbs the major standardized Medigap cost-sharing categories other than the Part B deductible. That characterization is a benefit-structure observation, not a plan-selection recommendation.

Plan K and Plan L introduce explicit cost sharing and annual out-of-pocket limit mechanics. The 2026 chart shows Plan K covering 50 percent of several cost-sharing categories, including Part B coinsurance or copayment, the first three pints of blood, Part A hospice cost sharing, skilled nursing facility coinsurance, and the Part A deductible, while Plan L covers 75 percent of those same categories. The source packet states that for Plans K and L, after the beneficiary meets the plan's out-of-pocket yearly limit and yearly Part B deductible, the Medigap plan pays 100 percent of covered services for the rest of the calendar year; for 2026, those out-of-pocket limits are $8,000 for Plan K and $4,000 for Plan L, and the yearly Part B deductible is $283. These plans are not full insulation instruments at the beginning of the year. They are cost-sharing designs with a defined annual transition point to full covered-service payment.

Plan M and Plan N apply different risk-sharing levers. The 2026 chart shows Plan M covering 50 percent of the Part A deductible while covering skilled nursing facility coinsurance and several other core categories at 100 percent, and Plan N covering the Part A deductible at 100 percent while structuring Part B coinsurance differently. The source packet states that Plan N pays 100 percent of the Part B coinsurance, but requires a copayment of up to $20 for some office visits and up to $50 for emergency room visits that do not result in an inpatient admission. Plan N also does not cover Part B excess charges in the 2026 standardized chart. Its architecture converts some premium-level risk transfer into point-of-service friction, preserving broad protection against many Medicare cost-sharing liabilities while leaving specific copayment and excess-charge exposures outside the policy.

The phrase "complete risk insulation" requires exact boundaries. No Medigap policy covers every possible healthcare expense. The source packet states that Medigap policies generally do not cover long-term care, vision or dental care, hearing aids, glasses, or private-duty nursing. The same source states that Medigap policies are not Medicare Advantage Plans, Medicare drug plans, Medicaid, employer group health plans, TRICARE, Veterans' benefits, long-term care insurance policies, or Indian Health Service, Tribal, and Urban Indian Health plans. Complete insulation therefore means insulation within a specified standardized benefit category, not universal healthcare indemnification. A plan that covers 100 percent of the Part A deductible insulates that deductible exposure; a plan that covers 100 percent of Part B excess charges insulates that excess-charge category; neither policy converts excluded long-term custodial care, dental services, hearing aids, or separate drug coverage into a Medigap benefit.

Part A deductible absorption is one of the most important standardized risk transfers because the Part A hospital deductible is organized by benefit period rather than by calendar year. The 2026 Medicare handbook states that inpatient hospital care is measured in benefit periods and that each time a new benefit period begins, the beneficiary must pay $1,736 in 2026 before Medicare starts paying; during a benefit period, days 1 through 60 require $0 per day after the deductible, days 61 through 90 require $434 per day, days 91 through 150 require $868 per lifetime reserve day, and after day 150 the beneficiary pays all costs. The same source states that a benefit period ends once the beneficiary has been out of the hospital for 60 days in a row, and that a new admission after those 60 days begins a new benefit period requiring another Part A deductible, potentially multiple times in a calendar year.

This benefit-period structure makes the Part A deductible more volatile than an ordinary annual deductible. A beneficiary with one hospital episode in a calendar year faces one Part A deductible for that benefit period. A beneficiary with distinct hospital episodes separated by a 60-day inpatient-free interval can face more than one Part A deductible in the same calendar year. The 2026 standardized Medigap matrix shows that Plans B, C, D, F, G, and N cover 100 percent of the Part A deductible, while Plan K covers 50 percent, Plan L covers 75 percent, Plan M covers 50 percent, and Plan A does not cover the Part A deductible. The actuarial effect of full Part A deductible coverage is to convert an episodic benefit-period liability into a premium-financed transferred risk. For high-benefit plans with 100 percent Part A deductible coverage, repeat benefit-period deductibles are absorbed by the policy rather than by household liquid reserves, subject to the policy's standardized terms.

Skilled nursing facility cost sharing adds a related secondary exposure. The Medicare handbook states that skilled nursing facility care is also measured in benefit periods; after the Part A deductible amount has been paid for the same benefit period, days 1 through 20 carry $0 daily cost sharing, days 21 through 100 require $217 per day in 2026, and days 101 and beyond require all costs. The standardized Medigap matrix shows that Plans C, D, F, G, M, and N cover skilled nursing facility care coinsurance at 100 percent, while Plans K and L cover 50 percent and 75 percent respectively, and Plans A and B do not cover that benefit. This feature matters because Medicare-covered skilled nursing facility exposure can extend beyond the acute hospital claim and into a separate daily coinsurance phase. A plan's SNF coinsurance treatment should therefore be read alongside its Part A deductible treatment.

Part B excess charges constitute a different kind of risk: balance billing above the Medicare-approved amount when a provider does not accept assignment, subject to federal limiting-charge rules. The 2026 Medicare source packet defines assignment as an agreement by a provider to accept the Medicare-approved amount as full payment and not bill more than the Medicare deductible and coinsurance. It defines an excess charge as the difference between the Medicare-approved amount and the higher amount a doctor or other provider is legally permitted to charge under Original Medicare. Medicare.gov states that, in many cases, the charge by a non-participating provider cannot exceed 15 percent above the Medicare-approved amount, and that this amount is called the limiting charge. (Medicare) The excess charge is therefore a statutory balance-billing margin, not an unlimited private invoice.

Plans F and G are the principal standardized excess-charge insulation mechanisms in the current matrix. The 2026 standardized chart shows that only Plans F and G cover Part B excess charges at 100 percent among the listed standardized plans. Plan F also covers the Part B deductible, while Plan G does not cover the Part B deductible for the modern newly eligible population. The benefit significance is direct: when a non-participating Medicare provider charges an allowable excess amount, a policy that covers Part B excess charges at 100 percent transfers that statutorily permitted balance-billing amount away from the household, subject to the policy terms and claim process. The source packet also states that, in most Medigap policies, the insurer receives Part B claim information directly from Medicare and pays the doctor whatever amount is owed under the policy, while other circumstances may require reimbursement processes based on policy limits.

The Part B excess-charge benefit must not be confused with ordinary Part B coinsurance. Original Medicare generally pays 80 percent of the Medicare-approved amount for many Part B-covered services after the Part B deductible, leaving the beneficiary's usual 20 percent coinsurance exposure. The excess-charge exposure arises only when the provider's legally permitted charge exceeds the Medicare-approved amount. Plans may cover Part B coinsurance but not excess charges, as Plan N demonstrates. Consequently, a household file can be well protected against the routine 20 percent coinsurance amount while still exposed to excess charges unless the selected standardized letter includes that benefit or state law otherwise restricts excess billing. The matrix must therefore contain separate rows for Part B coinsurance and Part B excess charges.

The 2020 pivot was created by the Medicare Access and CHIP Reauthorization Act of 2015 through amendments to the federal Medicare supplement statute. Section 1882 of the Social Security Act, codified at 42 U.S.C. § 1395ss, provides that on or after January 1, 2020, a Medicare supplemental policy that provides coverage of the Part B deductible may not be sold or issued to a newly eligible Medicare beneficiary; it defines newly eligible Medicare beneficiary to exclude individuals who had attained age 65 before January 1, 2020 or had certain Part A entitlement before that date. (U.S. Code) The statute further provides that, for a newly eligible beneficiary, references to standardized Plan C or Plan F are deemed references to Plan D or Plan G respectively, except as otherwise provided. (U.S. Code) The 2026 Medicare source packet implements this rule for consumers: Plans C and F are no longer available to people new to Medicare on or after January 1, 2020, while Plans D and G provide the same benefits except for coverage of the Part B deductible.

The MACRA pivot did not destroy grandfathered coverage. The 2026 source packet states that an individual eligible for Medicare before January 1, 2020 but not yet enrolled may be able to buy Plan C or Plan F, and that people already holding older standardized policies generally may keep them if they remain in force. The statutory logic was not to cancel existing blocks automatically, but to prevent new first-dollar Part B deductible coverage from being sold to newly eligible beneficiaries after the effective date. The policy rationale was utilization friction: Congress removed the ability of newly eligible beneficiaries to buy standardized Medigap coverage that pays the Part B deductible, thereby requiring some direct exposure to the Part B deductible before supplemental coverage begins. The uploaded 2026 Medicare chart identifies that deductible as $283 in 2026 for the K and L out-of-pocket note, while the separate 2026 Medicare cost fact sheet confirms the Part B deductible amount.

The high-deductible versions of Plans F and G add another layer of premium-risk tradeoff. The 2026 source packet states that Plans F and G also offer a high-deductible option in some states; under that option, the beneficiary must pay Medicare-covered costs, including coinsurance, copayments, and deductibles, up to $2,950 in 2026 before the Medigap policy pays anything, and Plan F cannot be purchased by people new to Medicare on or after January 1, 2020. CMS's current Medigap deductible announcements confirm that Plans F and G can be sold with a high-deductible option, that high-deductible Plan F is available only to those not new to Medicare before January 1, 2020, and that high-deductible Plan G is available to individuals new to Medicare on or after January 1, 2020. (Centers for Medicare & Medicaid Services) These designs alter timing of Medigap payment without altering the standardized nature of the underlying lettered benefit after the high deductible is satisfied.

Pricing remains outside the benefit matrix. The source packet states that costs can vary between policies offered by different companies for exactly the same coverage and may rise as the beneficiary ages; some states limit Medigap premium costs, and each policy covers only one person, requiring spouses to hold separate policies if both want Medigap coverage. Other source materials state that price is the only difference between policies with the same plan letter sold by different companies, while premiums can vary widely depending on company, plan, and residence. This is the practical power of the federal lettering matrix. It makes benefit comparison mechanical. It does not make premium comparison irrelevant. The consumer-protection function lies in separating benefit structure from price competition.

The standardized matrix also prevents category confusion with other coverage forms. The source packet states that Medigap cannot pay Medicare Advantage Plan deductibles, copayments, coinsurance, or premiums, and that a Medigap policy no longer provides benefits that supplement Medicare once the beneficiary is in a Medicare Advantage Plan. It further states that Medigap plans sold after 2005 do not include prescription drug coverage, and that Part D drug coverage must be handled through a separate Medicare drug plan if needed. Therefore, the lettered Medigap matrix is not a universal privatized overlay across every Medicare pathway. It attaches to Original Medicare cost sharing and, in modern policies, does not serve as drug coverage or managed-care cost-sharing protection.

The Household Medicare Diagnostic Matrix should therefore treat Section 9.1 as the structural pillar for standardized supplemental analysis. The matrix must first determine whether the household is in Original Medicare, because Medigap is a supplement to Original Medicare rather than an alternative delivery system. It must then identify the state standardization regime, because Massachusetts, Minnesota, and Wisconsin use different standardized structures. It must then identify the lettered plan, the availability of Part A deductible coverage, skilled nursing facility coinsurance coverage, Part B coinsurance treatment, Part B deductible eligibility under the post-

2020 rule, Part B excess charge coverage, foreign travel emergency coverage, high-deductible status, and any Plan K or Plan L out-of-pocket limit. The same matrix must exclude non-Medigap categories such as Medicare Advantage, Part D, Medicaid, employer group coverage, TRICARE, Veterans' benefits, and long-term care insurance from the Medigap row.

The actuarial conclusion is precise. Federal Medigap standardization transforms private supplemental insurance from an opaque benefit-design market into a controlled lettered matrix. That matrix allows the household file to isolate which Original Medicare liabilities are transferred and which remain. Full Part A deductible coverage neutralizes repeated benefit-period hospital deductible shocks where the plan letter provides that benefit. Full Part B excess charge coverage, available in the standardized matrix through Plans F and G, neutralizes the statutory excess-billing margin where the provider does not accept assignment and the limiting charge rule permits an amount above the Medicare-approved amount. (Medicare) The post-2020 prohibition on selling Part B deductible coverage to newly eligible beneficiaries preserves some point-of-service cost exposure while leaving high-benefit non-grandfathered designs such as Plan G available without first-dollar Part B deductible coverage.

The final synthesis for the Household Medicare Diagnostic Matrix is that Medigap risk transfer is both powerful and bounded. It can absorb standardized Original Medicare cost-sharing categories with high precision, but it cannot be treated as long-term care insurance, dental insurance, routine vision coverage, hearing aid coverage, drug coverage, or managed-care cost-sharing coverage. It is private commercial risk inside a public trust infrastructure, governed by federally standardized letter definitions, state oversight, and statutory benefit limits. Failure to map those definitions accurately can produce duplicate premiums, uncovered excluded services, exposure to Part B excess charges, repeated Part A benefit-period deductibles, or mistaken reliance on a policy that cannot operate with Medicare Advantage. The lettering matrix exists to prevent that confusion: the letter determines the standardized benefit package, the issuer determines price and underwriting treatment within legal limits, and the household's risk file determines whether the transferred categories match the actual liabilities created by Original Medicare.

9.2 The Statutory Medigap Open Enrollment Period

The Medigap Open Enrollment Period is the point at which a private supplemental insurance market is temporarily converted into a federally protected access corridor. The ordinary logic of voluntary commercial insurance permits carriers to classify risk, refuse applicants, impose price variation tied to health status, and preserve the insurer's capital pool from adverse selection. The Medigap open-enrollment rule suspends that ordinary market discretion for a tightly defined class of Medicare beneficiaries because Original Medicare leaves continuing cost-sharing exposure in the form of deductibles, coinsurance, copayments, and, in some cases, provider balance-billing categories analyzed in Section 9.1. Federal law therefore creates a brief statutory bridge between public entitlement and private supplementation: an individual who is age 65 or older and enrolled in Part B receives a one-time six-month period during which Medigap access is protected, private refusal is constrained, and medical underwriting cannot be used to deny coverage or impose health-status pricing discrimination.

The legal source of this Medigap open-enrollment protection is the Medicare supplement statute, not 42 CFR § 406.20 itself. Section 406.20 is a hospital-insurance eligibility regulation addressing basic requirements for premium Part A enrollment by individuals age 65 or over and certain disabled individuals; it does not create the six-month Medigap open-enrollment right. (eCFR) The operative federal Medigap rule is Social Security Act § 1882, codified at 42 U.S.C. § 1395ss, which provides that a Medicare supplement issuer may not deny or condition issuance or effectiveness of a Medigap policy, and may not discriminate in pricing because of health status, claims experience, receipt of health care, or medical condition, when the application is submitted before or during the six-month period beginning with the first month in which the individual is age 65 or older and enrolled for Part B benefits. (Legal Information Institute) The manuscript's statutory anchor is therefore the § 1395ss Medigap guaranteed-access framework, with 42 CFR Part 406 remaining relevant to Medicare entitlement timing only as background.

The purpose of the open-enrollment period is market-access equalization. Without a guaranteed window, the highest-need beneficiaries would often confront the greatest difficulty entering the supplemental market precisely when Original Medicare exposure becomes most economically significant. The 2026 official Medicare Medigap guide states that the best time to buy a Medigap policy is during the Medigap Open Enrollment Period, a six-month period that starts in the first month in which the beneficiary has Medicare Part B and is age 65 or older, and it emphasizes that this is a one-time enrollment period that does not repeat every year. Medicare's definition section states the same rule in categorical terms: the Medigap Open Enrollment Period is a one-time-only six-month period during which federal law allows purchase of any Medigap policy sold in the state, beginning with the first month the individual is covered under Part B and is age 65 or older.

The chronological architecture is a dual-trigger system. Age 65 alone does not open the federal Medigap window. Part B alone before age 65 does not necessarily activate the same federal age-65 Medigap open-enrollment protection, although state law may provide additional under-65 rights. The federal trigger requires simultaneous alignment: the individual must be 65 or older and enrolled in Medicare Part B. The clock begins on the first day of the first month in which both conditions exist. If Part B begins after age 65 because current-employment group health coverage supported a delayed Part B decision, the Medigap Open Enrollment Period begins when the later Part B enrollment occurs, not when the individual first reached age 65. The source packet explicitly notes that when employer coverage ends and Part B is obtained without late-enrollment penalty, the Medigap Open Enrollment Period starts when the household is ready to use it.

The irreversibility of the six-month block is its central actuarial hazard. The 2026 Medigap guide states that if an individual is 65 or older, the one-time Medigap Open Enrollment Period begins when Part B is elected, and it cannot be changed or repeated. Medicare.gov's current Medigap guidance likewise states that the six-month period starts the first month the individual has Part B and is age 65 or older, and that this one-time enrollment does not repeat every year like the annual Medicare Open Enrollment Period. (Medicare) This distinction must be treated as a structural boundary. Annual Medicare election periods may permit changes to Medicare Advantage or Part D coverage, but they do not recreate the federal Medigap open-enrollment safe harbor. Once the six-month Medigap window closes, the applicant generally returns to ordinary commercial underwriting rules unless another guaranteed-issue right or state-specific protection applies.

Inside the valid open-enrollment window, the access mandate is broad. The 2026 Medigap guide states that during the Medigap Open Enrollment Period an individual may enroll in any Medigap policy sold in the state, that an insurance company cannot refuse to sell any of the Medigap policies it offers, and that the company cannot use medical underwriting to decide whether to accept the application or deny coverage because of pre-existing health problems. The federal definition of medical underwriting in the source packet describes the process by which an insurance company uses medical history to decide whether to accept an application, whether to add a pre-existing condition waiting period if state law allows, and how much to charge for insurance. During the Medigap Open Enrollment Period, that risk-selection apparatus is legally constrained at the entry point.

The pricing protection is equally significant. The official Medigap guide states that during the Medigap Open Enrollment Period, an individual generally gets better prices and more choices among policies, and the insurance company cannot charge more for a Medigap policy because of health problems. Medicare's definition section confirms that during this period an applicant cannot be denied a Medigap policy or charged more due to past or present health problems. This does not mean every same-letter policy has the same premium across all carriers, all states, or all rating methods. The source packet separately states that each insurance company decides how to price its Medigap policies and that community-rated, issue-age-rated, and attained-age-rated methods may be used; the open-enrollment rule bars health-status discrimination, not every lawful pricing variable.

The open-enrollment window therefore creates health-status neutrality, not universal price uniformity. Section 9.1 explained that standardized same-letter benefits are identical across issuers in most states, while premiums may differ. The source packet repeats that the premium amount is the only difference between same-letter policies sold by different companies, and that premium differences can be substantial even for the same standardized coverage. During the Medigap Open Enrollment Period, however, the issuer cannot make a health-impaired applicant pay more simply because of past or present medical problems. The legal significance is profound: the window does not eliminate commercial pricing; it strips the carrier of health-condition pricing discrimination for the protected applicant class.

The pre-existing condition rule is more limited than the underwriting rule, and it must be stated with precision. The open-enrollment period bars denial and health-status pricing discrimination, but it does not always eliminate every temporary pre-existing condition waiting period. The 2026 Medigap guide states that coverage can start right away, but an insurance company may make the applicant wait for coverage related to a pre-existing condition in some cases. It defines a pre-existing condition as a health problem existing before the new insurance policy starts, and states that in some cases the Medigap company can refuse to cover out-of-pocket costs for those pre-existing health problems for up to six months, after which the Medigap policy will cover the pre-existing condition. Thus, the open-enrollment period guarantees access to the contract, while the pre-existing condition rule can temporarily delay supplemental payment for a narrowly defined prior condition unless offset rules eliminate the delay.

The lookback period is also capped. The official Medigap guide states that coverage for a pre-existing condition can be excluded only if the condition was treated or diagnosed within the six months before the Medigap policy coverage begins; this is the lookback period. Original Medicare remains operative during this waiting period. The source packet notes that Original Medicare will still cover Medicare-covered services for the condition even if the Medigap policy does not, but the beneficiary remains responsible for the Medicare coinsurance or copayment during the Medigap waiting period. The waiting period therefore does not suspend Medicare itself. It suspends the supplemental policy's obligation for certain out-of-pocket costs tied to the pre-existing condition during the permitted period.

Creditable coverage offsets sharply limit this waiting-period exposure. The 2026 Medigap guide states that waiting periods for pre-existing conditions can be avoided or shortened when a Medigap policy replaces certain other health coverage that counts as creditable coverage. It defines creditable coverage for Medigap purposes generally as other health coverage recently held before applying for the Medigap policy, and states that if the individual had at least six months of continuous prior creditable coverage, the Medigap company cannot make the applicant wait before covering the pre-existing condition. The same source states that many types of health care coverage can count for this purpose, but only if the break in coverage was no more than 63 days. This creates a day-for-day mitigation system: prior continuous coverage reduces or eliminates the Medigap pre-existing condition waiting period.

The creditable-coverage offset is conceptually different from the Part B delayed-enrollment safe harbor analyzed in Chapters 5 and 8. For Part B, the critical rule is group health plan coverage based on current employment. For Medigap pre-existing condition offsets, the source packet uses a broader formulation: creditable coverage is generally other health coverage recently held before applying for the Medigap policy, subject to the no-more-than-63-day break rule. The two uses of "creditable" should not be collapsed into one legal concept. A coverage source may fail as a Part B current-employment safe harbor while still requiring separate analysis for Medigap pre-existing condition offset purposes. The Household Medicare Diagnostic Matrix must keep those rows separate because they protect against different risks.

Guaranteed issue rights add a second, event-based layer of protection outside the initial Medigap Open Enrollment Period. The source packet states that if a Medigap policy is purchased when a guaranteed issue right, also called Medigap protection, exists, the insurance company must cover all pre-existing health conditions without a pre-existing condition waiting period. These rights are not the same as the six-month open-enrollment period. They arise from specified events, such as certain losses or changes in other coverage, and are governed by their own plan-letter and timing rules. The presence of guaranteed issue rights is therefore a separate diagnostic question after the open-enrollment window has expired. Absence of such a right can leave the applicant exposed to ordinary underwriting and market exclusion.

The consequences outside the open-enrollment window are explicit in the federal materials. The 2026 Medigap guide states that outside the Medigap Open Enrollment Period an individual may have to pay more for a policy, fewer policy options may be available, and there is no guarantee that a company will sell a Medigap policy unless the applicant meets medical underwriting requirements or has a guaranteed issue right. This is the commercial reversion point. After the protected six-month federal window, the supplemental market may again classify risk, deny applications, or price the contract differently where federal guaranteed-issue protections or state law do not intervene. The open-enrollment period is therefore not merely a convenience period. It is the primary federal access gate for health-status-neutral entry into the Medigap market.

Under-age-65 Medicare eligibility demonstrates the limits of the federal rule. The official Medigap guide states that some states have additional open-enrollment periods, including periods for people under 65, but that if an individual is under 65 and has Medicare because of disability or End-Stage Renal Disease, the individual might not be able to buy the desired Medigap policy, or any Medigap policy, until turning 65. It further states that federal law generally does not require companies to sell Medigap policies to people under 65, although some states require or permit such sales, sometimes with higher premiums or underwriting. The same source states that a person already holding Part B before age 65 will still receive a Medigap Open Enrollment Period upon turning 65, often with more policy options and lower premiums, and that during that age-65 Medigap window companies cannot refuse to sell any Medigap policy because of disability or other health problems or charge a higher premium based on health status than they charge other people who are 65.

This under-age-65 limitation reinforces the importance of the age-65 trigger. The federal Medigap open-enrollment rule is not a universal disability-market guarantee. It is a specific six-month protection tied to age 65 and Part B enrollment, with state law supplying additional protections in some jurisdictions. For beneficiaries who qualify for Medicare before 65, the Household Medicare Diagnostic Matrix must therefore identify both the federal under-65 limitation and the later age-65 reset. A beneficiary may have limited Medigap access before age 65, then acquire the full federal Medigap Open Enrollment Period at 65, even if Medicare Part B was already in effect before that birthday.

Employer coverage creates a distinct timing strategy problem, but the rule must remain non-advisory and factual. The source packet states that if a person has group health coverage through an employer or union because the individual or spouse is currently working, delaying Part B may be appropriate in some cases because benefits based on current employment often provide coverage similar to Part B and because starting Part B prematurely could cause the Medigap Open Enrollment Period to expire before a Medigap policy is useful. When employer coverage ends, the same source explains that the individual may have a chance to sign up for Part B without late-enrollment penalty, and the Medigap Open Enrollment Period will start when Part B begins. The actuarial issue is synchronization: the household must align the end of employment-based coverage, the start of Part B, and the six-month Medigap access window so that the guaranteed-entry period is not wasted.

Retiree coverage must be distinguished from current-employment coverage. The source packet notes that for people with retiree coverage, Medicare pays first after retirement, and retiree coverage is probably similar to coverage from a Medigap policy because both can fill some gaps in Medicare coverage such as coinsurance and deductibles. That observation does not make retiree coverage identical to Medigap or recreate the Medigap Open Enrollment Period later. The matrix should treat retiree coverage as a potential alternative supplemental structure whose presence may affect perceived need, but not as a mechanism for restarting the federal six-month Medigap window. The decisive Medigap trigger remains age 65 or older plus Part B enrollment, with the one-time nonrepeatable federal open-enrollment clock beginning at that point.

The underwriting exposure after expiration is not merely theoretical. Medical underwriting, as defined in the source packet, includes the insurer's use of medical history to decide whether to accept an application, whether to add a waiting period for pre-existing conditions if state law allows, and how much to charge. Outside the Medigap Open Enrollment Period, the source packet states that there is no guarantee a company will sell a policy if medical underwriting requirements are not met, unless a guaranteed issue right applies. The expiration of the federal window can therefore transform Medigap from a guaranteed-access product into a medically underwritten product, with consequences that may include denial, reduced plan availability, or higher premiums. This is the asset-erosion risk embedded in timing failure.

Guaranteed renewability should be distinguished from guaranteed issue. The source packet states that any new Medigap policy issued since 1992 is guaranteed renewable even if the beneficiary has health problems, meaning that the insurance company cannot cancel the policy as long as the policyholder remains enrolled and pays the premium. Guaranteed renewability protects a policy after it has been issued. Guaranteed issue or open enrollment controls access before issuance. A household that already secured a Medigap policy has a renewal protection; a household that missed the open-enrollment window and lacks a guaranteed issue right may not be able to obtain the policy in the first place. The matrix must therefore separate acquisition rights from continuation rights.

The section title's reference to elimination of pre-existing condition exclusions must therefore be read as a layered federal protection, not as an unconditional erasure of every waiting period. During Medigap Open Enrollment, companies cannot deny issuance or charge more due to health problems, but they may, in some cases, impose a pre-existing condition waiting period up to six months for conditions treated or diagnosed during the six-month lookback period. That waiting period can be reduced or eliminated by prior continuous creditable coverage, and if six months of continuous prior creditable coverage exists, the company cannot impose the waiting period. If a guaranteed issue right applies, the company must cover all pre-existing conditions without the waiting period. The federal protection is therefore robust but not simplistic.

The Household Medicare Diagnostic Matrix treats Section 9.2 as the core timing and underwriting-control pillar. The matrix must record the first month of Part B coverage, the first month the individual is age 65 or older, the six-month Medigap Open Enrollment Period start and end dates, whether the applicant is under 65 with Medicare due to disability or ESRD, whether state law provides additional rights, whether employer current-coverage timing supports delayed Part B, whether a guaranteed issue right exists, whether prior creditable coverage exists, whether any break in creditable coverage exceeded 63 days, and whether a pre-existing condition was treated or diagnosed during the six-month lookback period. Each variable changes the risk profile. The source packet confirms that the open-enrollment period cannot be changed or repeated, that outside it policy access may shrink or become more expensive, and that medical underwriting may defeat the application absent guaranteed issue rights.

The final actuarial conclusion is that the Medigap Open Enrollment Period is a one-time federal market-access asset. It converts a voluntary private insurance market into a temporary guaranteed-access channel by forbidding denial and health-status pricing discrimination for applicants who are 65 or older and enrolled in Part B. It does not last indefinitely, does not repeat annually, does not automatically protect every under-65 Medicare beneficiary in every state, and does not always erase pre-existing condition waiting periods unless creditable coverage or guaranteed issue rules eliminate them. Under the Household Medicare Diagnostic Matrix, the open-enrollment window is therefore not a passive date range. It is the decisive legal interval during which the household can secure standardized private supplemental protection without health-status gatekeeping. Failure to synchronize Part B activation, employer-coverage termination, and Medigap application timing can convert a lifetime guaranteed-entry opportunity into permanent underwriting exposure, narrowed policy availability, higher premium risk, and long-term household capital erosion.

9.3 Long-Term Actuarial Pricing Methodologies

Medigap premium development is the point at which federal benefit standardization meets private actuarial pricing. The standardized letter architecture described in Section 9.1 makes the underlying benefits of a same-letter Medigap policy identical across insurers in most states, but it does not make the premium identical, nor does it freeze the future premium path. The 2026 Medicare source packet states that the benefits in each lettered Medigap plan are the same no matter which insurance company sells the policy, and that the premium is the only difference between policies with the same plan letter sold by different companies. The same source states that the cost of Medigap policies can vary widely depending on the insurance company, plan, and location, and that there can be large premium differences for the same standardized coverage. The actuarial problem is therefore not whether Plan G from one issuer contains a different standardized benefit package from Plan G from another issuer. The problem is how the same standardized liability is priced over time.

The macroeconomic structure of Medigap pricing is anchored in the fact that supplemental coverage pays after Original Medicare has assigned cost sharing to the beneficiary. A Medigap insurer must price the expected transfer of deductibles, coinsurance, copayments, and other standardized benefit categories while also accounting for medical utilization, claims inflation, administrative expense, regulatory requirements, and the composition of the insured block. The source packet states that each insurance company decides how it sets the price, called the premium, for its Medigap policies, and that the pricing method affects how much the policyholder pays now and in the future. This sentence is the core actuarial warning. The initial premium is only the first data point. The rating methodology determines whether future increases arise only from inflation and other non-age factors, from the applicant's age at issue, or from the applicant's attained age as it advances through later retirement.

The 2026 Medicare materials identify three pricing methods for Medigap policies: community-rated, also called no-age-rated; issue-age-rated, also called entry-age-rated; and attained-age-rated. These categories are not cosmetic labels. They define the mechanical relationship between age and premium movement. Under a community-rated arrangement, the premium is generally the same for everyone, regardless of age or gender; under an issue-age-rated arrangement, the premium is based on the age of the applicant when the Medigap policy is purchased; under an attained-age-rated arrangement, the premium is based on the policyholder's current age, so the premium rises as the policyholder grows older. The Household Medicare Diagnostic Matrix must therefore treat pricing methodology as a long-term cash-flow variable, not as a footnote to plan-letter selection.

Community rating, also called no-age rating, is the most direct pooling model. The Medicare source packet states that under this method the same premium is generally charged to everyone regardless of age or gender, and that the premium is not based on the policyholder's age. Its social insurance resemblance is obvious: the rate cell spreads expected claims across a community rather than assigning a higher premium simply because one member of the pool is older than another. The example in the source packet shows a 65-year-old and a 72-year-old buying the same Medigap policy and paying the same monthly premium under the community-rated method. The actuarial implication is that the younger or lower-utilization portion of the insured pool helps stabilize the aggregate cost of older or higher-utilization segments, while the insurer prices the entire community block to meet expected claims and expenses.

Community rating does not mean static pricing. The source packet states that community-rated premiums may go up because of inflation and other factors, but not because of the policyholder's age. The relevant volatility is therefore collective rather than individual-age-driven. A policyholder does not move into a higher rate solely because of turning 70, 75, or 80, but the whole community block may be repriced if claims experience, medical cost inflation, regulatory requirements, administrative costs, or other permissible rating factors support an increase. This creates a flatter individual age curve but not an immunity from premium increases. The source packet reinforces this broader pricing reality by stating that other factors, including residence, medical underwriting, and discounts, can affect premium amounts. Community rating removes age as the individual annual step-up factor; it does not eliminate inflationary or block-level repricing.

The community-rated model therefore tends to be analytically attractive for households concerned about advanced-age premium acceleration, but its baseline cost may reflect the insurer's expectation that the rate will apply across a mixed-age population. The source packet does not provide a universal rule that community-rated policies always begin higher than other rating methods, nor does it provide a national numerical premium curve. The defensible actuarial conclusion is more precise: community rating prevents premium increases based on the individual's advancing age, while permitting increases due to inflation and other factors. In long-range household modeling, that means the projected premium path should contain medical inflation assumptions and possible block repricing, but not an individual attained-age ladder. A lower or higher initial premium in a specific market remains a carrier, state, residence, and underwriting fact rather than a federal constant.

Issue-age rating, also called entry-age rating, creates a different premium architecture. The 2026 Medicare source packet states that the premium is based on the age of the applicant at the time the Medigap policy is purchased. The same source states that premiums are lower for people who buy at a younger age and will not change as the policyholder gets older, although premiums may still increase because of inflation and other factors. The mathematical baseline is therefore the age at contract entry. A 65-year-old applicant and a 72-year-old applicant may pay different starting premiums for the same policy letter because the older applicant entered the policy at a later age, but once the policy is issued, the premium is not increased merely because that same individual becomes older.

This model offers a distinct kind of long-term predictability. The issue-age rate embeds the applicant's age at purchase into the original premium classification and then holds the individual's age factor fixed. The source packet example shows a 65-year-old buying a policy for a lower monthly premium than a 72-year-old buying the same policy, because the second applicant is older at purchase. That example illustrates the actuarial logic: the entry age determines the pricing cell, and later birthdays do not, by themselves, create a new age-based cell. For a household entering Medicare at 65 and expecting a long retirement horizon, issue-age rating can create a premium path in which the age component is locked at a lower entry point, while medical inflation and other permitted increases remain active.

Issue-age rating should not be mistaken for a guaranteed level premium. The source packet is explicit that issue-age-rated premiums may go up because of inflation and other factors, but not because of age. Therefore, an issue-age policy can still experience increases through insurer-wide or block-wide adjustments, medical cost inflation, utilization changes, geographic rating factors, discount expiration, or other permissible state-regulated pricing mechanisms. The matrix must not classify issue-age rating as premium certainty. It should classify it as age-factor stability. The difference is substantial. Age-factor stability removes the automatic birthday-driven component from the long-term curve, but it does not immunize the policy against systemic medical inflation or insurer repricing.

The term "mathematical minimization" is useful only if applied carefully. Issue-age rating can minimize the lifetime effect of age-based premium growth when compared with an attained-age structure because the age factor is determined at purchase rather than repeatedly recalculated. The source packet supports this conclusion by stating that issue-age premiums do not change as the policyholder gets older, while attained-age premiums are based on current age and go up as the policyholder ages. However, the official materials do not establish a universal rule that every issue-age policy will produce the lowest lifetime cost in every jurisdiction, every rating environment, or every market cycle. Premiums can vary widely by insurance company, plan, and location, and other pricing factors may affect the amount paid. The lawful conclusion is comparative, not absolute: issue-age rating reduces age-driven volatility, while leaving non-age inflationary forces intact.

Attained-age rating is the most visibly volatile of the three methods because it contains a direct chronological multiplier. The 2026 Medicare source packet states that attained-age premiums are based on the policyholder's current age, so the premium goes up as the policyholder grows older. It further states that attained-age premiums may be low for younger buyers, may be the least expensive at first, but can eventually become the most expensive, and may also go up because of inflation and other factors. This structure creates two distinct increase channels: an age-driven increase as the policyholder advances through successive age cells, and a systemic increase from inflation or other non-age factors. The combination is the attained-age volatility trap.

The chronological multiplier is conceptually simple. Each year of age can move the policyholder to a new rate basis because the premium is determined by current age rather than age at issue. The source packet's attained-age example shows a policyholder buying at 65 for a stated monthly premium, then paying a higher monthly premium at 66 and a still higher premium at 67. The exact dollar amounts in the example are not actual costs, and the source packet notes that the examples are intended to show how age affects premiums and why future cost should be examined. The structural point remains: under attained-age rating, the policyholder's birthday can itself become a premium-increase event.

The systemic overlay compounds the practical cash-flow effect. The source packet states that attained-age premiums may also increase because of inflation and other factors. Therefore, an attained-age policyholder may experience an age-based increase and an inflation-based increase within the same broad rating trajectory. This should not be described as mathematical compounding in the strict sense unless the actual filed rate schedule applies one increase on top of another in a particular manner; the official source does not provide a universal formula. The safe actuarial statement is that the attained-age model exposes the household to dual premium pressures: one from advancing age and another from the same medical inflation and other factors that can affect all rating methods. Over a long retirement horizon, that dual exposure can produce substantially greater premium volatility than a model that excludes individual age progression after issue.

The out-of-pocket shock phase in attained-age rating is a premium-liquidity phenomenon rather than a claim-liability phenomenon. A Medigap policy may continue to absorb standardized cost-sharing categories as designed, but the premium required to keep that protection may rise materially in later age bands. The source packet warns that attained-age policies may be least expensive at first but can eventually become the most expensive. The household therefore faces a paradox: the policy may be most needed at ages 75, 80, or 85 because medical utilization and concern about Original Medicare exposure often rise with age, while the premium path may be moving into its most burdensome phase. The risk is not that the standardized benefit changes because of age. The risk is that the price of maintaining the same standardized benefit becomes increasingly difficult to sustain.

The twenty-year comparison among the three methodologies should begin with identical-benefit control. If the selected letter plan is the same, the benefits are standardized in most states and do not change merely because the pricing method changes. The source packet states that benefits in each lettered plan are the same no matter which company sells it, and that the premium is the only difference between same-letter policies sold by different companies. Therefore, the proper comparison is not benefit richness. It is premium trajectory. Community rating removes individual age from the premium base but allows inflation and other factors. Issue-age rating fixes the age factor at contract entry but allows inflation and other factors. Attained-age rating moves with current age and also allows inflation and other factors.

Across a twenty-year horizon, community-rated and issue-age-rated structures generally offer flatter age-related curves because neither increases the premium solely due to the policyholder's advancing age. The source packet supports that conclusion directly: community-rated premiums are not based on age, and issue-age-rated premiums do not change as the policyholder gets older. Their future premium paths remain exposed to medical inflation, location-based differences, carrier-specific pricing decisions, underwriting outside protected periods, discount structures, Medicare SELECT features, and high-deductible options where applicable. Attained-age rating, by contrast, can begin with a lower premium for younger buyers but may eventually become the most expensive because it rises with age and may also rise because of inflation and other factors. The long-term question is therefore whether early premium savings are sufficient to compensate for later age-based escalation.

This comparison cannot be made responsibly through first-year premium alone. A low attained-age premium at age 65 may be financially efficient during the first few policy years but may create later affordability pressure as age-rated increases accumulate. A higher issue-age or community-rated premium may appear less attractive at the outset but may produce a flatter age-driven premium path. The official guide itself warns that the way the company sets the premium affects how much is paid now and in the future. It also states that other factors such as place of residence, medical underwriting, discounts, Medicare SELECT network requirements, and high-deductible options can affect the premium. A twenty-year projection must therefore include both the rating methodology and these external variables, rather than treating the first quoted price as a lifetime proxy.

Discounts and special designs add further complexity. The source packet states that Medigap policy cost may depend on whether the insurance company offers discounts, such as for women, non-smokers, married people, annual premium payment, electronic funds transfer, or multiple policies. It also states that costs may depend on whether medical underwriting is used or a different premium is charged when there is no guaranteed issue right or Medigap Open Enrollment Period, whether Medicare SELECT is sold and requires use of certain providers for full benefits, and whether a high-deductible option is offered for Plans F or G. These factors can distort a superficial comparison. A discounted first-year premium may not represent the long-term base cost. A Medicare SELECT policy may be lower because it imposes network conditions for full benefits. A high-deductible version may have a lower premium because the beneficiary must first absorb a defined amount of covered costs before the policy pays.

Medical underwriting is not part of the rating-method triad, but it interacts with premium access. During a valid Medigap Open Enrollment Period or a guaranteed issue right, the source packet states that medical underwriting does not apply. Outside those protected windows, the source packet warns that a company may use medical underwriting or charge a different premium when the applicant lacks a guaranteed issue right or is not in the Medigap Open Enrollment Period. This matters because long-term premium modeling may be constrained by the inability to switch later. A policyholder who later finds an attained-age premium trajectory burdensome may not necessarily be able to move to a different rating method without underwriting, denial risk, or higher premium exposure, depending on state law and guaranteed issue circumstances. The matrix should therefore treat the initial rating choice as potentially durable.

The household solvency analysis must also distinguish premium volatility from out-of-pocket volatility. A richer standardized plan can reduce claim-level uncertainty by absorbing deductibles, coinsurance, copayments, and excess charges within its covered categories, but it can increase premium burden. A high-deductible or lower-premium design can reduce monthly premium burden but leave more claim exposure before the policy pays. The 2026 source packet states that high-deductible Plans F or G require the beneficiary to pay the first $2,950 in 2026 of deductibles, copayments, and coinsurance for covered services not paid by Medicare before the Medigap policy pays anything, plus a separate deductible for foreign travel emergency care. This shows that rating methodology is only one axis. Deductible design, benefit letter, SELECT status, and premium rating method combine to shape the household cash-flow curve.

A rigorous pricing analysis should therefore model four layers. The first layer is the standardized benefit letter, because same-letter policies provide the same basic benefits in most states. The second layer is the rating method, because community-rated, issue-age-rated, and attained-age-rated structures determine how age affects premium development. The third layer is insurer and market adjustment, because premiums may rise from inflation and other factors under all three rating methods.

The fourth layer is non-rating modifiers, including location, discounts, underwriting status, Medicare SELECT features, and high-deductible options. The actuarial error is treating any one layer as controlling when the household's actual premium path emerges from all four.

The Matrix should also distinguish federal standardization from state rating regulation. The source packet establishes that benefits of same-letter plans are standardized, while pricing methods and premiums vary by company, plan, and location. It also states that some states limit Medigap premium costs, and that state insurance departments and SHIP programs can provide additional information about local policy availability and costs. Therefore, the manuscript should not claim that one national premium method dominates all markets. State law, local rating rules, insurer filings, closed and open blocks, and market composition can influence outcomes. The federal source supports an analytic framework, not a universal pricing forecast.

The term "structural volatility" is especially appropriate for attained-age contracts. The official materials identify an age-based increase mechanism and warn that such policies may eventually become the most expensive. This structural volatility can be obscured during the initial purchase period because the attained-age premium may be lower for younger buyers. In a 20-year projection, however, the policyholder who entered at 65 may reach ages 75, 80, and 85 while the rate schedule continues to respond to attained age. Inflation and other factors may also increase the premium during the same period. The model's risk is delayed visibility: a first-year affordability advantage may convert into late-retirement pressure at the very time when switching options may be limited by underwriting rules or loss of guaranteed issue protection.

Issue-age and community-rated models carry a different volatility profile. Their core protection is that premiums do not increase because the individual grows older, according to the source packet's descriptions of both models. Their residual volatility is systemic: inflation, claims experience, location, discounts, and other factors may still move premiums. They may present higher initial premiums in some markets, but the official source does not make that a universal rule. Their principal actuarial value lies in reducing or eliminating the birthday-driven premium component. For a household seeking premium predictability across advanced age, that age-curve distinction may be more important than a modest first-year premium spread. For a household with shorter expected holding period or different liquidity constraints, the first-year and intermediate-year premium pattern may carry different weight. This remains an educational risk-classification observation, not a plan selection instruction.

The Household Medicare Diagnostic Matrix uses Section 9.3 to convert Medigap pricing from a quoted-premium comparison into a long-term premium-risk audit. The matrix must record the standardized plan letter, rating methodology, initial premium, whether the premium is community-rated, issue-age-rated, or attained-age-rated, whether age will affect future premium movement, whether inflation and other factors may increase premiums, whether the insurer offers discounts, whether the policy is Medicare SELECT, whether a high-deductible option applies, whether underwriting could affect future switching, and whether the household's retirement cash-flow model can tolerate late-age premium escalation. The source packet supplies the necessary rule hierarchy: same-letter benefits are standardized; premium is the difference between same-letter policies; companies may use three pricing methods; and the pricing method affects present and future cost.

The final actuarial conclusion is that Medigap pricing methodology can transform the same standardized benefit into radically different lifetime cash-flow exposures. Community rating spreads age risk across the community and prevents individual age from driving premium increases, while leaving inflation and other factors active. Issue-age rating locks the age factor at contract purchase and avoids later age-based increases, while leaving the policy exposed to market-wide increases. Attained-age rating may begin with the lowest apparent premium but contains an age-based escalation mechanism that can combine with inflation and other factors, producing the greatest long-horizon volatility risk. Under the Household Medicare Diagnostic Matrix, the analytic failure is not choosing a wrong letter in isolation. It is failing to map the premium curve attached to that letter. A policy that insulates against Original Medicare cost sharing can still erode household assets if its premium trajectory is misclassified, if later switching is medically underwritten, or if early affordability masks late-retirement volatility.

Chapter 10: The Managed Care Paradigm: Medicare Advantage (Part C)

10.1 Replacement Infrastructure Frameworks

Medicare Advantage is not a supplemental wrap placed on top of Original Medicare. It is a federally authorized replacement infrastructure through which a beneficiary remains inside the Medicare statute but receives most Part A and Part B coverage through a private Medicare-approved plan rather than through the traditional federal fee-for-service payment pipeline. Medicare & You 2026 defines a Medicare Advantage Plan as another way to receive Medicare Part A and Part B coverage, offered by private companies approved by Medicare and required to follow Medicare rules; it also states that after enrollment in a Medicare Advantage Plan, the beneficiary still has Medicare but receives most Part A and Part B coverage from the plan, not Original Medicare. The legal architecture is codified in 42 CFR Part 422, where an MA organization is defined as a public or private entity organized and licensed by a state as a risk-bearing entity, with certification by CMS to meet MA contract requirements, and an MA plan is defined as health benefits coverage offered under a policy or contract by an MA organization to Medicare beneficiaries residing in the plan's service area. (Legal Information Institute)

The replacement character of Part C must be stated with precision. The beneficiary does not surrender Medicare entitlement, and statutory Medicare rights continue to exist inside a private delivery arrangement. The operational claims pathway, however, changes. Medicare & You states that the Medicare Advantage enrollee must use the Medicare Advantage Plan card to obtain Medicare-covered services, while keeping the red, white, and blue Medicare card because it may be needed later. Section 422.101 requires each MA organization to provide coverage, by furnishing, arranging for, or making payment for, all Part A and Part B services covered by Medicare for an enrollee entitled to both parts, except for specified hospice and related special rules. (Legal Information Institute) The beneficiary therefore moves from a federal claims adjudication model into a private plan administration model, while the federal floor of Medicare-covered benefits remains embedded in the Part C contract.

The financing layer is capitation-based rather than open-ended fee-for-service reimbursement. Medicare & You 2026 states that Medicare pays a fixed amount each month to the companies offering Medicare Advantage Plans, and that those companies must follow rules set by Medicare. The Part 422 payment regulation states that CMS makes advance monthly payments for coverage of original fee-for-service benefits for an individual in an MA payment area, with payment tied to bids, benchmarks, rebates, service-area variation, and risk adjustment. (eCFR) Section

422.300 describes the payment subpart as governing payments to MA organizations offering local and regional MA plans, including calculation of MA capitation rates and benchmarks, conditions under which payment is based on plan bids, adjustments including risk adjustment, collection of risk-adjustment data, and other payment rules. (eCFR)

This payment structure changes the institutional incentives. Original Medicare pays claims through the traditional fee-for-service system, which 42 CFR § 422.2 defines as Original Medicare through the traditional fee-for-service payment system. (Legal Information Institute) A Medicare Advantage plan instead receives a monthly federal payment stream and must administer a benefit package approved by CMS within the plan's network, utilization-management, cost-sharing, and provider-contracting framework. A coordinated care plan under § 422.4 includes a network of providers under contract or arrangement with the organization to deliver the CMS-approved benefit package, and the regulation expressly recognizes mechanisms to control utilization, including referrals from a gatekeeper and financial arrangements that offer incentives to providers to furnish high-quality and cost-effective care. (Legal Information Institute) The economic tension is structural: the MA organization receives a regulated prospective payment, while clinical consumption, network adequacy, member access, quality rules, appeals rights, and administrative costs must be managed inside that framework.

The phrase "private plan assumes 100 percent of downside loss" should not be overstated beyond the official source record. The federal materials support the conclusion that MA organizations are risk-bearing entities authorized to accept prepaid capitation and that CMS pays monthly amounts subject to bid, benchmark, rebate, risk-adjustment, and other payment rules. (Legal Information Institute) (eCFR) They do not support an unqualified assertion that every MA organization always bears every dollar of loss without exception in every contractual, regional, or risk-adjusted context. The source-controlled conclusion is stronger because it is narrower: Medicare Advantage transfers operational claims administration and material insurance risk to a private, state-licensed, CMS-certified risk-bearing organization under a prospective payment system, creating powerful incentives for network management, utilization review, benefit design discipline, and cost-sharing controls. (Legal Information Institute)

The managed care overlay appears immediately in the coverage rules. Medicare & You 2026 states that Medicare Advantage Plans provide almost all medically necessary services Original Medicare covers, while Original Medicare continues to cover hospice care, certain clinical research costs, and some new benefits from laws or Medicare policy decisions. The same source states that plans may require use of participating network providers, may have annual out-of-pocket limits for Part A and Part B covered services, may offer non-emergency out-of-network coverage at higher cost, may require prior authorization for certain services or drugs, and may require referrals to specialists. Thus, Part C is not simply a different payer name. It is a private administrative environment in which benefit access, provider access, prior approval, and cost exposure can be governed by plan-specific rules that may change annually with required notice.

The HMO model represents the most concentrated form of network governance in the ordinary Medicare Advantage taxonomy. Medicare & You 2026 states that in an HMO Plan, care is generally obtained from doctors, other health care providers, or hospitals in the plan's network, except for emergency care, out-of-area urgent care, and out-of-area dialysis. The same source states that some HMO Plans allow out-of-network services through a point-of-service option, but that the beneficiary usually pays more for such services. This design converts geographic and contractual network boundaries into a primary risk-control instrument. The plan can concentrate care inside a contracted provider panel, control referral channels, and use network composition to govern unit costs, clinical pathways, and utilization.

The primary-care gatekeeper structure should be described as common rather than universal. Medicare & You 2026 states that most HMO Plans require selection of a primary care doctor, while certain services, such as yearly screening mammograms, do not require a referral. Section 422.112 recognizes the gatekeeper architecture at the regulatory level: if an MA organization requires enrollees to obtain a referral in most situations before receiving specialist services, the organization must either assign a primary care provider for referral purposes or make other arrangements to ensure access to medically necessary specialty care. (Legal Information Institute) This is not merely an administrative inconvenience. It is a formal care-access architecture. Specialist care can be routed through primary care selection, referral generation, network status, and prior plan rules before the service is treated as payable under the managed care contract.

The out-of-network rule in the HMO paradigm is severe but not absolute in every circumstance. Medicare & You states that if an HMO enrollee obtains care outside the network without prior authorization, the enrollee may have to pay the full cost. Federal regulation also preserves mandatory exceptions. Section 422.100 requires timely and reasonable payment for certain services obtained from noncontracting providers, including 911-dispatched ambulance services, emergency and urgently needed services, post-stabilization services, temporary out-of-area renal dialysis, and services that were denied by the plan but later found on appeal to be services the enrollee was entitled to have furnished or paid for. (eCFR) Section 422.113 makes the

MA organization financially responsible for emergency and urgently needed services regardless of whether the services are obtained inside or outside the organization and regardless of prior authorization. (eCFR) The household risk is therefore concentrated in non-emergency, non-urgent, nonauthorized out-of-network care.

The HMO risk analysis must also account for network change. Medicare & You 2026 states that providers can join or leave a plan's network at any time during the year, that the plan can also change network providers during the year, and that the beneficiary generally cannot change plans during the year solely because a provider leaves, although the plan must still give access to qualified doctors and specialists and must provide notices and transition help in specified circumstances. Section 422.112 requires coordinated care plans to maintain and monitor a provider network supported by written agreements and sufficient to provide adequate access to covered services, including primary care providers, specialists, hospitals, skilled nursing facilities, home health agencies, and behavioral health providers. (Legal Information Institute) The legal safety valve is network adequacy, not provider immutability. A household that relies on a particular physician or facility must distinguish access to an adequate network from guaranteed permanence of a specific provider relationship.

The PPO model shifts the managed-care design from exclusionary gatekeeping to tiered financial friction. Medicare & You 2026 states that PPO Plans have network doctors, specialists, hospitals, and other providers, while also permitting use of out-of-network providers for covered services, usually at higher cost, if the provider agrees to treat the enrollee and has not opted out of Medicare for Part A and Part B items and services. Under 42 CFR § 422.4, a PPO plan must have a network of providers that have agreed to contractually specified reimbursement for covered benefits, and it must provide reimbursement for all covered benefits regardless of whether those benefits are provided within or outside the provider network. (Legal Information Institute) The PPO therefore preserves a contractual right to coverage outside the preferred network, but the right is paired with different cost-sharing rules and provider acceptance conditions.

The local-versus-regional PPO distinction is statutory rather than merely marketing-based. Section 422.2 defines an MA local plan as an MA plan that is not an MA regional plan, and defines an MA regional plan as a coordinated care plan structured as a PPO that serves one or more entire regions. (Legal Information Institute) The same definition requires a regional MA plan to have a network of contracting providers with agreed reimbursement for covered services and to pay for all covered services whether provided inside or outside the network. (Legal Information Institute) The geographic footprint therefore matters. A local PPO is tied to a local service area; a regional PPO is structured around one or more entire CMS-approved regions. Both remain managed-care contracts, but their network breadth, provider contracting strategy, and out-of-network exposure architecture can differ.

PPO flexibility is not the same as Original Medicare freedom of provider access. Medicare & You 2026 states that Original Medicare generally permits use of any doctor or hospital that accepts Medicare, while Medicare Advantage enrollees may need to use network doctors and other providers for non-emergency care, and some plans offer non-emergency out-of-network coverage at higher cost. Medicare & You also states that PPO enrollees do not need to choose a primary care doctor and, in most cases, do not need a referral to use a specialist, but costs for covered services are usually lower when in-network specialists are used rather than out-of-network specialists. The PPO tradeoff is therefore not provider freedom without friction. It is broader provider access in exchange for tiered cost sharing and possible assignment or provider-acceptance issues outside the network.

The official source packet does not support a universal statement that out-of-network PPO coinsurance "often" reaches a specific 30 to 50 percent range across all plans. It does support the broader structural conclusion that out-of-network care can cost more and that plan-specific cost sharing, deductibles, and network status materially affect household liability. Medicare & You 2026 states that out-of-pocket costs in a Medicare Advantage Plan depend in part on whether the service is obtained from a network provider or a provider that does not contract with the plan; if a non-emergency or non-urgent service is obtained from a non-network doctor, facility, supplier, or other provider, the plan may not cover the service or costs may be higher. Federal cost-sharing rules also establish maximum cost-sharing constraints for MA basic benefits; the official regulatory source states that for certain in-network basic benefits not otherwise specified and for out-of-network basic benefits, MA plans generally must not establish cost sharing exceeding 50 percent coinsurance or an actuarially equivalent copayment value. (Legal Information Institute) The lawful analysis is therefore that PPO out-of-network utilization can create substantial point-of-service financial exposure within regulated limits, not that every PPO applies a fixed national percentage.

The Private Fee-for-Service model is the Part C anomaly because it is neither a traditional HMO gatekeeper structure nor a standard PPO preferred-network model. Medicare & You 2026 states that a PFFS enrollee may go to any Medicare-approved doctor, other provider, or hospital that accepts the plan's payment terms, agrees to treat the enrollee, and has not opted out of Medicare for Part A and Part B items and services. Section 422.4 defines an MA private fee-for-service plan as an MA plan that pays providers at a rate determined by the plan on a fee-for-service basis without placing the provider at financial risk and that does not restrict enrollee choice among providers who are lawfully authorized to provide services and agree to accept the plan's terms and conditions of payment. (Legal Information Institute) The central risk is not a gatekeeper. It is provider acceptance of the private plan's terms.

The PFFS provider-access risk is episodic and practical. Medicare & You 2026 states that if a PFFS plan has a network, network providers have agreed to always treat plan members, while out-of-network doctors, hospitals, and other providers may decide not to treat the enrollee even if the provider has treated that enrollee before. The same source states that in a medical emergency, doctors, hospitals, and other providers must treat the enrollee, and that the PFFS plan decides the amount paid for services and provides annual cost-sharing information through the Annual Notice of Change and Evidence of Coverage. Thus, the point-of-service hazard in PFFS is not simply price. It is the possibility that a non-network provider will decline the plan's terms and conditions for the encounter.

The PFFS drug-coverage rule also differs from coordinated care plans. Section 422.4 states that MA organizations offering coordinated care plans must offer qualified Part D coverage in that plan or another MA plan in the same area, while PFFS organizations can choose to offer qualified Part D coverage in the PFFS plan. (Legal Information Institute) Medicare & You 2026 states the same operational rule: PFFS plans sometimes cover prescription drugs, and if a PFFS plan does not offer Medicare drug coverage, the enrollee can join a separate Medicare drug plan. This contrasts with many PPO or HMO configurations where Medicare drug coverage is commonly integrated and separate Part D enrollment may be constrained by plan type. The matrix must therefore track whether a PFFS file includes drug coverage or requires a separate Part D decision.

The Part C framework also contains a legal incompatibility with Medigap. Medicare & You 2026 states that it is illegal for someone to sell a Medigap policy to a person in a Medicare Advantage Plan unless the person is switching back to Original Medicare, and that Medigap cannot be used to pay Medicare Advantage copayments, deductibles, and premiums. This rule underscores the replacement nature of Part C. Medigap is a secondary supplement to Original Medicare; Medicare Advantage is the private pathway for receiving Part A and Part B benefits. A beneficiary file cannot solve Medicare Advantage network or cost-sharing exposure by layering Medigap on top of the plan. The risk-control instruments inside Part C are the plan's out-of-pocket maximum, provider network, prior authorization rules, cost-sharing design, appeals rights, and, where applicable, trial-right or enrollment-period protections.

The out-of-pocket maximum is the principal statutory cash-flow constraint inside Medicare Advantage, but it should not be mistaken for unlimited protection against every charge. Medicare & You 2026 states that Medicare Advantage Plans set a yearly limit on out-of-pocket costs for Part A and Part B covered services and that after the limit is reached, the enrollee pays nothing for Part A and Part B covered services for the rest of the year. The same guide states that Original Medicare has no yearly out-of-pocket limit unless supplemental coverage exists, while Medicare Advantage plans have yearly limits for covered Medicare services, which may include different in-network and out-of-network limits. The limitation is tied to covered Medicare services under the plan. Premiums, noncovered services, extra benefit charges, and services obtained outside plan rules may not behave like protected in-network covered cost sharing.

Coverage determinations and prior authorization convert medical necessity into an administrative file. Medicare & You 2026 states that an enrollee or provider can request an organization determination from the plan in advance to determine whether a service, drug, or supply is covered and how much the enrollee must pay, and that this sometimes functions as prior authorization before the plan covers the item or service. If coverage is denied, the plan must provide written notice and appeal rights. This is a major distinction from the traditional Original Medicare pathway, where the handbook notes that Original Medicare generally does not require prior approval to use a covered benefit and generally does not require a specialist referral. Medicare Advantage therefore relocates part of the risk from open provider access to administrative authorization timing.

The Household Medicare Diagnostic Matrix must treat Part C as a replacement infrastructure with multiple embedded risk rows. The first row identifies Part A and Part B entitlement, because Medicare Advantage enrollment requires both Part A and Part B, residence in the plan service area, and lawful presence or citizenship status under the 2026 handbook. The second row identifies plan type, including HMO, PPO, PFFS, MSA, and SNP categories. The third row identifies whether the plan is a coordinated care plan under § 422.4, because coordinated care plans may include networks, utilization controls, gatekeeper referrals, and provider incentives. (Legal Information Institute) The fourth row identifies the plan's service area, network status, provider availability, referral rules, prior authorization rules, and continuity-of-care implications when providers leave the network.

The matrix must then separate HMO, PPO, and PFFS hazards. For an HMO, the core risk is unauthorized non-emergency out-of-network utilization, because Medicare & You states that out-of-network care without authorization may leave the enrollee paying the full cost, subject to emergency, urgent, out-of-area dialysis, and other required exceptions. For a PPO, the core risk is tiered out-of-network cost sharing and provider willingness to treat, because PPO plans allow out-of-network covered services usually at higher cost if the provider agrees and has not opted out of Medicare. For PFFS, the core risk is acceptance of plan terms and conditions, because out-of-network providers may decide not to treat the enrollee even after prior treatment history, while network providers in a PFFS network have agreed to always treat plan members.

The final synthesis is that Medicare Advantage replaces the payment and delivery infrastructure of Original Medicare with a private, CMS-regulated, capitated or bid-based managed care system. The beneficiary retains Medicare status, but the operating environment becomes a private plan contract governed by 42 CFR Part 422, federal payment rules, service-area limits, network adequacy obligations, provider contracts, cost-sharing schedules, prior authorization processes, organization determinations, and appeal rights. (eCFR) (Legal Information Institute) The Household Medicare Diagnostic Matrix therefore treats Part C not as a supplement selection, but as a replacement architecture audit. Failure to map the plan type, network boundary, referral rule, out-of-network liability, PFFS provider-acceptance condition, drug-coverage status, and annual out-of-pocket limit can convert an ordinary physician visit, diagnostic test, hospital referral, or specialist consultation into an unhedged household liability. Within capitated private Medicare delivery, the decisive risk is not only whether a service is medically necessary. It is whether the service is obtained through the correct contractual channel, at the correct network tier, under the correct authorization rule, from a provider whose relationship with the plan supports payment at the point of care.

10.2 The Maximum Out-of-Pocket (MOOP) Mandate

The Maximum Out-of-Pocket mandate is the central financial safety valve inside the Medicare Advantage structure. Its statutory purpose is clearest when contrasted with Original Medicare. Under the 2026 Medicare handbook, Original Medicare generally requires the beneficiary to pay a portion of the cost for each covered service, and there is no yearly limit on what the beneficiary may pay out of pocket unless another coverage layer, such as Medigap, Medicaid, employer, retiree, or union coverage, applies. The same handbook states that for Part B-covered services under Original Medicare, the beneficiary usually pays 20 percent of the Medicare-approved amount after satisfying the annual Part B deductible, and that Original Medicare has no yearly out-of-pocket limit. Medicare Advantage reverses that particular exposure by placing a federal ceiling on annual Part A and Part B cost sharing inside a private plan contract. Medicare & You 2026 states that Medicare Advantage Plans set a yearly limit on what the enrollee pays out of pocket for services covered under Part A and Part B, and that once the plan's limit is reached, the enrollee pays nothing for Part A and Part B-covered services for the rest of the year.

The MOOP requirement is not a discretionary consumer feature or a marketing generosity category. It is a regulatory requirement embedded in the Part C benefit structure. Pursuant to 42 CFR § 422.100(f)(4), Medicare Advantage local plans must have an enrollee in-network maximum out-of-pocket amount for basic benefits that is no greater than the annual limit calculated by CMS using Medicare fee-for-service data projections, and Medicare Advantage organizations are responsible for tracking enrollee out-of-pocket spending and alerting enrollees and contracted providers when the in-network MOOP amount is reached. (eCFR) Under 42 CFR § 422.101, the basic benefit package requires the Medicare Advantage organization to provide coverage, by furnishing, arranging for, or making payment for, all services covered by Part A and Part B for an enrollee entitled to both parts, subject to Medicare coverage rules and plan service-area requirements. (eCFR) The MOOP mandate therefore converts a private managed-care arrangement into a bounded risk ecosystem for Medicare-covered medical services, while leaving noncovered and nonmedical exposures outside the protected accumulator.

The regulatory genesis is actuarial. CMS does not set the MOOP limit by arbitrary political preference. Section 422.100 defines Medicare fee-for-service data projections for MOOP purposes as projections of beneficiary out-of-pocket costs for the applicable contract year, based on recent Medicare fee-for-service data, including data for beneficiaries with and without diagnoses of End-Stage Renal Disease, consistent with generally accepted actuarial principles and practices. (eCFR) For 2024 and subsequent years, CMS annually calculates mandatory and lower MOOP limits by increasing or decreasing the prior year's limits to reflect specified percentiles of Medicare fee-for-service data projections, with the 95th percentile informing the mandatory MOOP and the 85th percentile informing the lower MOOP, subject to rounding rules and caps on annual increases where applicable. (eCFR) The regulatory objective is to limit maximum beneficiary exposure without making Medicare Advantage benefit packages actuarially unstable or discriminatory for high-cost conditions.

The 2026 CMS bid-review memorandum supplies the operative dollar architecture. CMS states that it followed §§ 422.100(f) and 422.101(d) to calculate the CY 2026 MOOP limits, using Medicare fee-for-service data projections and applying the applicable regulatory methodology. (mabenefitsmailbox.lmi.org) For 2026, the finalized Part C table establishes three in-network MOOP bands. Health Maintenance Organization and HMO point-of-service plans may use a lower MOOP range of $0 to $4,200, an intermediate range of $4,201 to $6,750, or a mandatory range of $6,751 to $9,250. Private Fee-for-Service plans use the same $0 to $4,200 lower range, $4,201 to $6,750 intermediate range, and $6,751 to $9,250 mandatory range. (mabenefitsmailbox.lmi.org) The statutory meaning is that $9,250 is the 2026 maximum in-network medical MOOP for the mandatory category, not a guaranteed plan-specific limit for every enrollee in every plan.

CMS's lower and intermediate MOOP categories create a regulated benefit-design spectrum rather than a single universal ceiling. The 2026 bid-review memorandum defines the mandatory MOOP category as the highest in-network MOOP amount allowed by CMS, defines the lower MOOP category as a voluntarily adopted lower in-network MOOP established by CMS in exchange for increased flexibility in cost-sharing requirements, and defines the intermediate MOOP category as a midpoint between lower and mandatory limits to encourage lower in-network MOOP amounts with some flexibility in cost-sharing requirements. (mabenefitsmailbox.lmi.org) The incentive is regulatory, not a direct consumer subsidy. A carrier that chooses a lower medical MOOP accepts a tighter catastrophic ceiling for enrollees, while CMS permits corresponding flexibility in specified cost-sharing standards. The plan must still comply with all applicable Part C cost-sharing, anti-discrimination, actuarial equivalence, bid, and benefit rules. (mabenefitsmailbox.lmi.org)

Preferred Provider Organization designs require a second accumulator because they contain both in-network and out-of-network covered-service pathways. Under 42 CFR § 422.100(f)(5), the local PPO in-network MOOP limits apply only to in-network providers, and local PPO plans must establish a combined enrollee MOOP amount for basic benefits provided in-network and out-of-network that is no greater than the total catastrophic limit applicable to regional plans under § 422.101(d)(3). (eCFR) The regulation further requires PPO plans to use the same MOOP type, lower, intermediate, or mandatory, for both the in-network MOOP and the combined in-and-out-of-network MOOP. (eCFR) For 2026, CMS's table sets PPO lower MOOP ranges at $0 to $4,200 in-network and $0 to $6,300 combined, intermediate ranges at $4,201 to $6,750 in-network and $4,201 to $10,100 combined, and mandatory ranges at $6,751 to $9,250 in-network and $6,751 to $13,900 combined. (mabenefitsmailbox.lmi.org)

The PPO dual-track design creates a material household accounting risk. An enrollee may reach an in-network MOOP while still having a higher combined in-network and out-of-network exposure ceiling that remains unresolved because out-of-network cost sharing is tracked in the broader combined ledger. Medicare & You 2026 states that Medicare Advantage out-of-pocket costs depend on whether services are received from a network provider or a provider that does not contract with the plan; if a non-emergency or non-urgent service is obtained from a provider outside the plan network, the plan may not cover the service or costs may be higher. The 2026 bid-review memorandum reinforces this distinction by requiring local and regional PPO plans to enter both in-network and combined MOOP amounts in the Plan Benefit Package, while HMOs generally enter only in-network amounts and PFFS plans use plan-type-specific MOOP structures. (mabenefitsmailbox.lmi.org) A household that treats the in-network MOOP as the universal spending ceiling can therefore underestimate the financial impact of authorized but higher-cost out-of-network utilization.

The MOOP accumulator protects covered medical cost sharing, not every expenditure associated with a Medicare Advantage contract. The Medicare Managed Care Manual states that the annual MOOP dollar limits include all cost sharing, specifically deductibles, coinsurance, and copayments, for Part A and Part B services, although a Medicare Advantage plan may also include supplemental benefits as services subject to the MOOP. (Centers for Medicare & Medicaid Services) Medicare & You 2026 similarly states that the plan's yearly out-of-pocket limit applies to all Part A and Part B-covered services and that once the limit is reached, the enrollee pays nothing for Part A and Part B-covered services. The accumulation rule is therefore categorical: the protected dollars are cost-sharing dollars assigned to covered Part A and Part B medical benefits under the plan's benefit design, not every dollar that leaves the household account.

The eligible-accumulation category includes the major medical liabilities that define Medicare Advantage catastrophic exposure. Hospital copayments, inpatient cost sharing, physician copayments, outpatient coinsurance, durable medical equipment coinsurance, Part B drug cost sharing, skilled nursing facility cost sharing, dialysis cost sharing, emergency and urgently needed service cost sharing, and other plan-imposed deductibles, coinsurance, or copayments for Medicare-covered Part A and Part B services are the kinds of medical cost-sharing amounts that fall inside the MOOP framework when they are plan-covered and properly owed by the enrollee. CMS's manual states that the annual MOOP includes all cost sharing for Part A and Part B services, and it separately requires plans to track enrollee out-of-pocket costs and notify enrollees when they reach or approach the plan's MOOP limit. (Centers for Medicare & Medicaid Services) Section 422.100 also requires plan cost sharing for specified basic benefits to comply with annual CMS limits and actuarial principles. (eCFR)

The phrase "diagnostic laboratory fees" requires careful legal classification. If a diagnostic service is a covered Part A or Part B basic benefit and the plan lawfully assigns deductible, copayment, or coinsurance to the enrollee, the enrollee's cost-sharing amount is part of the MOOP logic. If Original Medicare or the Medicare Advantage plan assigns no cost sharing for a specific preventive or laboratory category, there is no enrollee amount to accumulate. If a charge is for a noncovered service, an unauthorized out-of-network service outside applicable exceptions, a missed appointment fee, a lifestyle service, or a supplemental benefit outside the plan's MOOP inclusion rules, the charge does not automatically become protected merely because it was health-related. The Manual's accumulation rule is explicitly tied to cost sharing for Part A and Part B services, with supplemental-benefit inclusion permitted only where the plan elects and structures it that way. (Centers for Medicare & Medicaid Services)

The non-accumulation exclusions follow from the same definition. Monthly plan premiums, the Part B premium, the Part A premium where owed, optional supplemental benefit premiums, noncovered services, convenience items, lifestyle benefits, and charges for services obtained outside plan rules are not basic-benefit cost sharing merely because they appear in the household's healthcare budget. Medicare & You 2026 separates the plan premium and Part B premium from the plan's yearly limit on out-of-pocket costs for Part A and Part B-covered services, listing them as distinct cost factors in the Medicare Advantage cost discussion. The Medicare Managed Care Manual similarly defines the MOOP as including deductibles, coinsurance, and copayments for Part A and Part B services, while classifying Part D prescription drug benefits and supplemental benefits separately from basic benefits. (Centers for Medicare & Medicaid Services) A household that counts premiums toward the MOOP will overstate progress toward catastrophic medical protection.

Balance-billing language must be handled with precision in Part C. In Original Medicare, non-participating providers may in many cases charge a limiting charge above the Medicare-approved amount, as analyzed in Chapter 9. Medicare Advantage, by contrast, is administered under plan payment rules, provider contracts, noncontracting-provider protections, and plan-specific cost-sharing obligations. The 2026 Medicare handbook states that out-of-pocket costs in Medicare Advantage depend on whether the provider is in the network, whether the provider accepts assignment in certain plan types when out of network, and whether the service is non-emergency or non-urgent out-of-network care that the plan may not cover or may cover at higher cost. Amounts that are not plan-covered cost sharing for Part A and Part B basic benefits cannot be assumed to accumulate toward MOOP. The matrix must therefore separate lawful plan cost sharing from noncovered provider charges or unauthorized out-of-network liabilities.

The Part D firewall is the most important exclusion. Medicare Advantage plans often include Medicare drug coverage, but the medical MOOP and Part D out-of-pocket system are separate statutory and actuarial tracks. Medicare & You 2026 states that Medicare Advantage Plans set a yearly out-of-pocket limit for Part A and Part B-covered services, while Part D separately helps cover prescription drug costs and is administered by private insurers that follow Medicare rules. CMS's final 2026 Part D redesign materials state that the CY 2026 Part D annual out-of-pocket threshold is

$2,100, reflecting the Inflation Reduction Act redesign of the Part D benefit. (Centers for Medicare & Medicaid Services) The Medicare Managed Care Manual also states that special rules apply to collection of cost sharing related to Part D benefits offered in MA-PD plans, and those rules are found in the Prescription Drug Benefit Manual rather than the Part C benefit chapter. (Centers for Medicare & Medicaid Services)

The result is a two-ledger insurance contract for many Medicare Advantage enrollees. The medical ledger tracks Part A and Part B basic-benefit cost sharing toward the plan's medical MOOP. The prescription drug ledger tracks Part D covered-drug spending toward the Part D statutory out-of-pocket threshold. A plan document may present both inside one Evidence of Coverage, but federal law does not merge them into a single household catastrophic cap. Medicare & You 2026 states that most Medicare Advantage Plans include Part D and that some plan types may permit or require separate drug coverage rules, but the same handbook's medical-cost section identifies the annual out-of-pocket limit specifically for Part A and Part B-covered services. A household that reaches the Part D $2,100 covered-drug threshold has not automatically reached the Part C medical MOOP; a household that reaches the medical MOOP has not thereby eliminated Part D premium obligations, noncovered drugs, or drug charges outside the Part D protected structure. (Centers for Medicare & Medicaid Services)

The chronological reset rule is embedded in the annual nature of the benefit design. CMS annually calculates MOOP limits for the contract year, and the 2026 bid-review memorandum identifies the CY 2026 limits as contract-year values calculated from CMS methodology. (mabenefitsmailbox.lmi.org) Medicare & You 2026 describes Medicare Advantage Plans as setting a yearly limit, explains that once the limit is reached the enrollee pays nothing for Part A and Part B-covered services for the rest of the year, and separately states that annual coverage and cost changes take effect in January through the Annual Notice of Change and Evidence of Coverage framework. The MOOP accumulator is therefore not a lifetime ledger and not a rolling twelve-month medical deductible. It is a plan-year mechanism tied to the contract year and the plan's approved benefit package.

The calendar reset has meaningful actuarial consequences. A beneficiary who reaches the medical MOOP in September receives protection for additional covered Part A and Part B cost sharing only through the remaining part of that plan year. The following January begins a new contract-year accounting environment, with potentially new premiums, cost sharing, service areas, network composition, covered supplemental benefits, and medical MOOP amount reflected in the plan's Annual Notice of Change and Evidence of Coverage. Medicare & You 2026 states that Medicare Advantage rules can change each year and that the plan must notify enrollees about changes before the next enrollment year; it also states that Annual Notices of Change include changes in coverage and costs effective in January, while the Evidence of Coverage gives details about what the plan covers and how much the enrollee pays for the next year. The MOOP is therefore a strong annual barrier against catastrophic covered medical cost sharing, but it is not a multi-year reserve.

Mid-year plan transfer rules require more precision than the common assumption that accumulators always start over. The official Medicare Managed Care Manual states that during a contract year, when an enrollee switches to another plan of the same type offered by the plan, the accumulated annual contribution toward the MOOP limit in the previous plan to date is counted toward the MOOP limit in the new Medicare Advantage plan; where applicable, the transfer applies to both in-network and out-of-network MOOP. (Centers for Medicare & Medicaid Services) The same manual states that Medicare Advantage plans may extend transferability so that a contribution toward annual MOOP applies to a mid-year transfer into any Medicare Advantage plan type offered by the same Medicare Advantage organization, such as movement from an HMO to a PPO offered by that same organization. (Centers for Medicare & Medicaid Services) Thus, the source record does not support a categorical statement that all out-of-pocket progress is completely nontransferable in every mid-year plan change.

The corrected risk statement is sharper. MOOP transfer is not a universal federal portability right across all plan sponsors, all carriers, all plan types, and all mid-year enrollment events. CMS requires specified transfer treatment when the move is to another plan of the same type offered by the same plan or organization, and permits broader transferability across plan types within the same Medicare Advantage organization. (Centers for Medicare & Medicaid Services) A cross-organization move, a move into a plan that does not inherit the prior accumulator under CMS rules or plan policy, or a move into a different benefit design outside the permitted transfer structure can create a reset risk. Medicare & You 2026 confirms that Medicare Advantage Plans can charge different out-of-pocket costs and have different rules for services, and that plan rules, networks, coverage, costs, and service areas can change by enrollment year. For high-utilization households, the practical danger is not only a new provider network. It is the possibility of entering a new cost-sharing ledger before the prior year's protection has generated full economic value.

The transfer issue is especially important during Special Enrollment Periods, service-area moves, plan terminations, provider-network disruptions, and transitions between HMO, PPO, PFFS, SNP, and other Medicare Advantage structures. Medicare & You 2026 states that Medicare Advantage enrollment changes are available only at certain times, including Open Enrollment, Medicare Advantage Open Enrollment, and qualifying Special Enrollment Periods. The 2026 bid-review memorandum shows that each plan type has different MOOP data-entry structures: HMOs generally use in-network MOOP, local and regional PPOs require in-network and combined MOOP, and PFFS plans use PFFS-specific required MOOP amounts with optional in-network and out-of-network entries depending on network type. (mabenefitsmailbox.lmi.org) A mid-year transfer therefore requires a plan-type, sponsor, and accumulator audit, because the successor contract may not mirror the predecessor contract's in-network, out-of-network, or combined MOOP accounting.

The Medicaid and dual-eligible exception illustrates why MOOP should be viewed as a beneficiary-liability ledger rather than a theoretical plan-cost ledger. The Medicare Managed Care Manual states that for any dual eligible enrollee, Medicare Advantage plans must count toward the MOOP limit only those amounts the individual enrollee is responsible for paying, net of any state responsibility or exemption from cost sharing, and not merely the cost-sharing amounts established in the plan benefit package; as a result, for dual eligible enrollees not responsible for Medicare Parts A and B cost sharing, the MOOP limit will rarely, if ever, be reached, although plans must still track out-of-pocket spending. (Centers for Medicare & Medicaid Services) This rule demonstrates the legal nature of MOOP: it protects against enrollee responsibility for covered medical cost sharing, not abstract claim value.

The MOOP mandate also interacts with service-category cost-sharing ceilings. Under § 422.100(f)(6), Medicare Advantage plans must not impose cost sharing for specified basic benefits above levels annually determined by CMS to be discriminatory, and for 2026 and subsequent years, professional service categories are subject to cost-sharing limits that vary by MOOP type, with mandatory MOOP plans limited to 30 percent coinsurance or actuarially equivalent copayment, intermediate MOOP plans limited to 40 percent, and lower MOOP plans limited to 50 percent, subject to plan-payment minimums and other regulatory standards. (eCFR) CMS also applies generally accepted actuarial principles and practices in projections and calculations under the MOOP and cost-sharing rules. (eCFR) This means that MOOP is not the only protection against excessive point-of-service charges. It is the catastrophic ceiling layered above category-specific safeguards.

The Household Medicare Diagnostic Matrix treats Section 10.2 as the catastrophic medical-exposure pillar for Medicare Advantage. The matrix must record the plan type, in-network MOOP, combined MOOP if applicable, whether the plan uses lower, intermediate, or mandatory MOOP status, whether services are in-network, out-of-network, emergency, urgent, dialysis-related, authorized, or noncovered, whether the charge is a deductible, copayment, or coinsurance for a Part A or Part B basic benefit, whether Medicaid or another payer eliminates enrollee liability, whether the plan includes supplemental benefits in the MOOP, and whether a separate Part D accumulator applies. The source hierarchy is explicit: § 422.100 requires in-network MOOP, PPO combined MOOP, CMS annual calculation, and plan tracking; § 422.101 defines basic benefits as Part A and Part B covered services; and the Medicare Managed Care Manual explains that MOOP includes cost sharing for Part A and Part B services, while Part D and supplemental benefits occupy separate benefit categories. (eCFR) (eCFR) (Centers for Medicare & Medicaid Services)

The matrix must also resist the most common consumer-level compression error: treating every out-of-pocket dollar as MOOP-eligible. A monthly premium is not a medical cost-sharing accumulator. An optional supplemental benefit charge is not automatically a Part A or Part B basic benefit cost-sharing amount. A Part D drug copayment belongs to the Part D ledger, not the Part C medical MOOP ledger. An unauthorized out-of-network service that the plan does not cover cannot be made MOOP-eligible by retrospective classification. A lifestyle benefit, noncovered convenience service, or charge outside Medicare-covered medical care must be separately tested. Medicare & You 2026 anchors this distinction by tying the plan's yearly out-of-pocket limit to Part A and Part B-covered services, while separately listing premiums, deductibles, network status, extra benefits, and Part D coverage as distinct cost factors.

The final actuarial conclusion is that MOOP is a powerful but bounded federal risk-control device. It distinguishes Medicare Advantage from Original Medicare by imposing an annual catastrophic ceiling on covered Part A and Part B medical cost sharing, a ceiling that Original Medicare lacks unless supplemental protection exists. It also creates internal distinctions that can determine whether the ceiling functions as intended: lower versus intermediate versus mandatory limits, in-network versus combined PPO limits, Part A and Part B basic benefits versus Part D drug costs, medical cost sharing versus premiums, and transferable versus nontransferable accumulator scenarios. For 2026, CMS's final Part C limits place the mandatory in-network ceiling at $9,250 and the mandatory PPO combined ceiling at $13,900, with lower and intermediate MOOP categories available under CMS rules. (mabenefitsmailbox.lmi.org) Under the Household Medicare Diagnostic Matrix, failure to identify the exact MOOP type, service category, network track, calendar-year reset, Part D firewall, and mid-year transfer rule can convert a managed-care asset-protection feature into an unhedged source of cash-flow friction, particularly for high-utilization households whose liability emerges quickly and repeatedly inside a single contract year.

10.3 Utilization Management and Network Restrictions

Utilization management is the economic control surface of the Medicare Advantage paradigm. A Medicare Advantage organization receives federal payment through a private Part C contract and administers Medicare-covered benefits through plan rules, provider networks, cost-sharing structures, and coverage determination systems rather than through the ordinary Original Medicare fee-for-service channel. Medicare & You 2026 states that Medicare pays a fixed monthly amount to companies offering Medicare Advantage Plans, that those companies must follow Medicare rules, and that each plan may have different rules for how services are obtained, including referral requirements, network-use requirements for non-emergency or non-urgent care, and prior authorization for certain services or drugs. Under the Part C regulatory framework, a Medicare Advantage plan must provide coverage of basic benefits, meaning Part A and Part B services, by furnishing benefits directly, arranging for them, or paying for them, subject to the conditions and limitations in 42 CFR Part 422. (eCFR) Utilization management therefore should not be reduced to an arbitrary administrative obstacle. It is the operational mechanism by which a capitated or bid-based private delivery system manages clinical volume, protects the plan's contracted provider network, and converts broad Medicare entitlement into a controlled service pathway.

The tension between fee-for-service Medicare and capitated managed care is structural. Original Medicare generally allows access to any provider that accepts Medicare and, as Medicare & You 2026 explains, usually does not require a specialist referral and generally does not require prior approval to use a covered benefit. Medicare Advantage, by contrast, can require network providers, prior authorization, referrals, and plan-specific procedures before coverage attaches to a given service. Fee-for-service payment systems tend to finance volume after services are delivered, while managed care systems attempt to classify and authorize care before or during the service event. The economic reason is apparent: a private plan operating under federal payment rules must reconcile enrollee clinical demand, Medicare coverage obligations, medical necessity standards, network capacity, administrative costs, and quality expectations inside a finite contractual framework. Federal law permits management, but it increasingly confines management through coverage criteria, medical necessity rules, network adequacy standards, notification obligations, appeal rights, and oversight duties.

Prior authorization is the most visible instrument of administrative friction. Medicare & You 2026 states that for certain Medicare Advantage services or drugs, the enrollee may need plan approval, called prior authorization, before the plan covers them. The same handbook describes an organization determination as a decision that can be obtained in advance from the plan to find out whether a service, drug, or supply is covered and how much the enrollee will have to pay; sometimes this advance decision is required as prior authorization before the plan covers the item or service. The pre-service review pipeline therefore begins with a proposed medical service, moves through a plan-defined documentation channel, applies Medicare coverage and medical necessity criteria, and ends with approval, denial, a request for additional information, or, where urgency standards are met, a faster determination. When coverage is denied, Medicare & You 2026 states that the plan must provide written notice and appeal rights.

The federal standards governing prior authorization have become increasingly explicit. Under 42 CFR § 422.138, when a coordinated care plan uses prior authorization for basic or supplemental benefits, the plan must comply with the prior authorization section, and prior authorization may be used only to confirm diagnoses or other medical criteria that form the basis for coverage, to ensure that a basic benefit is medically necessary under § 422.101(c)(1), or to ensure that a supplemental benefit is clinically appropriate. (eCFR) That language matters because it narrows prior authorization from a free-standing cost-containment veto into a coverage-verification and medical-necessity instrument. CMS's 2024 Medicare Advantage and Part D final rule described the same reform as requiring coordinated care plan prior authorization policies to be used only to confirm diagnoses or other medical criteria or to ensure that an item or service is medically necessary, while also requiring continuity protections and annual utilization-management review. (Centers for Medicare & Medicaid Services)

Coverage criteria are not plan-invented from first principles. Pursuant to 42 CFR § 422.101, Medicare Advantage organizations must comply with CMS national coverage determinations, general coverage and benefit conditions included in Traditional Medicare laws unless superseded by MA-specific law, and written coverage decisions of local Medicare contractors with jurisdiction for the geographic area in which services are covered under the plan. (eCFR) Internal plan criteria may be used only when coverage criteria are not fully established in applicable Medicare statutes, regulations, NCDs, or LCDs, and those internal criteria must be publicly accessible and supported by current evidence in widely used treatment guidelines or clinical literature. (eCFR) Medical necessity determinations must be based on the applicable coverage and benefit criteria, whether the item or service is reasonable and necessary under section 1862(a)(1) of the Social Security Act, the enrollee's medical history, physician recommendations, clinical notes, and, where appropriate, involvement of the plan's medical director. (eCFR)

The 2026 prior authorization layer adds a specific denial-reason and transparency track. Beginning January 1, 2026, 42 CFR § 422.122 requires a Medicare Advantage organization that denies a prior authorization request, excluding drug requests as defined in the referenced rule, to provide the provider with a specific reason for the denial regardless of the method used to communicate the information. (eCFR) Beginning in 2026, the same regulation requires annual public reporting of prior authorization metrics, including lists of items and services requiring prior authorization, percentages of approvals and denials, approvals after appeal, extensions, expedited approvals and denials, and average and median decision times. (eCFR) CMS's Interoperability and Prior Authorization final rule separately explains that impacted payers, including Medicare Advantage organizations, must implement certain operational provisions generally beginning in 2026 and that beginning in 2026 payers must provide a specific reason for denied prior authorization decisions, while API requirements generally begin later. (Centers for Medicare & Medicaid Services)

Clinical review capacity is also regulated. Under 42 CFR § 422.137, a Medicare Advantage organization that uses utilization management policies and procedures, including prior authorization, must establish a utilization management committee led by the plan's medical director. The committee must include a majority of practicing physicians, at least one independent practicing physician free of plan conflict, at least one practicing physician with expertise in care of elderly or disabled individuals, and members representing various clinical specialties. (eCFR) The same regulation requires the committee to review all utilization management policies and procedures at least annually, including prior authorization, and that review must consider the services to which utilization management applies, Traditional Medicare coverage decisions and guidelines including NCDs, LCDs, and laws, and relevant current clinical guidelines. (eCFR) The Part C system therefore allows managed care controls, but it requires those controls to be clinically reviewed, documented, and tied to Medicare coverage standards rather than unsupported commercial rationing.

Prior authorization approval now has stronger continuity significance. Under 42 CFR § 422.138(c), if a Medicare Advantage organization approves a covered item or service through prior authorization, a pre-service determination, or a concurrent determination during inpatient or outpatient services, the organization may not later deny coverage on the basis of lack of medical necessity and may not reopen the decision except for good cause or reliable evidence of fraud or similar fault. (eCFR) CMS's 2024 final rule similarly states that approval for a course of treatment must be valid as long as medically reasonable and necessary to avoid disruptions in care, considering applicable coverage criteria, the patient's medical history, and the treating provider's recommendation. (Centers for Medicare & Medicaid Services) This rule reduces retroactive denial risk after approval, but it does not remove the pre-service obligation where plan rules require prior authorization before services are furnished.

The financial liability of non-compliance must be described with regulatory precision. Medicare & You 2026 states that if a Medicare Advantage enrollee obtains non-emergency health care outside an HMO network without authorization, the enrollee may have to pay the full cost. It also states that out-of-pocket costs depend on whether services are received from a network provider or a provider that does not contract with the plan; if a non-emergency or non-urgent service is obtained from a non-network provider, the plan may not cover the service or costs may be higher. The proper legal conclusion is not that every missing authorization automatically creates beneficiary liability in every plan type and every factual circumstance. Federal emergency and urgent-care rules, provider-contract rules, appeal rights, and plan documents can alter liability. The reliable conclusion is that failure to obtain required prior authorization can convert an otherwise medical service into a denied, delayed, or disputed claim, with potential provider or household financial exposure depending on the service, network status, plan type, notice rules, and appeals outcome.

Emergency and urgently needed services form a mandatory exception to ordinary authorization gates. Under 42 CFR § 422.113, a Medicare Advantage organization is financially responsible for emergency and urgently needed services regardless of whether the services are obtained inside or outside the organization and regardless of prior authorization. (eCFR) The regulation also defines urgently needed services as non-emergency covered services that are medically necessary and immediately required when the enrollee is temporarily outside the plan's service area or when the network is temporarily unavailable or inaccessible and it was not reasonable to obtain services through the plan. (eCFR) This exception prevents the managed care apparatus from requiring prior authorization in acute circumstances where delay would undermine safety. It also marks the boundary between legitimate network management and unlawful interference with emergency access.

Referral gates represent a distinct managed-care control separate from prior authorization. Medicare & You 2026 states that in many Medicare Advantage Plans, including HMOs, use of providers in the plan network is required, prior authorization may be required for certain services or drugs, and referrals may be required to use specialists. For HMO Plans specifically, the 2026 handbook states that a primary care doctor is required in most cases, a referral is required in most cases to use a specialist, and certain services such as yearly mammogram screenings do not require a referral. Under 42 CFR § 422.112, if a Medicare Advantage organization requires enrollees to obtain a referral in most situations before specialist services, the organization must either assign a primary care provider for referral purposes or make other arrangements to ensure access to medically necessary specialty care. (eCFR)

The primary care physician in a gatekeeper model functions as a clinical and administrative clearinghouse. The PCP channel organizes first-contact care, coordinates diagnostic routing, controls access to specialty panels where the plan requires referrals, and helps preserve the integrity of the network's utilization assumptions. From an actuarial perspective, the referral gate reduces unmanaged specialist entry, repetitive diagnostic sequences, duplicative consultations, and direct movement into higher-cost service environments without a primary clinical screen. Under § 422.112, however, the gatekeeping mechanism cannot be used to deny access to medically necessary specialty care. The plan must provide or arrange necessary specialty care, must maintain an ongoing source of primary care for enrollees who accept it, and must establish written standards for timely access to care and medical necessity determinations. (eCFR)

Self-referral in a referral plan can nullify coverage only when the plan documents and applicable law support that outcome. The strictest version appears in the HMO rule. Medicare & You 2026 states that if non-emergency health care is obtained outside the HMO network without authorization, the full cost may fall on the enrollee, and it emphasizes the importance of following plan rules such as obtaining prior approval when required. In an in-network specialist context, a missing referral may create denial or claim-processing exposure if the plan's Evidence of Coverage requires referral documentation before the specialist visit. The institutional rule is that referral compliance is part of the plan's coverage pathway. A service can be medically appropriate and still administratively defective if the plan requires a PCP referral and the required referral is absent, subject to the plan's member-protection rules, provider liability rules, exceptions, and appeal rights.

Network adequacy supplies the regulatory counterweight to utilization control. The relevant numerical network adequacy standards are not contained solely in 42 CFR § 422.112. Section 422.112 establishes access-to-services obligations, including PCP panels, specialty care access, network-unavailable out-of-network coverage at in-network cost sharing, timely appointment standards, and continuity-of-care requirements. (eCFR) The detailed time-and-distance and minimum-provider methodology is codified in 42 CFR § 422.116. Under § 422.116, network-based Medicare Advantage plans must demonstrate adequate contracted provider networks sufficient to provide access to covered services, and beginning with contract year 2024, new or expanding service-area applicants must demonstrate compliance as part of the CMS application process, with CMS permitted to deny an application based on network evaluation. (eCFR)

The time-and-distance rules are mathematical access standards. Section 422.116 requires Medicare Advantage plans to meet maximum time and distance standards and contract with a specified minimum number of each provider and facility-specialty type; those criteria vary by county type. (eCFR) The regulation classifies county environments, including large metro, metro, micro, rural, and counties with extreme access considerations, and CMS annually publishes a Health Service Delivery Reference file identifying minimum provider and facility number requirements, provider and facility time-and-distance standards, and ratios used for network reviews. (eCFR) For example, the base time and distance table in § 422.116 lists primary care at 10 minutes and 5 miles in large metro counties, 15 minutes and 10 miles in metro counties, 30 minutes and 20 miles in micro counties, 40 minutes and 30 miles in rural counties, and 70 minutes and 60 miles in counties with extreme access considerations. (eCFR)

The provider-specialty list is broad because network adequacy is not satisfied merely by contracting with hospitals and primary care offices. Section 422.116 identifies provider-specialty types such as primary care, cardiology, dermatology, endocrinology, gastroenterology, general surgery, gynecology and obstetrics, nephrology, neurology, oncology, ophthalmology, orthopedic surgery, podiatry, psychiatry, pulmonology, rheumatology, urology, clinical psychology, and clinical social work; it also identifies facility-specialty types including acute inpatient hospitals, cardiac services, critical care, outpatient surgical services, skilled nursing facilities, diagnostic radiology, mammography, physical therapy, occupational therapy, speech therapy, inpatient psychiatric facility services, outpatient infusion and chemotherapy, and outpatient behavioral health. (eCFR) The network is therefore reviewed as a multi-dimensional clinical infrastructure, not as a single directory count.

Minimum provider counts are also quantitative. Section 422.116 states that for certain provider and facility specialties, CMS calculates the minimum number by multiplying the minimum ratio by the number of beneficiaries required to cover, dividing the result by 1,000, and rounding up to the next whole number. (eCFR) The same regulation states that provider-specialty ratios represent the minimum number of providers per 1,000 beneficiaries, while the acute inpatient hospital ratio represents beds per 1,000 beneficiaries. (eCFR) Separately, Medicare Advantage plans must ensure that at least 85 percent of beneficiaries in micro, rural, or extreme-access counties have access to at least one provider or facility of each specialty type within published time-and-distance standards, and at least 90 percent of beneficiaries in large metro and metro counties have such access. (eCFR) These thresholds establish a population-access standard rather than an individualized guarantee that every specialist will be located immediately adjacent to every beneficiary.

Network adequacy does not make provider networks static. Medicare & You 2026 states that providers can join or leave a plan's network at any time during the year, that the plan can also change network providers during the year, and that the enrollee usually cannot change plans during the year solely because a provider leaves, although the plan must still provide access to qualified doctors and specialists. The same source states that if the network changes, the plan must help the enrollee choose a new provider to continue managing care, help continue needed care already in progress, and notify the enrollee about enrollment periods and possible options for changing plans. Section 422.112 adds the regulatory backstop: when an in-network provider or benefit is unavailable or inadequate to meet medical needs, the plan must arrange for and cover medically necessary covered benefits outside the provider network at in-network cost sharing. (eCFR)

The network disruption trap is therefore not theoretical. A major multi-specialty group, hospital system, behavioral health provider panel, oncology group, or diagnostic facility can leave a network after the plan year has begun. Medicare & You 2026 confirms that network participation can change during the year and that such changes generally do not automatically permit plan switching, except through available enrollment periods or qualifying special circumstances. Federal rules provide notice and access protections, but those protections may require re-routing care, transferring records, obtaining new referrals, re-submitting prior authorization requests, confirming continuity-of-care rules, or invoking an organization determination or appeal. For a high-utilization household, the economic injury is not only the possibility of a denied claim. It is the administrative time cost, care interruption risk, and cash-flow uncertainty created when a previously stable treatment pathway must be rebuilt inside a changed network.

The network-disruption analysis must be linked back to utilization management because the two systems interact. A new network specialist may require a new PCP referral. A continuing treatment plan may require confirmation that prior authorization remains valid under the successor provider relationship. A facility change may alter site-of-service cost sharing. A service available in Original Medicare without prior approval may require Medicare Advantage authorization before the plan pays. Medicare & You 2026 states that Medicare Advantage costs and rules can change each year, that plans must notify enrollees before the next enrollment year, and that Annual Notice of Change and Evidence of Coverage materials provide the relevant annual rules, coverage, and cost details. The household file must therefore track both the network map and the administrative map. A provider listed in the network is not the same as a fully authorized service.

The Household Medicare Diagnostic Matrix treats Section 10.3 as the utilization-management and network-adequacy control pillar for Part C. The matrix must identify whether the plan type uses a gatekeeper structure, whether a PCP is required, whether specialist referrals are required, whether the service is subject to prior authorization, whether the requested service is a basic benefit or supplemental benefit, whether Medicare NCDs or LCDs govern the coverage criteria, whether internal plan criteria are publicly accessible and evidence-based, whether the UM committee has reviewed the applicable policy, whether emergency or urgent-service exceptions apply, whether the provider is in network, whether the plan's network is adequate under federal time-and-distance and minimum-provider standards, and whether an in-network service is unavailable or inadequate, triggering the out-of-network in-network-cost-sharing protection under § 422.112. (eCFR) (eCFR) (eCFR)

The final synthesis is that utilization management is the internal friction system of privatized public coverage. It allows a Medicare Advantage organization to manage service flow, prevent unmanaged specialty utilization, channel care through contracted networks, and require administrative proof that a service meets Medicare coverage and medical necessity standards. Federal law simultaneously limits that friction through NCD and LCD conformity, publicly accessible internal criteria when Medicare criteria are incomplete, medical director responsibility, utilization-management committee review, specific denial reasons, public reporting metrics, emergency and urgent-care protections, appeal rights, and network adequacy standards. (eCFR) (eCFR) (eCFR) (eCFR) Under the Household Medicare Diagnostic Matrix, a valid Medicare entitlement can still become a denied, delayed, or financially disputed service if the beneficiary file fails to map prior authorization, referral gates, network status, service-area limits, continuity-of-care protections, and appeal pathways before care is delivered. The operational risk inside Part C is therefore not only clinical need. It is the conversion of clinical need into an authorized, network-compliant, medically necessary, administratively documented, and federally protected covered service.

MODULE V: THE FOUR PHASES OF THE PRESCRIPTION DRUG PARADIGM (PART D)

Chapter 11: Actuarial Flow of the Part D Benefit Design

11.1 The Stage-by-Stage Allocation Matrix

The modern Medicare Part D benefit is governed by a statutory accounting system that measures prescription-drug liability through True Out-of-Pocket cost accumulation rather than through a simple tally of total pharmacy spending. TrOOP is not equivalent to total drug cost, plan liability, manufacturer liability, or household premium expenditure. It is the regulated ledger that determines when a Part D enrollee crosses from ordinary cost-sharing status into catastrophic protection. Under 42 CFR § 423.100, incurred costs for Part D purposes include specified costs for covered Part D drugs not paid under the plan because of deductible or cost-sharing rules before the enrollee satisfies the out-of-pocket threshold, but only when those costs are paid by the enrollee or by another permitted person or entity in a manner not reimbursed through insurance, a group health plan, or another third-party payment arrangement, subject to the regulation's special post-2025 rules. (eCFR)

The term TrOOP therefore describes a federal allocation engine, not merely a beneficiary checkbook. CMS's TrOOP guidance states that payments count only when they are for specified drug costs, are made by or on behalf of the person enrolled in a Medicare drug plan, and are not covered by other insurance. Payments that count include deductible amounts and copayments or coinsurance for covered prescriptions, along with certain payments made by permitted outside sources, while payments that do not count include the share paid by the Medicare drug plan, monthly drug plan premiums, drugs purchased outside the United States and its territories, drugs not covered by the plan, excluded drugs even if covered as supplemental benefits, over-the-counter drugs or most vitamins, and payments made or reimbursed by group health plans, other insurance, and several other third-party arrangements. The resulting ledger is highly selective. It advances the beneficiary through the Part D year only when the payment belongs to the statutory cost-sharing universe.

The post-Inflation Reduction Act structure must be stated with historical accuracy. The familiar coverage gap, commonly called the donut hole, no longer governs the modern defined standard Part D benefit after 2024. The current Part D regulation states that the coverage gap is the period between the initial coverage limit and the out-of-pocket threshold during the years 2006 through 2024, and 42 CFR § 423.104

states that for 2025 and each subsequent year there is no coverage gap. (eCFR) (eCFR) The post-2025 benefit design therefore moves from deductible status into initial coverage, and then from initial coverage into catastrophic status once the annual out-of-pocket threshold is reached. The historic four-stage vocabulary survives as institutional memory, but the operative non-LIS standard benefit for 2026 contains no donut-hole phase.

The current dollar threshold also requires exact correction. The $2,000 figure is the 2025 statutory baseline established by the Inflation Reduction Act redesign. For calendar year 2026, CMS states that the annual Part D out-of-pocket threshold is $2,100, reflecting the original 2025 $2,000 cap adjusted by the annual percentage increase in average expenditures for covered Part D drugs. (Centers for Medicare & Medicaid Services) The 2026 Medicare handbook states the same beneficiary-facing rule: yearly out-of-pocket costs for covered Part D drugs are capped at $2,100 in 2026, and after that cap is reached no copayment or coinsurance is owed for covered Part D drugs for the rest of the calendar year. Section 11.1 therefore treats $2,100 as the operative 2026 threshold, while recognizing $2,000 as the 2025 redesign baseline.

The annual deductible phase is the first formal boundary in the standard Part D allocation matrix. CMS's Final CY 2026 Part D Redesign Program Instructions state that the 2026 defined standard deductible is $615 and that the enrollee pays 100 percent of gross covered prescription drug costs until that deductible is met. (Centers for Medicare & Medicaid Services) The appendix to the same CMS instructions lists the 2026 deductible phase as 100 percent beneficiary cost sharing with a $615 deductible. (Centers for Medicare & Medicaid Services) During this phase, the plan has not yet entered ordinary post-deductible cost-sharing operation for the drug claim, although the enrollee receives the benefit of negotiated prices for covered Part D drugs under 42 CFR § 423.104(g). (eCFR) The deductible is therefore a front-end attachment point: the covered drug cost is still being adjudicated through the Part D system, but the enrollee bears the full covered-drug cost up to the deductible limit.

Every properly paid beneficiary dollar in the deductible phase performs two accounting functions. First, it satisfies the plan deductible, subject to the plan's approved benefit design and the defined standard structure. Second, because the payment is for a covered Part D drug cost not paid by the plan due to application of the deductible, it enters the incurred-cost ledger that moves the enrollee toward the annual out-of-pocket threshold under 42 CFR § 423.100. (eCFR) The distinction matters because a payment for a noncovered drug, a drug not treated as covered through a coverage determination or appeal, an excluded drug, an over-the-counter item, or a premium charge does not become TrOOP merely because it was paid at a pharmacy. CMS's TrOOP guidance states that only formulary drugs, or nonformulary drugs treated as being on the formulary through coverage determination, exception, or appeal, and obtained through an allowed pharmacy channel, count toward TrOOP.

The initial coverage phase begins after the deductible is satisfied. Under the 2026 defined standard design, CMS states that the enrollee pays 25 percent coinsurance for covered Part D drugs in the initial coverage phase. The sponsor typically pays 65 percent of the cost of applicable drugs and selected drugs, 75 percent of the cost of all other covered Part D drugs, the manufacturer typically covers 10 percent of applicable-drug cost through the Manufacturer Discount Program, and CMS pays a 10 percent selected-drug subsidy during a price applicability period. (Centers for Medicare & Medicaid Services) This formula is the post-IRA redistribution of drug liability. It is no longer a simple split between beneficiary and plan; it is a four-cornered allocation among beneficiary, plan sponsor, manufacturer, and federal subsidy mechanisms depending on whether the drug is applicable, non-applicable, or selected.

The beneficiary-facing version of the initial coverage phase may appear as fixed copayments, tiered copayments, coinsurance, or an actuarially equivalent plan-specific design rather than the pure defined standard 25 percent coinsurance formula. The 2026 Medicare handbook states that actual drug costs vary based on prescriptions, formulary status, drug tier, drug benefit phase, pharmacy type, and Extra Help status. The governing regulation permits standard prescription drug coverage to use coinsurance equal to 25 percent of actual cost or actuarially equivalent average expected coinsurance of no more than 25 percent, and permits approved tiered copayments consistent with the applicable regulatory requirements. (eCFR) Thus, a beneficiary may experience the initial coverage phase through a fixed copayment for one tier and a coinsurance percentage for another, but the actuarial engine remains the same: covered drug claims continue to accumulate toward the out-of-pocket threshold through the permitted TrOOP components.

The manufacturer-discount rule is one of the most important post-IRA corrections. Under the former coverage gap structure, CMS's older TrOOP guidance identified manufacturer discounts under the Medicare Coverage Gap Discount Program as payments that could count toward TrOOP. That older framework corresponds to the donut-hole period through 2024. The current regulation, however, states that for 2025 and subsequent years, incurred costs include certain reimbursed costs through insurance, group health plans, or other third-party arrangements, but do not include payments by a manufacturer under the Manufacturer Discount Program. (eCFR) Therefore, under the modern 2026 Part D redesign, the manufacturer's 10 percent initial coverage discount for applicable drugs affects total liability allocation, but it should not be treated as beneficiary TrOOP. The TrOOP ledger is narrower than the total financing stack.

The end of the initial coverage phase is no longer controlled by a historical initial coverage limit. The regulation states that for 2025 and each subsequent year there is no initial coverage limit, and the same regulation states that for 2025 and later there is no coverage gap. (eCFR) CMS's 2026 instructions state that the initial coverage phase ends when the enrollee reaches the annual out-of-pocket threshold of $2,100 for 2026. (Centers for Medicare & Medicaid Services) The modern horizon is therefore a direct TrOOP horizon: after deductible satisfaction, the beneficiary remains in initial coverage until the statutory out-of-pocket threshold is reached, without passing through a separate donut-hole claim architecture. This creates a more linear cost path than the prior benefit design, although plan formularies, tiers, negotiated prices, pharmacy networks, and utilization controls can still produce considerable month-to-month variability before the threshold is reached.

The elimination of the coverage gap fundamentally changed the cash-flow profile of Part D. Prior designs created a mid-year psychological and financial cliff because the beneficiary could move into a coverage gap after the initial coverage limit and encounter a distinct cost-sharing regime before catastrophic coverage. The current eCFR language terminates that concept for 2025 and subsequent years by eliminating both the initial coverage limit and the coverage gap. (eCFR) CMS's 2026 redesign instructions carry that structure forward by presenting only three standard non-LIS phases: deductible, initial coverage, and catastrophic. (Centers for Medicare & Medicaid Services) This is the central structural stabilization enacted through the Inflation Reduction Act redesign. The prior donut-hole interruption is replaced by a continuous accumulation model that moves the enrollee toward a statutory out-of-pocket ceiling.

The catastrophic phase is the terminal annual protection stage. Under 42 CFR § 423.104, after an enrollee's incurred costs exceed the annual out-of-pocket threshold, cost sharing is zero dollars for 2024 and each subsequent year. (eCFR) CMS's 2026 instructions state that in catastrophic coverage the enrollee pays no cost sharing for covered Part D drugs; sponsors typically pay 60 percent of covered Part D drug costs, manufacturers typically pay a 20 percent discount for applicable drugs, and CMS pays a reinsurance subsidy equal to 20 percent for applicable drugs and 40 percent for non-applicable drugs and selected drugs during the applicable period. (Centers for Medicare & Medicaid Services) The beneficiary's liability drops to zero, but the system's liability does not disappear. It is redistributed among sponsor liability, manufacturer discount liability where applicable, and federal reinsurance.

The catastrophic window must therefore be described as beneficiary risk insulation, not total system cost elimination. Once the 2026 $2,100 annual out-of-pocket threshold is reached, the Medicare handbook states that no copayment or coinsurance is owed for covered Part D drugs for the rest of the calendar year. The Medicare & You text also states that the yearly out-of-pocket Part D drug cap applies to covered Part D drugs and that once the cap is reached no copayment or coinsurance applies for the rest of the calendar year. The phrase "covered Part D drugs" remains critical. Noncovered drugs, excluded drugs, drugs outside the formulary unless obtained through exception or appeal, premiums, Part D IRMAA, and other non-TrOOP items do not become free merely because the catastrophic threshold has been reached.

The calendar-year reset is the second major temporal rule. The 2026 Medicare handbook describes the Part D out-of-pocket cap as applying to covered Part D drugs for the rest of the calendar year once the cap is reached. CMS's 2026 redesign instructions also state that when TrOOP is administered on a calendar-year basis, no 2025 TrOOP accumulation can apply for 2026 and the TrOOP accumulator resets on January 1, 2026 using the 2026 defined standard deductible and annual out-of-pocket threshold. (Centers for Medicare & Medicaid Services) The allocation matrix therefore resets every January 1 for ordinary calendar-year Part D administration. A beneficiary who reached catastrophic coverage in November does not remain in catastrophic status indefinitely; the deductible and TrOOP ledger restart for the next calendar year unless an unusual non-calendar-year employer group waiver plan rule applies under CMS guidance.

The Medicare Prescription Payment Plan does not alter this phase progression. Medicare & You 2026 states that the payment option spreads out-of-pocket costs for covered drugs across the calendar year, may help manage expenses, but does not save money or lower drug costs. CMS guidance on the program states that participation does not affect how the enrollee moves through the Part D benefit or what counts toward TrOOP, and TrOOP-eligible costs remain treated as incurred based on the date each Part D claim is adjudicated. (Centers for Medicare & Medicaid Services) The program is therefore a liquidity mechanism, not a benefit redesign. It can smooth monthly cash flow, but it does not lower the deductible, reduce the $2,100 statutory threshold, change the manufacturer-discount allocation, or merge Part D costs into Part C medical MOOP accounting.

Mid-year plan movement creates administrative friction, but the official rule is transferability rather than forfeiture. CMS's TrOOP guidance states that when a person switches Medicare drug plans during the year, the TrOOP balance transfers to the new Medicare drug plan, and Medicare has established processes for transferring that balance, with periodic updates for late claims and possible use of the most recent Explanation of Benefits if discrepancies arise. The Part D Coordination of Benefits Manual states that sponsors must track TrOOP and correctly apply it to the TrOOP limit, and that the TrOOP threshold and gross covered drug spending are calculated annually and must be transferred between Part D sponsors when a beneficiary disenrolls and re-enrolls before the end of the coverage year. (Centers for Medicare & Medicaid Services) The correct risk statement is therefore not that TrOOP is lost. It is that the transfer mechanism can produce short-term reconciliation lag, claims reprocessing, or documentation demands during the administrative handoff.

The transfer pipeline is itself a federal data process. CMS's manual describes the NCPDP Financial Information Reporting standard and the CMS Part D Transaction Facilitator, which identifies enrollment changes, generates transactions to prior sponsors, collects monthly gross covered drug costs and TrOOP amounts, and forwards year-to-date accumulated data to the current plan of record. (Centers for Medicare & Medicaid Services) This system exists because the TrOOP ledger is beneficiary-specific and calendar-year-specific, while plan membership may change inside that year. If the data move cleanly, the new plan can place the beneficiary in the correct deductible, initial coverage, or catastrophic status. If data lag or discrepancies occur, the beneficiary file may temporarily experience pharmacy-counter confusion, higher apparent cost sharing, or later adjustment. The administrative risk is timing and reconciliation, not legal non-transferability.

The stage-by-stage allocation matrix also interacts with formulary control. Medicare & You 2026 states that drug costs vary based on whether prescriptions are on the plan's formulary, what tier a drug is in, which benefit phase applies, and which pharmacy is used. Under 42 CFR § 423.100, a covered Part D drug is a Part D drug included on the formulary or treated as included because of a coverage determination or appeal, and obtained at a network pharmacy or an out-of-network pharmacy in accordance with the applicable rules. (eCFR) This means that the TrOOP horizon cannot be modeled merely from a retail receipt. The underlying drug must be a covered Part D drug in the plan's adjudication system, and pharmacy channel rules must be satisfied. A nonformulary drug paid entirely out of pocket outside the exception or appeal pathway does not necessarily advance the statutory ledger.

The Household Medicare Diagnostic Matrix treats Section 11.1 as the Part D pharmaceutical cash-flow pillar. The matrix must identify the plan deductible, the defined standard deductible for the calendar year, the covered status of each drug, the formulary tier, the pharmacy channel, the benefit phase at the time of dispensing, the beneficiary-paid cost sharing, permitted third-party TrOOP payments, excluded payments, manufacturer-discount status, selected-drug subsidy status, the current

TrOOP accumulator, the calendar-year reset date, any Medicare Prescription Payment Plan participation, and any mid-year plan transfer reconciliation. CMS's 2026 instructions supply the principal annual values: $615 deductible, 25 percent defined standard beneficiary coinsurance in initial coverage, $2,100 annual out-of-pocket threshold, zero beneficiary cost sharing in catastrophic coverage, and the post-IRA liability distribution among sponsor, manufacturer, and federal reinsurance. (Centers for Medicare & Medicaid Services)

The final actuarial conclusion is that the redesigned Part D benefit is no longer a four-phase system with a donut-hole discontinuity. It is a three-phase annual allocation matrix: deductible, initial coverage, and catastrophic. The beneficiary pays 100 percent of covered drug costs up to the 2026 $615 deductible under the defined standard design, then generally proceeds through initial coverage with plan-specific copayments or coinsurance that corresponds to the 25 percent defined standard architecture, and finally reaches catastrophic protection when TrOOP reaches the 2026 annual threshold of $2,100. (Centers for Medicare & Medicaid Services) The historical $2,000 cap remains the 2025 baseline, but the 2026 statutory threshold is $2,100 after indexing. (Centers for Medicare & Medicaid Services) Under the Household Medicare Diagnostic Matrix, failure to distinguish total drug cost from TrOOP, covered drugs from noncovered drugs, premiums from cost sharing, manufacturer discounts from beneficiary-incurred costs, and transfer lag from transfer loss can convert a routine prescription pattern into avoidable cash-flow volatility. The modern Part D system is more protective than the historic donut-hole structure, but it remains mathematically exacting: the household's pharmaceutical risk is governed by the drug's covered status, the phase of the benefit, the statutory TrOOP ledger, and the calendar year in which the claim is adjudicated.

11.2 Modernized Legislative Changes and Out-of-Pocket Caps

Medicare Part D began as a voluntary outpatient prescription drug benefit added to Title XVIII of the Social Security Act through the Medicare Prescription Drug, Improvement, and Modernization Act of 2003. Public Law 108-173 described its purpose as amending Title XVIII to provide a voluntary program for prescription drug coverage under Medicare, and the codified Part D statute states that qualified prescription drug coverage under prescription drug plans and MA-PD plans first became effective on January 1, 2006. (GovInfo) The original statutory architecture was not designed as a seamless household asset shield. It was a partially subsidized private-plan framework that distributed liability among the beneficiary, the Part D sponsor, the federal treasury, and later the pharmaceutical manufacturer, while preserving federal fiscal limits through deductibles, initial coverage boundaries, an annual out-of-pocket threshold, and a catastrophic reinsurance layer. The early standard benefit therefore placed the beneficiary file inside a multi-threshold system: an annual deductible, a 25 percent coinsurance structure above the deductible, an initial coverage limit, a coverage gap, and a catastrophic phase. The Social Security Act's Part D standard benefit provisions show the original 2006 deductible at $250, the initial coverage limit at $2,250, and the annual out-of-pocket threshold at $3,600, with later-year amounts subject to statutory update formulas. (Social Security)

The historical design reflected fiscal containment as much as insurance protection. A beneficiary obtained access to negotiated prices and a subsidized private drug benefit, but the statutory design deliberately preserved significant mid-year cost exposure before catastrophic protection attached. The coverage gap was the most visible expression of that cost-containment compromise. Under the current Social Security Act text, the historic coverage-gap provisions still show the long phase-down of beneficiary exposure after the Affordable Care Act amendments: generic-drug gap coinsurance moved from 93 percent in 2011 down by seven percentage points each year before reaching 25 percent in 2020 and subsequent pre-redesign years, while applicable-drug gap percentages moved through 97.5 percent, 95 percent, 90 percent, 85 percent, and 75 percent by 2019 and subsequent years, before interaction with manufacturer discounts. (Social Security) This gradual closure reduced the most extreme cash-flow shock, but it did not eliminate the underlying structural discontinuity. The pre-2025 system still contained a named coverage-gap phase between initial coverage and catastrophic protection, requiring households to model a separate exposure tier rather than a single continuous path to a hard annual cap.

The social-policy weakness of the legacy architecture was the cash-flow cliff. Prescription drug coverage is not an isolated retail purchase for many Medicare beneficiaries; it is a continuity-of-care instrument for chronic disease management, cardiovascular stabilization, oncology adherence, endocrine control, transplant maintenance, behavioral health continuity, and prevention of avoidable acute utilization. A benefit design that causes point-of-sale cost sharing to change sharply during a plan year can create a nonclinical trigger for medication deferral, dose stretching, therapy substitution, or abandonment. Federal sources do not need to use the language of household asset erosion to establish the mechanism. The statutory tables themselves show that the original benefit contained a large gap between the initial coverage limit and catastrophic protection, and the later phase-down rules show that Congress and CMS repeatedly modified the design to reduce that exposure. (Social Security) The policy failure was not that Part D lacked value. The failure was that its earlier benefit geometry made the timing of claims as important as the medical need for the drug.

The Inflation Reduction Act restructurings replaced that legacy geometry. CMS states that the Inflation Reduction Act of 2022 made changes to the defined standard Part D drug benefit, that the 2026 program instructions implement those IRA-related changes, and that the redesigned structure includes an indexed annual out-of-pocket threshold, revised liability for enrollees, sponsors, manufacturers, and CMS, and the selected drug subsidy program. (Centers for Medicare & Medicaid Services) The eCFR now states the decisive legal break: for 2025 and each subsequent year there is no initial coverage limit, and for 2025 and each subsequent year there is no coverage gap. (eCFR) The definition of "coverage gap" in 42 CFR § 423.100 is correspondingly historical, identifying the coverage gap as the period between the initial coverage limit and the out-of-pocket threshold during the years 2006 through 2024. (eCFR) Thus, the donut hole is no longer a current benefit phase under the modern standard Part D design. It is a legacy phase that ended after 2024.

The modern continuous-protection shift is not rhetorical. It is a mechanical replacement of the old coverage-gap tier with a direct progression from deductible to initial coverage to catastrophic coverage. For 2026, CMS states that the defined standard deductible is $615, that the enrollee pays 100 percent of gross covered prescription drug costs until the deductible is met, that initial coverage uses 25 percent beneficiary coinsurance for covered Part D drugs, and that the initial coverage phase ends when annual out-of-pocket spending reaches $2,100. (Centers for Medicare & Medicaid Services) Medicare & You 2026 states the beneficiary-facing version: annual out-of-pocket costs for drugs covered by the plan are capped at $2,100 in 2026, and once that limit is reached, no copayment or coinsurance is owed for covered Part D drugs for the rest of the calendar year. The $2,000 figure remains important as the 2025 baseline, but the operative 2026 threshold is $2,100 because the statute indexes the cap after 2025. (Centers for Medicare & Medicaid Services)

The hard annual out-of-pocket cap is the central asset-protection reform. Before the redesign, catastrophic coverage still permitted beneficiary cost sharing. The current eCFR memorializes that pre-2024 rule by showing that, for years preceding 2024, catastrophic cost sharing was the greater of specified copayments or 5 percent coinsurance. For 2024 and each subsequent year, once incurred costs exceed the annual out-of-pocket threshold, cost sharing is $0. (eCFR) The modern statutory event is therefore binary. Before the threshold, the beneficiary may owe deductible, copayment, or coinsurance depending on phase, formulary tier, pharmacy channel, and plan design. After the threshold, the beneficiary's cost-sharing liability for covered Part D drugs terminates for the remainder of the calendar year. Medicare & You 2026 confirms that the $2,100 cap is reached through beneficiary out-of-pocket spending plus certain payments made by other people or entities, including

Medicare's Extra Help program, and then copayments and coinsurance for covered Part D drugs stop for the rest of the calendar year.

The cap is "hard" only for the covered Part D drug universe. It does not eliminate premiums, Part D IRMAA, noncovered drugs, excluded drugs, over-the-counter products, or costs outside the plan's covered-drug rules. CMS's TrOOP guidance states that plan premiums do not count toward True Out-of-Pocket costs, that drugs not covered by the plan do not count, that excluded drugs and most over-the-counter drugs or vitamins do not count, and that payments by certain other third-party arrangements generally do not count. Current 42 CFR § 423.100 defines covered Part D drug status through formulary inclusion, treatment as included through a coverage determination or appeal, and proper pharmacy channel rules. (eCFR) The hard cap therefore protects covered Part D drug cost sharing, not every pharmacy-counter or premium-related dollar. The Household Medicare Diagnostic Matrix must preserve that distinction because the cap's power depends on whether the claim is legally inside the Part D benefit.

The liability rebalancing behind the cap is as important as the consumer-facing protection. CMS states that in the 2026 initial coverage phase, the enrollee pays 25 percent coinsurance for covered Part D drugs, the sponsor typically pays 65 percent of applicable drugs and selected drugs and 75 percent of all other covered Part D drugs, the manufacturer typically covers 10 percent of applicable-drug cost through the Manufacturer Discount Program, and CMS pays a 10 percent subsidy for selected drugs during a price applicability period. (Centers for Medicare & Medicaid Services) In catastrophic coverage, CMS states that the enrollee pays no cost sharing, sponsors typically pay 60 percent of covered Part D drug costs, manufacturers typically pay a 20 percent discount for applicable drugs, and CMS pays reinsurance equal to 20 percent for applicable drugs and 40 percent for other covered Part D drugs that are not applicable drugs, including selected drugs during a price applicability period. (Centers for Medicare & Medicaid Services) This is the fiscal center of the redesign. The beneficiary is removed from catastrophic cost sharing, but the claim remains financed through sponsor liability, manufacturer discount liability where applicable, and federal reinsurance.

This reallocation also changes insurer accountability. Under the legacy catastrophic model, plan liability in catastrophic coverage was substantially lower than under the modern redesign, while federal reinsurance played a dominant financing role. CMS's Manufacturer Discount Program final guidance explains that the IRA eliminated beneficiary catastrophic cost sharing beginning in 2024, increased plan liability in the catastrophic phase for 2024, and, beginning in 2025, eliminated the coverage gap, introduced manufacturer discounts in initial and catastrophic phases, lowered the annual cap on enrollee out-of-pocket costs, and changed plan and government reinsurance liability in catastrophic coverage. (Centers for Medicare & Medicaid Services) The redesigned allocation increases the private sponsor's share in catastrophic coverage while reducing beneficiary exposure and creating manufacturer discount obligations outside the old donut-hole structure. The public budget is not removed from the system, but federal reinsurance is redesigned and paired with higher plan responsibility and manufacturer participation.

The Manufacturer Discount Program replaces the Coverage Gap Discount Program and illustrates how the donut-hole system was dismantled rather than merely renamed. CMS states that, effective January 1, 2025, Part D coverage is available only for applicable drugs covered by a Manufacturer Discount Program agreement with CMS, that manufacturers must provide discounts in the initial and catastrophic coverage phases, and that the Coverage Gap Discount Program ended on December 31, 2024 and was replaced by the Manufacturer Discount Program. (Centers for Medicare & Medicaid Services) The eCFR similarly distinguishes the old Coverage Gap Discount Program from the new Manufacturer Discount Program and defines the Coverage Gap period as a 2006 through 2024 construct. (eCFR) The legal transformation is therefore exact: manufacturer discount obligations no longer depend on a mid-year donut-hole phase. They are embedded in the post-deductible benefit structure itself.

The indexing rules prevent the cap from becoming a static nominal dollar amount divorced from national prescription-drug spending growth. Section 423.104 establishes that the annual out-of-pocket threshold was $2,000 for 2025 and, for 2026 and each subsequent year, equals the previous year's amount increased by the annual percentage increase and rounded to the nearest $50. (eCFR) The same regulation defines the annual percentage increase for Part D drug expenditures as the annual percentage increase in average per capita aggregate expenditures for Part D drugs in the United States for Part D eligible individuals, based on the 12-month period ending in July of the previous year, and it specifies trend and multiplicative update components. (eCFR) CMS's 2026 program instructions apply that formula to produce the $2,100 threshold from the 2025 $2,000 baseline. (Centers for Medicare & Medicaid Services) The cap is therefore a statutory indexed ceiling, not a permanently frozen $2,000 nominal number.

The deductible is indexed through the same general statutory tradition of annual parameter adjustment. Section 423.104 states that the annual deductible was $250 for 2006 and that later-year deductibles are increased by the annual percentage increase and rounded to the nearest multiple of $5. (eCFR) CMS sets the 2026 defined standard deductible at $615. (Centers for Medicare & Medicaid Services) This indexing matters because the deductible phase remains the beneficiary's first point-of-service exposure. The redesign caps total annual covered-drug cost sharing, but it does not remove the front-end deductible for plans using a deductible, subject to plan-specific designs and exceptions such as drugs covered before the deductible. Medicare & You 2026 states that some plans have no deductible and that some plans with deductibles cover certain tiers before the deductible, while covered-drug copayments or coinsurance after the deductible depend on tier and other plan factors.

The modern "leveling" of formulary-tier pricing must be stated as a regulatory discipline, not a guarantee of identical copayments across plans. Section 423.104 permits actuarially equivalent standard coverage and tiered copayments, but tiered copayments must be consistent with the 25 percent actuarial standard and approved under CMS processes; the regulation further provides that tiered cost sharing may not exceed levels annually determined by CMS to be discriminatory. (eCFR) Medicare & You 2026 states that the amount paid for a covered drug depends on whether the drug is on the formulary, what tier applies, which benefit phase applies, and which pharmacy is used. The post-IRA system therefore does not flatten every plan's tier design into one national schedule. It imposes a hard annual out-of-pocket endpoint and regulatory guardrails around tiered cost sharing, thereby limiting extreme annual exposure while leaving plan-specific formularies, tiers, preferred pharmacy structures, utilization management, and negotiated pricing relevant inside the year.

Indexed copay behavior is clearest in the catastrophic phase. Under the older statute, catastrophic cost sharing used either specified copayments or 5 percent coinsurance, and those copayments were indexed through 2023. Current § 423.104 states that for 2024 and each subsequent year, cost sharing after the annual out-of-pocket threshold is $0. (eCFR) This is not merely lower catastrophic cost sharing; it is a categorical elimination of beneficiary cost sharing in catastrophic coverage. The resulting modernization shifts the household's modeling problem away from indefinite post-threshold coinsurance and toward the timing of when the annual TrOOP threshold will be reached, whether each claim is a covered Part D drug, whether costs are properly credited to the ledger, and whether liquidity tools such as the Medicare Prescription Payment Plan smooth payment timing without altering the total annual obligation. Medicare & You 2026 states that the payment option spreads covered-drug out-of-pocket costs across the calendar year but does not save money or lower drug costs.

Low-Income Subsidy alignment adds a separate equity layer to the redesign. CMS states that the Inflation Reduction Act expanded the full Low-Income Subsidy, also called Extra Help, to certain individuals with limited resources and income up to 150 percent of the federal poverty level starting January 1, 2024. (Centers for Medicare &

Medicaid Services) Medicare & You 2026 states that Extra Help assists with Medicare drug costs such as premiums, deductibles, and coinsurance, and that individuals who qualify for Extra Help and join a Part D plan or MA-PD plan do not pay a Part D late enrollment penalty. The official handbook also states that Extra Help may permit more frequent plan changes and that automatic qualification can arise through full Medicaid, state Medicaid payment of Part B premiums or other Medicare costs, or Supplemental Security Income benefits. The LIS expansion therefore aligns with the hard cap by reducing point-of-service friction for vulnerable cohorts before the cap is reached, while the cap limits total covered-drug cost sharing for the broader population.

The redesigned benefit also changes creditable-coverage analysis outside Part D. CMS states that enhancements to the Part D defined standard benefit under the IRA make the prior simplified creditable-coverage determination methodology no longer reflective of actuarial equivalence with the richer defined standard benefit; for 2026 only, certain non-retiree-drug-subsidy group health plans may use either the existing simplified methodology or a revised methodology, and the revised methodology requires coverage designed to pay at least 72 percent of participants' prescription drug expenses rather than 60 percent. (Centers for Medicare & Medicaid Services) This is a secondary consequence of modernization. A richer federal Part D baseline makes some non-Medicare drug coverage harder to classify as creditable. The Household Medicare Diagnostic Matrix must therefore connect the out-of-pocket cap to the Part D late-enrollment-penalty row, because outside coverage that once appeared comparable may require renewed actuarial testing against the post-IRA standard.

The elimination of the donut hole also changes the interpretation of historical plan documents, educational materials, and household spreadsheets. Any model still projecting a separate 2025 or 2026 coverage-gap phase is obsolete. The current regulation is unambiguous: no initial coverage limit and no coverage gap exist for 2025 and subsequent years. (eCFR) The continuing relevance of the old coverage-gap term is historical, not operational. The old sequence, deductible, initial coverage, coverage gap, catastrophic, should be replaced for current non-LIS standard modeling by deductible, initial coverage, catastrophic. This does not make drug spending trivial. It makes the boundary conditions clearer. The household must still account for formulary exclusions, tier placement, specialty coinsurance, pharmacy network selection, utilization management, Part D IRMAA, premiums, and the calendar-year reset. But the mid-year donut-hole cliff no longer belongs in the current benefit phase map.

The Household Medicare Diagnostic Matrix treats Section 11.2 as the modernization pillar for pharmaceutical risk. The matrix must record whether the drug year is being modeled under pre-2025 or post-2024 law, whether a coverage-gap phase exists for the applicable year, the annual deductible, the current out-of-pocket threshold, the plan's tier and cost-sharing structure, the covered-drug status of each medication, the TrOOP-recognized payer category, the Extra Help status of the beneficiary, any selected-drug subsidy implications, Manufacturer Discount Program applicability, and the calendar-year reset. CMS's 2026 instructions supply the operative modern figures and liability architecture: $615 deductible, 25 percent beneficiary coinsurance in defined standard initial coverage, $2,100 annual out-of-pocket threshold, zero beneficiary cost sharing in catastrophic coverage, 60 percent typical sponsor liability in catastrophic coverage, 20 percent typical manufacturer discount on applicable drugs in catastrophic coverage, and federal reinsurance of 20 percent or 40 percent depending on drug category. (Centers for Medicare & Medicaid Services)

The final synthesis is that the Inflation Reduction Act modernization stabilized the Part D benefit by replacing a legacy split-tier exposure system with an indexed hard-cap model. The original MMA framework created a voluntary prescription drug benefit effective in 2006, but it also embedded significant beneficiary cost exposure through an initial coverage limit, a coverage gap, and post-threshold catastrophic cost sharing. (U.S. Code) The modern framework eliminates the coverage gap after 2024, removes catastrophic beneficiary cost sharing beginning in 2024 and thereafter, and sets a hard indexed annual out-of-pocket cap beginning with $2,000 in 2025 and $2,100 in 2026. (eCFR) Under the Household Medicare Diagnostic Matrix, failure to recognize those modern statutory boundaries converts a forward-looking retirement cash-flow model into an obsolete projection based on defunct insurance phases. The contemporary Part D file must be analyzed as an indexed annual risk corridor: front-end deductible exposure, plan-specific initial coverage cost sharing, TrOOP accumulation, Extra Help mitigation where applicable, manufacturer and sponsor liability reallocation, and zero beneficiary cost sharing for covered Part D drugs after the annual threshold is reached.

11.3 The Medicare Prescription Payment Plan Mechanics

The Medicare Prescription Payment Plan is the cash-flow leveling mechanism created to solve a problem that the modern Part D out-of-pocket cap, by itself, could not fully eliminate. The Inflation Reduction Act redesigned Part D to impose a hard annual limit on covered-drug cost sharing, but high-utilization beneficiaries can still encounter severe point-of-sale compression before that limit is reached. A household using one or more high-cost covered Part D drugs may exhaust the annual statutory out-of-pocket corridor early in the year, even though the annual liability is bounded. The

Medicare Prescription Payment Plan therefore operates as a monthly installment infrastructure: it changes the timing of payment, not the legal amount of Part D cost sharing owed. Medicare & You 2026 states that the program works with current drug coverage to spread out-of-pocket costs for covered drugs across January through December, may help manage expenses, but does not save money or lower drug costs. CMS likewise explains that, beginning in 2025, Part D sponsors must offer enrollees the option to pay out-of-pocket prescription drug costs in monthly amounts during the plan year instead of paying those amounts at the pharmacy counter. (Centers for Medicare & Medicaid Services)

The cap reference must be reconciled precisely. The initial statutory implementation year, 2025, used a $2,000 annual out-of-pocket threshold, and CMS's final part one guidance used that $2,000 amount in the statutory formula examples. (Centers for Medicare & Medicaid Services) For the 2026 plan year, the indexed Part D out-of-pocket cap is $2,100, and the 2026 handbook states that covered-drug out-of-pocket costs are capped at $2,100 for the year. Accordingly, a 2025 example divides $2,000 across the remaining months; a 2026 example divides $2,100 across the remaining months. The program remains identical in concept: participation does not reduce the annual TrOOP liability, does not subsidize covered prescriptions, and does not change the catastrophic threshold. It converts pharmacy-counter shocks into monthly invoices.

Under the statutory smoothing formula codified for 2026 and later, the first-month maximum monthly cap is calculated by taking the annual out-of-pocket threshold, subtracting Part D incurred costs already accumulated before participation begins, and dividing the result by the number of months remaining in the plan year, including the month for which the cap is being calculated. (Federal Register) If participation is elected before the plan year starts, the first active month has no prior TrOOP to subtract and uses all twelve months in the divisor. For 2025, that produced a baseline first-month cap of $166.67, equal to $2,000 divided by twelve. (Centers for Medicare & Medicaid Services) For 2026, the analogous full-year baseline is $175.00, equal to the $2,100 cap divided by twelve. That figure is a maximum first-month bill, not a guaranteed bill; if actual covered-drug out-of-pocket costs for the first month are lower than the maximum monthly cap, the sponsor must bill the lesser actual amount rather than the cap. (Federal Register)

The subsequent-month calculation is dynamic, not level-payment amortization in the conventional consumer-credit sense. For each later month, the maximum monthly cap equals the sum of any remaining out-of-pocket costs owed from prior months that have not yet been billed, plus any additional out-of-pocket costs incurred during the new month, divided by the number of months remaining in the plan year, including the month being billed. (Federal Register) CMS's guidance emphasizes that the calculation can vary by person and by month because it depends on prior incurred costs, new out-of-pocket costs, and the number of months left in the plan year; if the participant remains in the program through the end of the plan year, monthly bills through the December payment equal the total out-of-pocket costs incurred under the program for the year. (Centers for Medicare & Medicaid Services) This is why monthly bills can rise after a new high-cost prescription, fall when no additional claims occur, and change again if later claims are adjusted.

The progressive compounding effect is administrative rather than interest-bearing. Federal rules prohibit the sponsor from charging late fees, interest payments, or other fees associated with payment mechanisms under the program. (Centers for Medicare & Medicaid Services) What compounds is not interest. What compounds is the remaining unpaid covered-drug cost-sharing balance when new covered-drug claims are added to an already deferred balance. If an April fill generates a high covered-drug cost and the participant is billed only the maximum monthly cap, the unpaid remainder is carried forward. If additional claims occur in May, the May cap recalculates using the prior remaining balance plus the new May out-of-pocket amount, divided over the remaining months. CMS's examples show this recalculation structure month by month, with the maximum monthly cap increasing or decreasing as new out-of-pocket costs are incurred and as the divisor shrinks later in the calendar year. (Centers for Medicare & Medicaid Services)

The pharmacy-counter experience is the most visible operational change. For a valid program participant, the covered Part D claim is adjudicated so that the participant pays zero dollars at the point of sale for the participant-responsibility amount included in the program. The Part D sponsor pays the pharmacy both the sponsor's normal portion and the amount the participant otherwise would have paid at the counter. CMS's final guidance states that participants pay $0 at the point of sale instead of ordinary out-of-pocket cost sharing, and that sponsors must pay the pharmacy the enrollee's cost-sharing amount in addition to the sponsor portion. (Centers for Medicare & Medicaid Services) The 2026 Federal Register codification states that each PDP sponsor and each MA-PD organization must provide the option to pay $0 cost sharing at the point of sale and then pay plan cost sharing in capped monthly amounts. (Federal Register)

The claims-processing architecture uses a coordinated electronic mechanism. CMS requires an additional BIN or PCN unique to the Medicare Prescription Payment Plan to process the final patient-responsibility amount after applicable other payers have processed the claim. (Federal Register) This prevents the payment plan from being treated as separate insurance and keeps the Part D sponsor as the source of both the primary claim payment and the payment-plan amount sent to the pharmacy. CMS also requires that the payment plan not affect the amount paid to pharmacies or the timing of such payments, and it prohibits sponsors from imposing program implementation fees on pharmacies or holding pharmacies responsible for unpaid participant balances. (Federal Register) The pharmacy is therefore a dispensing and transaction-processing node, not a collection agency for the deferred balance.

The post-service invoicing loop is separate from premium collection. Medicare & You 2026 states that a participant continues to pay any plan premium separately and receives a bill from the health or drug plan for prescription drugs instead of paying the pharmacy. The 2026 codified rule requires a bill for the Medicare Prescription Payment Plan to be separate from any premium-collection bill, and the billing period is a calendar month. (Federal Register) Required billing content includes the program statement, effective date of participation, last payment received, any balance carried over from the prior month, itemized out-of-pocket prescription costs for the month, the amount due under the monthly cap calculation, the remaining total out-of-pocket cost-sharing balance, nonpayment next steps, opt-out information, dispute procedures, and Low-Income Subsidy information. (Federal Register)

Participation does not slow TrOOP advancement. The Federal Register rule states that participation must have no impact on true out-of-pocket accumulation and that costs incurred under the program are treated as incurred based on the date each Part D claim is adjudicated. (Federal Register) CMS's final guidance gives the same operational rule: a participant's TrOOP-eligible costs are still treated as incurred once the relevant prescription drug claim has been adjudicated, and the ordinary PDE data accessed through plan-to-plan processes contain the information needed if a mid-year plan change occurs. (Centers for Medicare & Medicaid Services) This is the central actuarial distinction. The household may physically pay a deferred installment in later months, but the federal Part D benefit ledger advances when the covered claim is adjudicated, not when the installment check clears.

Program participation also does not alter PDE reporting or real-time benefit tool liability displays. The final 2026 rule requires Prescription Drug Event records to reflect participant and plan liability as if the Medicare Prescription Payment Plan did not apply, and it requires real-time benefit tools to show cost-sharing information without being distorted by the payment-plan transaction layer. (Federal Register) The result is a clean separation between benefit accounting and cash-flow timing. Part D benefit phase, TrOOP accumulation, manufacturer discount treatment, plan liability, federal reinsurance, and the statutory out-of-pocket cap remain benefit-system variables. Installment billing is a receivable-management function layered on top of those variables.

Nonpayment activates a controlled administrative sequence. For 2026 and later, when a participant fails to pay a program bill, the Part D sponsor must provide a grace period of at least two months after notifying the participant of the missed payment; the grace period begins on the first day of the month after the initial notice is sent. (Federal Register) The participant must be allowed to pay the overdue balance during the grace period to remain in the program. If nonpayment occurs with fewer than two full calendar months left in the year, the grace period carries into the next calendar year, and the sponsor must allow the participant to opt into the program for the next year while the grace period remains active. (Federal Register) These protections preserve continuity before termination of participation can occur.

Termination from the payment plan is not disenrollment from Part D. Federal rules prohibit a Part D sponsor from disenrolling a Part D enrollee from the drug plan because of failure to pay any amount billed under the Medicare Prescription Payment Plan, and they also prohibit declining future Part D plan enrollment based on failure to pay a monthly payment-plan amount. (Federal Register) If a participant is terminated from the payment plan, the sponsor may continue billing outstanding amounts, but the participant resumes paying new out-of-pocket cost sharing directly at the pharmacy for later covered Part D drugs until the annual out-of-pocket threshold is reached. (Centers for Medicare & Medicaid Services) Thus, nonpayment can remove the smoothing protection, but it cannot be used as an independent basis to strip the beneficiary of the underlying Part D contract.

Outstanding balances can restrict later access to the smoothing mechanism, but the restriction is sponsor-specific. The codified rule permits a sponsor to preclude a person from opting into the Medicare Prescription Payment Plan in a subsequent year only if an overdue balance remains owed to that sponsor. A different Part D sponsor, without the same sponsor relationship, cannot preclude participation based on a debt owed to another sponsor. (Federal Register) If the overdue balance is later paid, the sponsor must promptly permit opt-in after payment. (Centers for Medicare & Medicaid Services) The financial consequence is therefore narrower than a universal Medicare exclusion but still material: an unpaid program debt can impair future cash-flow smoothing within the same sponsor framework and can force pharmacy-counter payment of new out-of-pocket costs in later years until the debt barrier is cleared.

The Matrix consequence is exact. The Household Medicare Diagnostic Matrix must treat the Medicare Prescription Payment Plan as a liquidity and billing variable, not as a drug-cost reduction benefit. Its row should record the applicable calendar-year out-of-pocket threshold, the date of opt-in, the first-month divisor, accumulated TrOOP before participation, covered Part D drug status, additional monthly out-of-pocket claims, remaining unpaid balance, monthly cap, separate premium obligation, installment bill due date, grace-period status, dispute pathway, and sponsor-specific preclusion exposure. The 2026 value must be entered as $2,100, while the 2025 baseline value must be entered as $2,000. (Centers for Medicare & Medicaid Services) The program stabilizes timing, but only if the household file correctly models dynamic recalculation rather than assuming a fixed, equal monthly payment for the entire year.

The final synthesis is that the Medicare Prescription Payment Plan is a federal cash-flow smoothing instrument built into modern Part D. It prevents the pharmacy counter from becoming the single concentrated collection point for high early-year covered-drug cost sharing. It does not lower the cost of covered drugs, does not change formulary status, does not reduce the annual TrOOP cap, does not alter catastrophic protection, does not merge premiums into the out-of-pocket threshold, and does not delay TrOOP accumulation. It replaces immediate point-of-sale collection with plan-sponsored monthly receivables, governed by a first-month formula, a subsequent-month recalculation formula, separate billing, no interest or late fees, grace-period protections, and sponsor-specific preclusion rules. Under the Household Medicare Diagnostic Matrix, failure to map this algorithm can convert a tool of cash-flow stabilization into a source of unexpected invoices, recalculated balances, late-year budget strain, and avoidable loss of future smoothing access.

Chapter 12: Formulary Architecture and Utilization Governance

12.1 Structural Formulary Tiers and Chemical Classifications

The Medicare Part D formulary is the statutory and actuarial map through which a private prescription drug plan sponsor converts the general promise of outpatient drug coverage into an enforceable list of covered compounds, pricing tiers, pharmacy conditions, and utilization controls. A formulary is not a passive catalog. It is a federally reviewed clinical-financial instrument that determines whether a medication is covered, what tiered cost-sharing position applies, whether the claim may be filled without additional administrative screening, and whether the pharmacy transaction is credited into the beneficiary's annual Part D cost architecture. The official 2026 Medicare handbook describes the formulary as a plan's list of covered drugs and explains that Part D plans generally place drugs into different levels called tiers, with different costs attached to different tiers. The same handbook warns that actual drug costs depend on formulary status, tier placement, benefit phase, pharmacy channel, and Extra Help status, which means that formulary architecture is one of the principal determinants of household pharmaceutical cash flow.

The assignment label's reference to 42 CFR Part 423 Subpart V must be reconciled precisely. Subpart V of Part 423 governs Part D communication requirements, not the core substantive formulary design rules; the current Part 423 table of contents identifies Subpart V as "Part D Communication Requirements" and locates it at §§ 423.2260 through 423.2276. (Legal Information Institute) The substantive formulary requirements are principally located in 42 CFR § 423.120, which governs access to covered Part D drugs, formulary requirements, Pharmacy and Therapeutics Committee obligations, adequate formulary standards, transition supplies, and formulary change limitations. (eCFR) Drug utilization management is addressed under Subpart D, including § 423.153, and formulary and tiering exception rights are principally located in Subpart M, including § 423.578. (eCFR) Subpart V remains relevant as the communication and disclosure layer because plan materials must accurately convey formulary, tier, utilization-management, and exception information, but the legal machinery of formulary construction resides elsewhere in Part 423.

The federal purpose of formulary regulation is to permit managed drug purchasing without permitting discriminatory benefit design. A Part D sponsor may use a formulary, but the formulary cannot be an unreviewed commercial preference list designed solely to shift cost away from the sponsor. Under § 423.120, a plan using a formulary must develop and review that formulary through a Pharmacy and

Therapeutics Committee. That committee must include a majority of practicing physicians or practicing pharmacists, at least one independent practicing physician and one independent practicing pharmacist free of conflict relative to the plan and pharmaceutical manufacturers, and at least one practicing physician and pharmacist with expertise in the care of elderly or disabled individuals. (eCFR) The committee must base clinical decisions on scientific evidence and standards of practice, consider safety and efficacy advantages, review exceptions and utilization-management policies, evaluate treatment protocols at least annually, document formulary and utilization-management decisions, and review and approve all clinical prior authorization criteria, step therapy protocols, and quantity limit restrictions applied to covered Part D drugs. (eCFR)

This P&T Committee framework is the formal clinical check against pure fiscal rationing. The sponsor's actuarial incentive is to control drug spending through tiering, preferred formulary placement, pharmacy contracting, generic substitution, biosimilar adoption, and utilization edits. The federal regulatory counterweight requires expert clinical review, conflict management, evidence-based decision making, CMS approval, and adequate coverage across therapeutic categories and classes. Section 423.120 requires an adequate formulary to include, within each therapeutic category and class of Part D drugs, at least two Part D drugs that are not therapeutically equivalent and bioequivalent, with different strengths and dosage forms available, unless the category or class contains only one Part D drug. (eCFR) The same rule requires adequate coverage of drug types commonly needed by Part D enrollees as recognized in national treatment guidelines and CMS approval of the formulary. (eCFR) The formulary therefore performs two simultaneous functions: it narrows the universe of covered drugs for administrability and contracting leverage, while federal law prevents that narrowing from becoming clinically inadequate or condition-targeted discrimination.

Protected-class coverage illustrates the same policy balance. The 2026 Medicare handbook states that all plans must cover a wide range of prescription drugs that people with Medicare take, including most drugs in certain protected classes, such as drugs used to treat cancer, HIV/AIDS, depression, psychosis, seizures, or to prevent organ transplant rejection. These classes are not merely ordinary formulary categories. They represent high-clinical-risk domains where under-coverage could destabilize serious illness, induce avoidable acute care, or create discriminatory effects against individuals with complex diagnoses. Section 423.120 recognizes categories and classes of clinical concern and permits utilization-management exceptions for protected-class drugs only within defined boundaries, including quantity limitations due to safety and, subject to CMS review and approval, certain prior authorization and step therapy requirements for enrollees not already on existing therapy, with antiretroviral medications receiving additional protection. (eCFR)

The tiering system is the visible price architecture layered onto the formulary. Federal law does not require every Part D plan to use identical tier names, identical tier numbers, or a uniform five-tier structure. Medicare's public-facing explanation states generally that Part D plans place drugs into tiers, that each tier has a different cost, and that drugs in lower tiers generally cost less than drugs in higher tiers. Medicare.gov's consumer education similarly describes tiering through examples, including lower-cost generic tiers, brand-name tiers, non-preferred brand tiers, and a specialty tier for very high-cost drugs. (Medicare) The correct institutional statement is therefore that tier labels are plan-design conventions approved through the Part D bid and formulary process, not a single federally mandated national nomenclature. Nevertheless, the common tier continuum is stable enough to support household modeling when treated as a plan-specific risk grid rather than a universal statutory table.

The lowest tier is commonly reserved for preferred generic drugs. These medications usually represent the plan's lowest cost-sharing position because they are chemically equivalent or therapeutically substitutable options that the sponsor has selected for preferred placement through formulary and contracting analysis. In a household cash-flow model, this tier often behaves like the least volatile outpatient drug category because point-of-sale liability is commonly expressed as a fixed copayment or low coinsurance. The actuarial role of the preferred generic tier is to steer routine maintenance therapy toward the lowest available net-cost channel while preserving covered-drug access. The clinical risk is not the tier itself, but improper substitution or failure to confirm that the generic alternative is clinically appropriate for the beneficiary's diagnosis, dosage form, prior response, allergy profile, or therapeutic narrowness. The P&T Committee's evidence and safety review obligations under § 423.120 supply the formal mechanism through which such substitutions must be evaluated. (eCFR)

The second tier is often used for non-preferred generic drugs or, in other plan designs, for preferred brand-name drugs. This variability is why plan-specific formulary review is indispensable. A model that assumes Tier 2 always means the same chemical or economic class will misprice household exposure. If Tier 2 functions as a non-preferred generic tier, the plan is still placing the drug in a generic category but signaling that the selected molecule, dosage form, release mechanism, or manufacturer relationship does not qualify for the lowest cost-sharing position. If Tier 2 functions as a preferred brand tier, the plan is identifying a brand product that has enough clinical or contracting value to receive favorable placement above generic tiers. The official Medicare handbook's rule is categorical rather than numerically rigid: a lower tier generally costs less than a higher tier, and the applicable formulary must be reviewed because each plan has its own drug list.

The third tier commonly captures preferred brand-name drugs where the plan has accepted higher ingredient cost in exchange for clinical value, contract concessions, or formulary strategy. From an actuarial standpoint, this tier marks the transition from low-cost maintenance-drug economics into more significant plan-sponsor liability and beneficiary cost-sharing exposure. A preferred brand may carry a fixed copayment in some designs or coinsurance in others. The household effect depends not only on the tier, but also on the deductible, the initial coverage phase, whether the beneficiary has reached the annual out-of-pocket threshold, and whether the drug is subject to prior authorization, step therapy, or quantity limits. The 2026 Medicare handbook places these variables in the same cost matrix, stating that actual cost varies based on formulary status, tier, benefit phase, pharmacy channel, and Extra Help.

The fourth tier generally contains non-preferred drugs, often non-preferred brands, higher-cost generics, or drugs for which the sponsor has identified preferred therapeutic alternatives. This tier is not merely a higher price rung; it is the formulary's behavioral nudge. A non-preferred placement tells the pharmacy system, prescriber, and beneficiary file that the plan will cover the drug under ordinary formulary rules, but at less favorable cost sharing than available alternatives. The non-preferred tier therefore converts the plan's therapeutic and contracting judgment into point-of-service financial friction. The beneficiary may still have coverage, but the household's monthly prescription budget can become volatile if a maintenance drug moves from a preferred tier to a non-preferred tier, if a brand-name price increase raises coinsurance exposure, or if a generic or biosimilar entry causes the plan to increase cost sharing for the original product while continuing to cover the lower-cost alternative. The Medicare handbook expressly notes that a plan may change a drug list during the year if it follows Medicare guidelines and gives examples involving new therapies, new drugs, new medical information, manufacturer price increases, and generic or biosimilar alternatives.

The fifth or sixth tier is the specialty tier, a formally regulated category reserved for high-cost Part D drugs. Unlike ordinary plan-specific tier labels, the specialty tier has a defined regulatory threshold mechanism. Section 423.104 defines a specialty tier as a formulary cost-sharing tier dedicated to high-cost Part D drugs whose ingredient cost for a 30-day equivalent supply exceeds the specialty-tier cost threshold. CMS determines the threshold using prescription drug event data, including 30-day equivalent ingredient cost calculations and a top-one-percent methodology. (eCFR)

For placement on a specialty tier, the sponsor's claims data must generally demonstrate that more than 50 percent of the plan's prescription drug events for the drug, adjusted for 30-day equivalent supplies, exceed the specialty-tier cost threshold; for newly approved drugs without claims history, the sponsor must estimate that the ingredient-cost portion of negotiated prices will exceed the threshold more than 50 percent of the time, subject to the applicable formulary and change requirements. (eCFR) Federal rulemaking later identified the current specialty-tier threshold as $950 while explaining that the CY 2027 threshold would increase to $1,080. (Centers for Medicare & Medicaid Services)

Specialty-tier placement is often the point at which the household's financial exposure shifts from predictable copayment behavior to coinsurance-linked volatility. Section 423.104 permits up to two specialty tiers and sets maximum allowable cost sharing for specialty-tier drugs. A plan with the full defined standard deductible is limited to 25 percent coinsurance for the specialty tier; a plan with no deductible may use up to 33 percent coinsurance; and plans with deductibles between zero and the defined standard deductible use a regulatory formula for maximum coinsurance. (eCFR) The actuarial implication is straightforward. A fixed copayment establishes a known point-of-sale obligation, while coinsurance makes the beneficiary's obligation a percentage of the drug's adjudicated cost, at least until the annual Part D out-of-pocket threshold is reached. In 2026, the annual Part D out-of-pocket threshold is $2,100, after which no copayment or coinsurance is owed for covered Part D drugs for the rest of the calendar year.

Step therapy is the first major operational hurdle inside utilization governance. It is a clinical sequencing protocol that requires use of one or more lower-cost or preferred alternatives before the plan will cover a more expensive or non-preferred drug. In its strongest form, step therapy is not merely a price signal. It is a coverage condition. Section 423.578 treats a step therapy requirement as a cost utilization tool that may cause a Part D drug not to be covered until the plan's coverage policy requirements are met. (eCFR) Medicare's public-facing materials define step therapy in simpler terms, stating that it involves trying a less expensive similar drug before a plan covers the prescribed drug. The actuarial purpose is volume redirection: the plan attempts to route initial therapy toward generics, biosimilars, preferred brands, or clinically accepted first-line agents before permitting access to higher-cost therapy.

Step therapy can be clinically rational when the preferred first-line therapy is safe, effective, and consistent with accepted treatment standards. It can become financially and medically destabilizing when the beneficiary has already failed the preferred therapy, experienced adverse effects, requires a different route of administration, has contraindications, or has a diagnosis for which the preferred step is not clinically appropriate. Federal law addresses that tension through P&T Committee review and the exception process. The P&T Committee must review and approve step therapy protocols applied to covered Part D drugs. (eCFR) When a step requirement prevents coverage of a necessary drug, the exception process must address an exception to the coverage policy that causes the drug not to be covered because of a cost-utilization tool, including step therapy, dosage limitations, or therapeutic substitution. (eCFR)

Quantity limits are the second major utilization-management device. A quantity limit restricts how much of a drug the plan will cover over a specified period, such as a dosage amount, frequency, or days' supply. The Medicare handbook describes quantity limits as rules under which a plan covers only a certain amount of a drug over a certain number of days. Quantity limits may be grounded in FDA labeling, safety concerns, drug-drug interaction risk, duplicate therapy prevention, abuse potential, waste reduction, or cost control. Section 423.120 expressly requires the P&T Committee to review policies guiding quantity limits and to approve all quantity-limit restrictions applied to covered Part D drugs. (eCFR) In protected-class contexts, the regulation also recognizes utilization-management processes that limit drug quantity due to safety. (eCFR)

The financial effect of a quantity limit is often hidden until the pharmacy claim rejects. If the prescriber writes for a dosage or days' supply that exceeds the plan's limit, the claim may adjudicate for a smaller covered amount, reject pending documentation, or require an exception request. A household spreadsheet that multiplies a known copayment by twelve months can therefore become obsolete when the dose changes, when a titration schedule exceeds the limit, when a maintenance drug is converted from thirty-day to ninety-day supply, or when a specialty compound requires individualized dosing. Quantity limits are especially relevant for medications with weight-based dosing, variable dose escalation, rescue dosing, or multiple daily administrations. The legal point is not that quantity limits are forbidden; it is that they must be clinically reviewed, tied to coverage policy, disclosed in plan materials, and subject to exception review where the limit is not clinically appropriate for the beneficiary's condition.

Prior authorization is the third major utilization hurdle and often the most documentation-intensive. Prior authorization requires the prescriber to submit information before the plan will cover the drug under ordinary terms. Medicare's public materials state that before certain prescriptions can be filled, the prescriber may need to contact the plan to verify that the drug is medically necessary, and that the plan may need more information from the prescriber before covering the drug. In Part D practice, the required information may include diagnosis codes, laboratory values, disease severity, prior therapy history, contraindications, duration of therapy, prescriber specialty, FDA-labeled indication, compendia support where relevant, and documentation showing that formulary alternatives are ineffective or unsafe. Section 423.120 requires P&T Committee review and approval of all clinical prior authorization criteria applied to covered Part D drugs. (eCFR)

Prior authorization serves two actuarial functions. First, it screens for indication integrity, preventing coverage where the drug is prescribed outside the plan's covered condition criteria or where another Medicare coverage pathway, such as Part B rather than Part D, controls payment. Second, it reduces utilization leakage by preventing automatic access to high-cost drugs when the plan's formulary contains preferred alternatives. The clinical risk is administrative delay. A medically necessary drug can become temporarily inaccessible if the prescriber's documentation is incomplete, if laboratory evidence is not current, if the pharmacy claim is submitted before authorization, or if the plan applies a coverage criterion inconsistent with the prescriber's clinical judgment. The exception and coverage determination system therefore becomes the legal safety valve that converts clinical disagreement into an adjudicable administrative record.

The formal exception process is the mechanism by which formulary rigidity is tempered by individualized medical necessity. CMS states that a tiering exception is used to obtain a non-preferred drug at the lower cost-sharing terms applicable to drugs in a preferred tier, while a formulary exception is used to obtain a Part D drug not included on the formulary or to request waiver of a utilization-management requirement such as step therapy, prior authorization, or quantity limits. (Centers for Medicare & Medicaid Services) Section 423.578 requires each sponsor that uses a formulary to establish and maintain CMS-approved exceptions procedures for off-formulary drugs, and the sponsor must grant an exception whenever it determines that the drug is medically necessary and would be covered but for being off formulary. (eCFR)

The burden of proof in an exception request falls heavily on the prescribing clinician's supporting statement. For a non-formulary drug exception, the prescriber must support medical necessity by showing that all covered Part D drugs on any formulary tier for the same condition would not be as effective, would have adverse effects, or both. (eCFR) For a tiering exception, the prescriber must establish that the preferred alternative drugs for the condition would not be as effective, would have adverse effects, or both. (eCFR) The plan may require follow-up written support and additional medical documentation when an oral statement is provided. (eCFR) This structure prevents the exception system from becoming a preference-based override. It is a medical-necessity pathway, not a convenience pathway.

A successful exception changes the financial and coverage ledger. If a non-formulary drug is approved, the enrollee's costs for that drug are treated as included for purposes of calculating and meeting the annual out-of-pocket threshold. (eCFR) If a tiering exception is approved, the sponsor must provide the drug at the cost-sharing level that applies to preferred alternative drugs, and where alternative drugs exist on multiple tiers, cost sharing is assigned at the lowest applicable tier under the regulation's requirements. (eCFR) The sponsor may not create a special formulary tier or unique cost-sharing requirement applicable only to drugs approved through the non-formulary exception process. (eCFR) Thus, an exception does not merely permit the fill. It determines whether the drug enters the Part D benefit ledger as a covered drug, whether cost sharing is reduced, and whether the transaction advances the beneficiary toward the annual catastrophic threshold.

The exception process has limits. Beginning in 2022, if a Part D sponsor maintains one or two specialty tiers, the sponsor may design its tiering exception process so that drugs on the specialty tier are not eligible for tiering exceptions to non-specialty tiers. (eCFR) This limitation is crucial for household risk modeling. A specialty-tier drug may be clinically necessary and covered, but still remain locked in percentage-based specialty cost sharing until the annual Part D out-of-pocket cap is reached, unless the plan design or applicable law provides a different result. For a household dependent on specialty therapy, the relevant question is therefore not merely whether the drug is on the formulary. The full diagnostic question is whether the drug is on a specialty tier, whether the tier allows exceptions, whether the drug carries utilization edits, whether the drug's ingredient cost accelerates TrOOP accumulation, and whether the annual cap will be reached early enough to stabilize later-year cash flow.

Formulary change rules add another layer of mid-year risk. Medicare & You 2026 states that plans can make formulary changes during the year if they follow Medicare guidelines, and that a plan may notify affected enrollees of formulary changes involving drugs already being taken. Section 423.120 requires notice for negative formulary changes and specifies content that must identify the affected drug, whether the plan is removing the drug, moving it to a higher cost-sharing tier, or adding or making more restrictive prior authorization, step therapy, or quantity limit requirements; the notice must also state the reason for the change, identify appropriate alternative drugs on the formulary in the same or lower tier and expected cost sharing, and explain how to obtain a coverage determination, including exceptions. (eCFR) The operational danger is tier drift: a drug that was priced safely in January can become materially more expensive or administratively restricted later in the year if lawful formulary change procedures are satisfied.

The transition process is a temporary protection against abrupt loss of access, not a permanent entitlement to prior coverage. Section 423.120 requires a transition process for enrollees prescribed Part D drugs not on the new plan's formulary, including drugs that are technically on formulary but require prior authorization or step therapy. The transition process applies to new enrollees following annual election, newly eligible Medicare enrollees from other coverage, individuals who switch plans after the contract year begins, and current enrollees affected by formulary changes. (eCFR) It must ensure access to a temporary supply within the first 90 days of coverage under the new plan and written notice within three business days after adjudication of the temporary fill. (eCFR) This protects continuity during administrative transition, but it does not eliminate the need for a formulary exception, alternative therapy, or successful prior authorization before the temporary bridge expires.

The Household Medicare Diagnostic Matrix must treat formulary analysis as a multi-row risk audit rather than a simple covered-or-not-covered binary. The first row identifies whether the drug is a covered Part D drug, because noncovered or excluded drugs do not behave like ordinary formulary claims. The second row records formulary placement, including tier number, tier label, and whether the tier uses copayment or coinsurance. The third row identifies whether the drug is generic, preferred generic, non-preferred generic, preferred brand, non-preferred drug, biological product, biosimilar, interchangeable biological product, selected drug, or specialty-tier drug. The fourth row records utilization edits: prior authorization, step therapy, quantity limit, therapeutic substitution, generic substitution, or dose restriction. The fifth row records exception status, including prescriber support, medical necessity rationale, preferred alternative failure, adverse effect evidence, and whether the requested relief is a tiering exception, formulary exception, or utilization-management exception. The sixth row records annual Part D phase status and TrOOP progress, because the same specialty-tier coinsurance exposure that destabilizes the first quarter may terminate after the statutory out-of-pocket threshold is reached.

The final synthesis is that formulary architecture is the operational face of Part D actuarial governance. The formulary determines covered-drug access; the tier determines point-of-service financial intensity; the specialty tier determines whether high-cost therapy is governed by percentage coinsurance within federal limits; utilization-management edits determine whether the pharmacy claim can proceed without additional documentation; and the exception process determines whether clinical necessity can override formulary exclusion, unfavorable tiering, or administrative restrictions. Federal law does not prohibit plan sponsors from managing drug utilization. It requires that management to operate through CMS-approved formulary standards, P&T Committee review, adequate therapeutic coverage, protected-class safeguards, transition protections, disclosure obligations, and appealable exception processes. Failure to map these structures converts a theoretical household prescription budget into an obsolete model vulnerable to tier drift, claim rejection, sudden coinsurance escalation, unfilled prescriptions, and preventable cash-flow shock. Under the Household Medicare Diagnostic Matrix, Section 12.1 supplies the primary structural pillar for formulary tiering, chemical classification, step therapy, quantity limits, prior authorization, and exception appeals; it is the analytic manual for stabilizing household wealth against systemic pharmaceutical risk inside a privatized public drug benefit.

12.2 The Appeals and Grievances Pipeline

The Medicare Part D appeals and grievances structure is the administrative due-process system that converts a pharmacy denial, formulary restriction, tiering dispute, reimbursement refusal, or utilization-management rejection into a legally reviewable federal record. Its first doctrinal requirement is classification. A grievance is not the same instrument as an appeal. A grievance is an administrative complaint about operational conduct, quality of care, access friction, waiting times, customer service, plan staff behavior, or other dissatisfaction that does not itself decide whether a drug must be covered or paid. Medicare & You 2026 describes complaint, or grievance, channels for concerns about quality of care and other services, while separately defining an appeal as the action available when a beneficiary disagrees with a coverage or payment decision by Medicare or a Medicare plan. Under federal Part D grievance procedures, the grievance generally must be filed no later than 60 calendar days after the precipitating event or incident, and CMS operational guidance states that plans generally respond within 30 days, with expedited grievance handling required within 24 hours in specified urgent contexts. (eCFR) (CMS)

The coverage-determination pipeline is different because it adjudicates entitlement to payment or coverage. A Part D coverage determination is the plan sponsor's first formal decision about drug benefits. Medicare & You 2026 states that a coverage determination is the first decision a Medicare drug plan, not the pharmacy, makes about benefits, including whether the plan covers a drug, whether the plan's coverage requirements have been met, or how much the enrollee must pay; the same source states that an exception request for a non-formulary drug, a waiver of a coverage rule such as prior authorization, or lower cost sharing for a higher-tier drug is also processed through the coverage-determination structure. CMS guidance describes an initial determination as a decision by the plan or delegated entity concerning payment or provision of an item, service, or drug, and it directs plans to follow Part 423 Subpart M for Part D coverage determinations and appeals. (CMS) Thus, a grievance complains about process or treatment; a coverage determination determines the drug-coverage liability itself.

The practical border between the two categories can be delicate. CMS guidance explains that a general complaint about a drug not appearing on the formulary may be a grievance or inquiry, but when an enrollee states that a drug was rejected at the pharmacy and is needed, or that a drug is covered for the prescribed indication, the matter should be treated as a coverage request. The same guidance provides that if a person states an intent to file a grievance after a denial of drug coverage, the dispute should be treated as an appeal of the denial rather than left in the grievance channel. (CMS) This classification rule is central to wealth preservation because a grievance does not itself compel formulary payment, reimbursement, or tier correction. A household file that places a coverage denial into the grievance lane can lose time while the drug claim remains unpaid or unavailable.

Once the plan issues an adverse coverage determination, Level 1 begins through plan redetermination. CMS states that if a Part D plan sponsor denies a request in whole or in part, the enrollee, the enrollee's prescriber, or the enrollee's representative may appeal to the plan sponsor by requesting a standard or expedited redetermination. CMS's current Part D redetermination page states that redetermination requests must be filed with the plan sponsor within 65 calendar days from the date of the notice of coverage determination. (CMS) The regulatory mechanics explain the apparent 65-day convention: 42 CFR § 423.582 provides a 60-calendar-day filing period after receipt of the written coverage determination notice, and receipt is presumed to occur five calendar days after the notice date unless evidence shows otherwise. (Legal Information Institute) Accordingly, the handbook or plan-facing operational shorthand may state 65 days from the notice date, while the regulatory rule is 60 days after presumed receipt.

The Level 1 decision clock is short because the subject matter is clinical access, not ordinary civil debt. CMS states that once the plan sponsor receives the redetermination request, it must decide and provide written notice as quickly as the enrollee's health requires, but no later than 72 hours for expedited requests or seven calendar days for standard requests; payment redeterminations require written notice and payment where appropriate within 14 calendar days after the request is received. (CMS) Section 423.590 confirms those timelines and adds a critical internal-review safeguard: a person who was not involved in the original coverage determination must conduct the redetermination, and when the issue is a denial based on lack of medical necessity, the redetermination must be made by a physician with appropriate medical expertise. (Legal Information Institute) The administrative appeal therefore is not simply a customer-service escalation. It is a regulated second look inside the plan sponsor's own structure.

Failure to meet the Level 1 decision deadline has legal consequences. Under § 423.590, if the Part D plan sponsor fails to issue the redetermination within the standard or payment timeframes, that failure constitutes an adverse redetermination decision, and the sponsor must forward the request to the Independent Review Entity within 24 hours after expiration of the adjudication timeframe. The same automatic forwarding rule applies when the plan fails to complete an expedited redetermination within 72 hours. (Legal Information Institute) This rule is a consumer-protection device. It prevents a plan sponsor from defeating review by administrative inaction. Delay becomes denial for purposes of escalation, and the federal review network is activated.

Level 2 moves the dispute from internal plan review to external independent adjudication. CMS states that an enrollee, enrollee representative, or prescriber may request standard or expedited reconsideration of a plan denial of coverage or payment, or review of a plan dismissal, by filing with the designated Part D Independent Review Entity. CMS's current Part D reconsideration page states that the request must be filed with the IRE within 65 calendar days from the date of the plan sponsor's redetermination decision notice, and that all requests must be written, including requests submitted by fax. (CMS) The regulation again frames the timing as 60 calendar days after receipt of the written redetermination, with receipt presumed five calendar days after the date of the written redetermination unless evidence shows otherwise. (Legal Information Institute) The administrative shorthand and the regulation therefore align through the same date-of-notice plus presumed-receipt structure.

The IRE's role is not advisory. It is the federally designated external review body for Part D denials after the plan's redetermination. Section 423.600 requires the IRE to solicit the views of the prescribing physician or other prescriber when an appeal is filed or forwarded, and it requires a written account of those views to be contained in the IRE record. For non-formulary drug disputes, the regulation requires a prescriber determination that all covered Part D drugs on any formulary tier for the same condition would not be as effective for the individual, would have adverse effects, or both. (Legal Information Institute) This evidentiary requirement shows why the clinical record is the core of the appeal. General dissatisfaction with price rarely carries the dispute; documented therapeutic failure, contraindication, adverse reaction, or medical necessity does.

The IRE operates under strict decision windows. CMS states that once the IRE receives a benefit request, it must decide and provide written notice as quickly as the enrollee's health requires, but no later than 72 hours for expedited requests or seven calendar days for standard benefit requests; for payment disputes, the IRE must decide, provide written notice, and instruct the plan to make payment where appropriate within 14 calendar days after receiving the request. (CMS) Medicare.gov states the same public-facing timelines for drug appeals: seven days for standard benefit appeals, fourteen days for payment appeals, and seventy-two hours for fast appeals. (Medicare) The IRE stage therefore becomes the most important early external checkpoint for formulary denials, prior authorization disputes, tiering exceptions, and reimbursement refusals.

If the Level 2 decision remains adverse, Level 3 introduces a monetary jurisdictional gate. The dispute moves to the Office of Medicare Hearings and Appeals only if the amount remaining in controversy satisfies the annual threshold. CMS states that for calendar year 2025 the Part D ALJ amount in controversy threshold is $190, and for calendar year 2026 the threshold is $200. (CMS) CMS's 2026 Part D appeals flow chart confirms that the ALJ hearing threshold is at least $200 for 2026 and states that the amount-in-controversy requirement is adjusted annually in accordance with the medical care component of the Consumer Price Index. (CMS) The AIC threshold operates as an access filter. A low-dollar dispute may end at the IRE even when the legal issue is meaningful, while an expensive specialty-drug dispute may move into formal hearing jurisdiction because the claim value exceeds the federal minimum.

The filing window for Level 3 is tightly regulated. Medicare.gov states that a party has 60 days from the date of the Part D IRE decision to ask for a Level 3 appeal through OMHA. (Medicare) Section 423.2014 similarly requires the request for an ALJ hearing or review of an IRE dismissal to be filed within 60 calendar days from the date the enrollee receives written notice of the IRE reconsideration or dismissal, with good-cause extensions available under the regulatory standards. (Legal Information Institute) The request must be complete and directed to the office specified in the IRE notice. The administrative record at this stage generally includes the plan's coverage determination, the redetermination record, the IRE reconsideration, prescriber statements, medical records, formulary evidence, and any supporting clinical documentation submitted during the lower levels.

The Level 3 hearing is structurally different from the plan's internal review. Medicare.gov explains that an ALJ hearing allows the appeal to be presented to a new person who independently reviews the facts, listens to testimony, and makes a decision; hearings are usually held by telephone or video-teleconference, with in-person hearings available if the ALJ finds good reason. (Medicare) Federal rulemaking confirms the de novo character of ALJ review in the Part D context, meaning the adjudicator conducts a new review rather than merely asking whether the plan sponsor acted reasonably under its internal guideline. (Federal Register) The practical effect is important: the household file gains access to an independent federal adjudicator who may evaluate the entire clinical and pharmaceutical record under Medicare law rather than under the plan sponsor's initial claims posture.

The ALJ stage, however, is not a simple litigation opportunity without procedural cost. The request must be timely, complete, and supported; the AIC threshold must be satisfied; and the record must be clinically coherent. A specialty-drug denial may meet the $200 threshold immediately, while a modest tiering dispute may fail to qualify unless claims are aggregated where allowed or the annual cost exposure is sufficient. Medicare.gov states that the request can be made by using the OMHA hearing form, submitting a written request containing identifying and appeal information, or filing through the OMHA electronic appeal portal; it also permits an on-the-record review in certain circumstances when no hearing is sought. (Medicare) From an actuarial perspective, Level 3 is where administrative proficiency becomes asset protection: a missing laboratory report, absent prescriber statement, vague diagnosis, or undocumented failure of alternatives can convert a medically appropriate therapy into an unrecovered out-of-pocket liability.

Level 4 is review by the Medicare Appeals Council, a component of the Departmental Appeals Board. Medicare.gov states that a party may move to Level 4 if OMHA does not issue a timely decision or if the party disagrees with the OMHA decision, and that the request for Council review must be made within 60 days after receipt of the OMHA decision. (Medicare) Council review is not the same as another initial pharmacy review. The Council examines the ALJ decision, the hearing record, legal conclusions, procedural regularity, and the adequacy of the administrative reasoning. Under § 423.2100, when the Council reviews an ALJ or attorney adjudicator written decision, it undertakes de novo review. (Legal Information Institute) In practical terms, the Council is the final administrative tribunal before federal judicial review.

The Council stage should be understood as legal and procedural consolidation. It can affirm, reverse, modify, or remand depending on the administrative record and applicable law. The prescriber's clinical statement remains important, but the argument often shifts toward whether the lower adjudicator properly applied Part D coverage rules, formulary exception standards, evidence requirements, procedural timelines, and medical-necessity principles. Medicare.gov directs appellants to follow the ALJ decision instructions and submit a written request or Council review form identifying the disputed items, service dates, reasons for disagreement, and date of the ALJ decision. (Medicare) The household risk at Level 4 is delayed finality. While a case is moving through the Council, the pharmacy counter may continue to require payment unless the drug has been furnished, the plan has implemented a favorable decision, or separate interim protections apply.

Level 5 is federal district court judicial review, the final avenue in the ordinary Part D appeals sequence. Medicare.gov states that judicial review may be requested if the Appeals Council does not issue a timely decision, if the party disagrees with the Council's Level 4 decision, and if the case meets a minimum dollar amount; the request for judicial review must generally be made within 60 days after receipt of the Council's decision. (Medicare) CMS's 2026 Part D appeals flow chart states that the Federal District Court amount in controversy threshold is at least $1,960 for 2026. (CMS) That threshold is materially higher than the ALJ threshold and reflects the federal judiciary's role as the terminal review body rather than as an ordinary claims-processing forum.

The federal-court threshold creates a significant access barrier for household-level Part D disputes. A single low-cost generic denial is unlikely to support judicial review. A high-cost specialty therapy, oncology agent, immunologic compound, or chronic rare-disease medication may satisfy the threshold more readily. Yet even where the dollar threshold is satisfied, federal litigation requires legal sophistication, procedural compliance, and substantial time. CMS's general federal district court guidance states that an action must be filed within 60 calendar days after receipt of the Council decision, with receipt generally presumed five days after the date of the notice unless evidence shows otherwise. (CMS) This final stage underscores why the first three levels are economically decisive. Most retirement households cannot treat federal litigation as a routine pharmaceutical access tool.

The full Part D appeals pipeline is therefore a five-level federal recourse network. The coverage determination begins the formal drug-coverage record. Level 1 plan redetermination gives the sponsor a regulated internal opportunity to correct or defend its denial. Level 2 IRE reconsideration moves the dispute to external independent review and requires prescriber views to enter the record. Level 3 OMHA review permits ALJ or attorney adjudicator consideration if the $200 2026 amount-in-controversy threshold is met. Level 4 Medicare Appeals Council review creates final administrative review of the ALJ decision or dismissal. Level 5 federal district court review is available only after administrative exhaustion and satisfaction of the $1,960 2026 judicial threshold. CMS's official flow chart tracks the same structure from coverage determination through redetermination, IRE reconsideration, OMHA hearing, Medicare Appeals Council review, and federal district court review. (CMS)

This structure must be coupled directly to formulary governance. A prior authorization denial, step therapy refusal, quantity-limit dispute, non-formulary rejection, specialty-tier issue, reimbursement denial, at-risk drug management determination, or tiering exception dispute becomes financially meaningful only when it is placed into the correct procedural lane. Medicare & You 2026 states that an appeal is available when a plan denies a requested drug, payment for a drug already obtained, a requested cost-sharing change, or continued payment for a needed item or drug. Medicare & You also states that if a network pharmacy cannot fill a prescription, the pharmacist should provide a notice explaining how to contact the drug plan to request a coverage determination, and that expedited requests are available when the plan determines, or the prescriber states, that waiting may put life or health at risk. A pharmacy rejection is therefore not the end of the claim. It is often the beginning of the formal record.

The Household Medicare Diagnostic Matrix treats Section 12.2 as the primary operational pillar for the "Appeals & Formal Recourse" rows. The matrix must record the adverse action date, notice date, presumed receipt date, grievance versus appeal classification, coverage-determination status, redetermination deadline, expedited eligibility, prescriber statement status, IRE filing deadline, IRE decision deadline, AIC calculation, OMHA eligibility, Medicare Appeals Council filing date, federal-court threshold status, and whether the claim involves benefits not yet received or reimbursement for drugs already purchased. The distinction between a 72-hour expedited review, a seven-day standard benefit review, and a fourteen-day payment review is not clerical. It determines whether the household is confronting immediate clinical interruption, near-term pharmacy access, or retrospective cash recovery.

The wealth-preservation consequence is direct. Modern Part D includes a 2026 annual out-of-pocket cap for covered Part D drugs, but that cap protects only drugs that are recognized and adjudicated inside the Part D benefit structure. A drug denied as non-formulary, restricted by prior authorization, blocked by step therapy, limited by quantity rules, or rejected for payment may require out-of-pocket payment outside the expected household model until the denial is reversed, the alternative drug is accepted, or the claim is otherwise resolved. The appeals pipeline is therefore a capital-protection mechanism. It prevents a plan-level denial from becoming a permanent liquidation event without federal review.

The final synthesis is that mastery of the Part D appeals and grievances system is not merely clinical navigation. It is administrative asset defense. A grievance preserves accountability for operational misconduct, but it does not substitute for a coverage appeal. A coverage determination establishes the first appealable drug-benefit decision. A redetermination must be filed within the 65-day notice-date convention, corresponding to the 60-day-after-receipt regulatory rule, and the plan must decide within 72 hours, seven days, or fourteen days depending on urgency and payment status. The IRE supplies independent review under the same expedited, standard, and payment clocks. OMHA introduces the 2026 $200 ALJ amount-in-controversy threshold. The Medicare Appeals Council supplies final administrative review. Federal District Court review requires the 2026 $1,960 amount-in-controversy threshold and the capacity to pursue formal judicial proceedings. A household strategy that fails to track these deadlines and thresholds leaves prescription-drug wealth exposure unprotected against adverse coverage decisions, administrative delay, and claim denial. Under the Household Medicare Diagnostic Matrix, the appeals record is not paperwork; it is the legal ledger through which a denied medication either returns to covered status or remains an unhedged charge against non-sheltered household assets.

Chapter 13: Serious Illness Transitions and Hospice Care Integration

13.1 Hospice Isolation Architecture

The Medicare hospice benefit occupies a singular position inside the federal health-insurance architecture because it does not behave like ordinary acute-care coverage, ordinary Medicare Advantage managed care, ordinary Part D prescription drug administration, or ordinary supplemental cost-sharing protection. Hospice is a Part A benefit under the Hospital Insurance program, designed for individuals who are terminally ill, meaning the medical prognosis is a life expectancy of six months or less if the illness runs its normal course. CMS's Medicare Benefit Policy Manual states that eligibility to elect hospice requires entitlement to Part A and certification of terminal illness, and it specifies that only care provided by, or under arrangements made by, a Medicare-certified hospice is covered under the Medicare hospice benefit. (CMS) The official Medicare Hospice Benefits booklet in the source packet states the same beneficiary-facing principle: hospice is a program of care and support for people who are terminally ill and their families, with a focus on comfort rather than cure, and with services generally organized around physical care, counseling, drugs, equipment, supplies, and whole-person support for terminal illness and related conditions.

The hospice carve-out is the legal and administrative mechanism by which end-of-life care is isolated from the ordinary Medicare Advantage managed-care environment. A Medicare Advantage plan may remain technically active, premiums may continue, and non-hospice benefits may remain relevant, but the hospice benefit itself is paid through Original Medicare rather than through the plan's ordinary managed-care payment pathway. Medicare & You 2026 states that Original Medicare will be billed for hospice care even when the beneficiary is enrolled in a Medicare Advantage Plan, and that switching back to Original Medicare is not required for hospice to be covered. The Medicare Advantage section of the same handbook explains that Medicare Advantage Plans provide almost all medically necessary services Original Medicare covers, but Original Medicare covers the cost for hospice care and certain other limited categories. This is the core isolation architecture: the managed-care plan remains present, but terminal-illness-related hospice liability exits the plan's ordinary network, prior authorization, and capitation structure.

The systemic purpose of the carve-out is protective. Medicare Advantage is built around private-plan administration, service-area rules, contracted networks, referral structures, prior authorization protocols, and negotiated cost controls. Hospice, by contrast, is organized around an interdisciplinary hospice plan of care, palliative symptom management, caregiver support, and certification of terminal prognosis.

The source booklet states that once hospice begins, Original Medicare covers everything needed related to the terminal illness and related conditions, even if the beneficiary remains enrolled in a Medicare Advantage Plan or other Medicare health plan. The design prevents the most vulnerable phase of serious illness from being forced entirely through a private plan's ordinary network architecture. It does not eliminate all financial exposure, but it moves terminal-illness-related palliative care into a dedicated federal benefit channel.

The eligibility trigger is certification, not mere serious illness. CMS's Medicare Benefit Policy Manual requires clinical certification that the individual is terminally ill, based on the judgment of the hospice medical director or physician member of the interdisciplinary group and the individual's attending physician, if there is one, regarding the normal course of the illness. The manual further states that no one other than a medical doctor or doctor of osteopathy may certify or recertify terminal illness, and that the fact that a beneficiary lives longer than expected is not, by itself, cause to terminate benefits. (CMS) The corresponding regulation, 42 CFR § 418.22, requires certification that the prognosis is for life expectancy of six months or less if the terminal illness runs its normal course and requires a physician narrative explaining the clinical findings supporting that prognosis. (eCFR)

The dual certification rule is most exact at the first election period. For the initial 90-day period, the Medicare Benefit Policy Manual states that certification must be obtained no later than two calendar days after hospice care is initiated, by the end of the third day, from the hospice medical director or physician member of the hospice interdisciplinary group and from the individual's attending physician if there is one. (CMS) The official hospice booklet states that, at the start of the first 90-day benefit period, the hospice doctor and regular doctor, if one exists, must certify terminal illness with a life expectancy of six months or less. The regulatory requirement is therefore clinical and documentary. Hospice is not activated merely by preference, frailty, custodial need, or family hardship. It requires formal medical certification tied to the terminal prognosis standard.

The benefit-period sequence is also precise. Hospice care is given in benefit periods: two 90-day benefit periods followed by an unlimited number of subsequent 60-day benefit periods. The eCFR rule at 42 CFR § 418.21 identifies the sequence as an initial 90-day period, a subsequent 90-day period, and an unlimited number of subsequent 60-day periods, available in order. (eCFR) The official hospice booklet states that a benefit period starts when hospice care begins and ends when the applicable 90-day or 60-day period ends; after the first 90-day period, the hospice medical director or other hospice doctor must recertify terminal illness at the start of each later benefit period. This sequence is not a six-month hard cutoff. It is a prognosis-based continuing entitlement framework, provided recertification remains clinically supportable.

The palliative-curative boundary is the deepest legal feature of the hospice election. The hospice benefit is not merely an additional service package layered onto full curative Medicare coverage for the same terminal condition. By electing hospice, the beneficiary chooses a care model focused on palliation, comfort, symptom management, and psychosocial support rather than treatment intended to cure the terminal illness. The official hospice booklet states that once hospice begins, the benefit will not cover treatment intended to cure the terminal illness and related conditions, while the beneficiary retains the right to stop hospice care at any time. The Medicare Benefit Policy Manual states the waiver rule more legally: for the duration of the hospice election, the individual waives Medicare payments for hospice care provided by a hospice other than the designated hospice, unless arranged by the designated hospice, and for Medicare services related to treatment of the terminal condition or a related condition except through specified hospice and attending-physician pathways. (CMS)

This waiver does not mean the beneficiary loses Medicare for all other illnesses. The hospice booklet states that after hospice begins, covered services for conditions not related to the terminal illness remain available, and Original Medicare pays for covered benefits for health problems that are not part of the terminal illness and related conditions, subject to ordinary deductibles and coinsurance. The Medicare Benefit Policy Manual likewise states that Medicare services for a completely unrelated condition remain available if the patient is eligible for such care. (CMS) The controlling distinction is relatedness. Hospice reorganizes payment for the terminal illness and related conditions, while unrelated conditions remain in ordinary Medicare or Medicare Advantage channels according to the applicable coverage pathway.

The hospice benefit's financial mechanics are built around a bundled hospice payment system rather than ordinary item-by-item patient cost sharing for terminal-condition care. The Benefit Policy Manual states that covered hospice services must be reasonable and necessary for palliation and management of the terminal illness and related conditions, must be consistent with a plan of care established and periodically reviewed by the attending physician, medical director, and hospice interdisciplinary group, and are paid to the hospice on a per diem basis according to the level of care. (CMS) Covered hospice levels include routine home care, continuous home care during brief periods of crisis, inpatient respite care, and general inpatient care for pain control or acute or chronic symptom management that cannot be managed in other settings. (CMS) The financial implication is that the hospice provider, not the beneficiary's ordinary Medicare Advantage plan, becomes the organizing payment entity for terminal-illness-related palliative services.

The covered service package is broad but conditional. The official hospice booklet lists doctor services, nursing care, medical equipment such as wheelchairs or walkers, medical supplies such as bandages and catheters, prescription drugs for pain and symptom control, hospice aide and homemaker services, physical and occupational therapy, speech-language pathology services, social worker services, dietary counseling, grief and loss counseling, short-term inpatient care, respite care, and other Medicare-covered services needed to manage the terminal illness and related conditions as recommended by the hospice team. Medicare & You 2026 similarly lists pain relief and symptom management items and services, medical, nursing, and social services, drugs, durable medical equipment, aide and homemaker services, and spiritual and grief counseling. These benefits are not free-floating entitlements. They must be tied to the terminal illness or related conditions and coordinated through the designated hospice plan of care.

The cost-sharing structure is sharply different from ordinary Part A and Part B cost sharing. Medicare & You 2026 states that the beneficiary pays nothing for hospice care, may owe a copayment of up to five dollars per prescription for outpatient drugs for pain and symptom management, and owes five percent of the Medicare-approved amount for inpatient respite care. The hospice booklet and related Medicare materials state that there is no deductible for hospice care, although monthly Part A and Part B premiums, where applicable, are not erased by hospice election. (Medicare) The Benefit Policy Manual further specifies that respite care coinsurance is equal to five percent of Medicare's payment for a respite care day, subject to a maximum tied to the inpatient hospital deductible for the applicable hospice coinsurance period. (CMS) Thus, hospice can dramatically reduce terminal-illness-related cost exposure, but it does not become a universal zero-cost long-term-care entitlement.

The outpatient drug rule is a major Part D interface. Drugs for pain and symptom management related to the terminal illness are part of the hospice benefit, with the limited hospice drug copayment exposure described above. Medicare & You 2026 states that hospice coverage includes drugs for pain and symptom management and that the beneficiary may pay up to five dollars per outpatient prescription for those drugs. The hospice booklet states that prescription drugs not for the terminal illness or related conditions are not included in the hospice benefit, but may be covered by Medicare drug coverage, with a possible copayment. This creates a two-channel drug architecture. Terminal-related palliative medications belong to hospice Part A. Unrelated outpatient medications may remain in Part D or another drug coverage structure. Misclassification can create denied claims, duplicate pharmacy rejections, and avoidable out-of-pocket payment.

The Medicare Advantage residual channel must be analyzed with equal precision. If a beneficiary was in a Medicare Advantage Plan before hospice and remains in that plan while paying any plan premiums, the hospice booklet states that the plan covers medically necessary extra services, such as dental or vision benefits, and covered services for health problems unrelated to the terminal illness. The same booklet states that unrelated services may be obtained through Original Medicare or through the Medicare Advantage Plan, and if the plan includes drug coverage, the plan covers drugs not related to the terminal illness. Medicare & You 2026 confirms the same arrangement: when hospice care begins, the Medicare Advantage Plan may still cover services that are not part of the terminal illness or related conditions. The plan is not extinguished; it is financially displaced for terminal-related hospice care.

Billing relatedness is the operational hinge. CMS's Medicare Claims Processing Manual states that when a beneficiary elects hospice, the Common Working File maintains hospice entitlement information, and Medicare contractors use that hospice status to examine and adjudicate claims. For professional claims, attending physician services may use modifier GV when furnished by an attending physician not employed or paid under arrangement by the hospice; services unrelated to the terminal condition use modifier GW. The same manual states that professional claims for hospice beneficiaries submitted without GV or GW are denied, and that services unrelated to the terminal condition may be billed for non-hospice Medicare payment using GW on professional claims or condition code 07 on institutional claims. (CMS) The prompt's institutional-modifier framing therefore requires correction: institutional claims use condition code 07 for non-terminal condition treatment; professional claims use the GV and GW modifier logic.

This claims architecture is a safeguard and a trap. It is a safeguard because it prevents terminal-condition services from being fragmented across unmanaged, non-hospice providers while hospice is responsible for the plan of care. It is a trap because a provider who does not understand hospice status may submit an otherwise covered service through the wrong channel, omit required coding, fail to document unrelatedness, or seek payment from the wrong payer. The Claims Processing Manual states that covered Medicare services unrelated to the terminal condition may be processed in the normal manner when coded appropriately with GW or condition code 07, but contractors may conduct prepayment or post-payment review to validate unrelatedness. (CMS) For the household, the coding issue is not an internal billing detail. It can determine whether a claim is paid, routed to hospice, denied, or temporarily pushed into direct liability.

Room and board is the most commonly misunderstood exclusion. The hospice booklet states that the hospice benefit does not cover room and board, but if the hospice team determines that short-term inpatient or respite care is needed and arranges it, Medicare will cover the facility stay, with a possible small respite copayment. Medicare & You 2026 states that Medicare-certified hospice care is usually provided in the home or another facility where the person lives, such as an assisted living facility or nursing home, but Medicare does not pay room and board in a facility unless the hospice medical team decides short-term inpatient care is needed to manage pain and other symptoms in a Medicare-approved facility. This is the essential custodial-care boundary. Hospice may bring clinical and support services into the place of residence, but it does not transform rent, assisted living charges, nursing-facility room charges, or long-term custodial lodging into a Medicare-covered benefit.

Respite care is the narrow room-and-board exception most relevant to caregiver exhaustion. The hospice booklet states that inpatient respite care can be arranged by the hospice provider in a Medicare-approved facility such as a hospice inpatient facility, hospital, or nursing home, and that the stay can last up to five days each time, on an occasional basis. Medicare & You 2026 similarly states that inpatient respite care is covered in a Medicare-approved facility so that a caregiver can rest, for up to five days each time, arranged by the hospice provider. The distinction is crucial. Short-term, hospice-arranged respite care is a covered hospice service with limited cost sharing. Long-term custodial room and board is not. A household that assumes hospice pays for indefinite facility residency may face immediate and severe private-pay exposure.

Unarranged care is the second major liability gate. The hospice booklet states that once hospice begins, the beneficiary must get hospice care from the chosen hospice provider, and the hospice team must give or arrange all care for the terminal illness and related conditions. It further warns that care from any provider not set up by the hospice medical team is not covered under the hospice benefit, except for the continuing role of the chosen attending medical professional where applicable. The same booklet warns that hospital outpatient care, inpatient care, or ambulance transportation may generate full-cost exposure if obtained without hospice-team coordination in circumstances where hospice arrangement is required. This rule is difficult for families because medical crises often feel like ordinary emergency events. Under hospice, the designated hospice team becomes the first coordination node for terminal-related crises unless emergency circumstances or unrelated conditions change the coverage analysis.

The curative-treatment exclusion reinforces the same principle. The hospice booklet states that once hospice begins, the benefit will not cover treatment intended to cure the terminal illness or related conditions, while the beneficiary retains the right to stop hospice care at any time. The Benefit Policy Manual states that an individual may revoke the hospice election at any time in writing, that the hospice cannot revoke the election on the patient's behalf, and that upon revocation the individual resumes Medicare coverage of benefits waived when hospice was elected. (CMS) Revocation is therefore the legal path back to ordinary curative coverage for the terminal condition. While hospice remains elected, curative terminal-condition treatment outside the hospice framework is not simply a different treatment preference; it is a payment-boundary violation unless the election is revoked or the service falls within an allowed exception.

The hospice right to change provider and right to stop hospice care further illustrate that the carve-out is an elected status, not a custodial lock-in. The hospice booklet states that the beneficiary has the right to change hospice provider once during each benefit period and the right to stop hospice care at any time; if care is stopped, the hospice provider asks for a form with the date care will end. The booklet also states that a person in a Medicare Advantage Plan when hospice begins can stay in that plan while receiving hospice as long as plan premiums continue, and may continue plan coverage after hospice ends if premiums have been paid. These rights are important for household planning. They preserve exit and continuity options, but they do not erase the need to coordinate services carefully during the hospice election.

Quality and fraud protections also belong in the isolation architecture. The hospice booklet warns that scammers may attempt to enroll people in hospice who do not need it, and it states that the doctor is the only one who can certify terminal illness with a life expectancy of six months or less. The booklet also identifies rights to care meeting professionally recognized standards and the right to contact a Beneficiary and Family Centered Care Quality Improvement Organization when quality concerns are unresolved with the hospice provider. The diagnostic lesson is that hospice enrollment should be treated as a formal clinical, financial, and legal election requiring valid certification, designated provider selection, plan-of-care review, and complaint pathways, not as a generic home-care label.

The Household Medicare Diagnostic Matrix must place hospice in its own isolated risk column. The first row identifies Part A entitlement and terminal prognosis certification. The second row records the election date, designated hospice provider, attending physician, hospice medical director or hospice physician certification, and benefit-period status. The third row separates terminal-illness-related and related-condition services from unrelated conditions. The fourth row tracks payer responsibility: hospice Part A for related palliative services, Original Medicare or Medicare Advantage for unrelated services depending on channel and plan rules, Part

D for unrelated drugs where applicable, and private household liability for noncovered room and board or unarranged care. The fifth row records cost sharing: no ordinary hospice deductible, up to five dollars for outpatient pain and symptom-management prescriptions, five percent coinsurance for inpatient respite care, ordinary cost sharing for unrelated Medicare-covered services, and full-cost exposure for excluded or unarranged services where coverage requirements fail.

The wealth-preservation implication is severe. Families often hear "hospice is covered" and infer that every cost associated with end-of-life living arrangements, custodial assistance, facility room charges, emergency transport, specialist consultations, prescription drugs, and caregiver relief is absorbed by Medicare. The source documents reject that inference. Medicare covers hospice care for terminal illness and related conditions through a Medicare-approved hospice provider, generally in the home or place of residence, but it does not cover ordinary room and board in the home, assisted living facility, nursing home, or long-term hospice residence unless short-term inpatient or respite care is arranged under the hospice rules. It covers terminal-related palliative drugs through hospice, but unrelated drugs may remain in Part D. It pays hospice through Original Medicare even when the beneficiary remains in Medicare Advantage, but the plan's residual responsibilities apply only to extra benefits and unrelated services within the applicable rules.

The final synthesis is that hospice isolation architecture is a federal risk-partitioning system. It removes terminal-illness-related palliative care from ordinary managed-care payment operations and places it under Original Medicare Part A through a Medicare-certified hospice, subject to certification, election, benefit-period, plan-of-care, and relatedness rules. It protects against uncontrolled terminal-condition cost sharing by covering hospice services through the designated hospice, but it also creates strict liability gates around curative treatment, unarranged terminal-related care, room and board, unrelated conditions, non-hospice providers, and claims coding. Under the Household Medicare Diagnostic Matrix, the hospice carve-out row is not merely a care-preference entry. It is a wealth-preservation control designed to separate covered palliative care from uncovered custodial housing, unrelated medical care, residual Medicare Advantage benefits, Part D drug claims, and uncoordinated crisis services. Mastery of the CMS hospice protocols is therefore essential for preventing serious illness from becoming a sudden, unclassified liquidation event against household non-sheltered assets.

13.2 Primary Statutory Responsibilities for End-of-Life Benefit Allocation

The Medicare hospice benefit is not merely a clinical service category. It is a statutory payment allocation rule embedded inside the Hospital Insurance title of Medicare. Pursuant to Section 1812(a)(4) of the Social Security Act, hospice care is identified as a discrete Part A benefit available for terminally ill individuals who meet the statutory election and certification requirements; Section 1812(d) then supplies the election architecture by providing that Medicare payment for hospice care may be made during two 90-day periods and an unlimited number of subsequent 60-day periods, but only if the individual elects hospice care from a particular hospice program instead of certain other Medicare benefits. (Social Security) This statutory structure prevents hospice from being absorbed into ordinary managed-care administration as a routine Part C service line. Hospice is its own election-based Part A entitlement, financed and adjudicated through the Original Medicare hospice system after the election becomes effective.

The hospice election statement is therefore not a ceremonial consent form. It is a legal switch that changes the federal payment channel for terminal-illness-related care. CMS Product No. 11303, the official Medicare Hospice Benefits booklet, states that hospice eligibility requires Part A, certification by the hospice doctor and regular doctor, if one exists, that the person is terminally ill with a life expectancy of six months or less, acceptance of comfort care instead of curative care, and a signed statement choosing hospice care instead of other Medicare-covered treatments for the terminal illness and related conditions. Once that election is made, the beneficiary does not simply add a new care team to existing managed-care rules. The election waives ordinary Medicare payment for services related to treatment of the terminal condition or equivalent to hospice care unless those services are furnished by, or under arrangements made by, the elected hospice program, with a statutory exception for certain attending-physician services. (Social Security)

This allocation rule explains why Original Medicare becomes the primary payer for hospice even during Medicare Advantage enrollment. Medicare & You 2026 states directly that Original Medicare is billed for hospice care even if the beneficiary is enrolled in a Medicare Advantage Plan, and the beneficiary is not required to switch back to Original Medicare for hospice coverage. The official hospice booklet states the same rule with broader operational detail: once hospice care begins, Original Medicare covers everything needed related to the terminal illness, even if the individual remains enrolled in a Medicare Advantage Plan or other Medicare health plan. This is the statutory reversion doctrine. The enrollee remains in the Part C plan unless disenrollment occurs, but the plan's ordinary capitation-funded risk structure no longer carries the hospice-care liability for the terminal diagnosis.

The capitation carve-out is codified in 42 CFR § 422.320. That regulation requires a Medicare Advantage organization to inform eligible enrollees about hospice availability when hospice programs are available in the service area or referral to outside hospice programs is common, and it further provides that a hospice-electing beneficiary continues Medicare Advantage enrollment unless disenrollment occurs. The retained enrollment, however, is financially limited: the enrollee remains entitled to receive through the Medicare Advantage plan only benefits other than those that are the responsibility of the Medicare hospice. (Legal Information Institute) The regulation then states the payment rule: no payment is made to the MA organization on behalf of a Medicare enrollee who has elected hospice care, except for the rebate portion and any monthly prescription drug payment, and this no-payment rule applies from the first day of the month after the hospice election month until the first day of the month after the election ends. (Legal Information Institute)

The actuarial logic is exact. CMS removes the hospice liability from the plan's capitated risk rate because the hospice program, not the Medicare Advantage organization, becomes the federally designated payment recipient for hospice care. Section 422.320 provides that during the hospice election CMS reduces monthly capitation to the beneficiary rebate amount, or zero for plans with no beneficiary rebate, plus any Part D monthly payment, and CMS pays through the original Medicare program both the hospice program for hospice care and the MA organization, provider, or supplier for other Medicare-covered services furnished to the enrollee. (Legal Information Institute) The Medicare Managed Care Manual explains the same rule institutionally: an MA enrollee who elects hospice may remain enrolled, the plan receives a reduced capitation rate, the plan remains responsible for supplemental benefits, CMS pays the hospice program for hospice care, and CMS pays for other Medicare-covered services through Original Medicare subject to usual payment rules. (CMS)

The operational claim pathway follows that payment architecture. Hospice providers do not route terminal-illness-related hospice per-diem claims through a private plan's ordinary network gate. They submit hospice election and claim transactions to the Medicare contractor system. CMS's Medicare Claims Processing Manual states that when a beneficiary elects hospice, the hospice must complete a Notice of Election on the institutional claim format, and a timely Notice of Election must be submitted to and accepted by the A/B Medicare Administrative Contractor for Home Health and Hospice, identified in CMS manuals as the A/B MAC (HHH), within five calendar days after the hospice admission date. (CMS) The same manual specifies that if the hospice fails to file timely and no exception applies, Medicare will not cover and pay the days from admission through the accepted filing date, and those days become provider liability rather than beneficiary liability. (CMS) This is a direct federal claims-processing corridor, not a private-plan authorization route.

The relatedness doctrine supplies the boundary between the hospice payer channel and residual managed-care or Original Medicare channels. The Social Security Act waiver applies to services determined, under Secretarial guidelines, to be related to the treatment of the condition for which the terminal diagnosis was made or equivalent to hospice care. (Social Security) CMS Product No. 11303 states that after hospice begins, covered services for conditions not related to the terminal illness remain available, but the beneficiary remains responsible for applicable deductibles and coinsurance for those unrelated Medicare-covered services. The same booklet states that the hospice provider can be asked for a list of items, services, and drugs determined not related to the terminal illness and related conditions, and that the list must include the reasons those items are not related and must be furnished to non-hospice providers or Medicare if requested.

The presumption of relatedness is not a casual administrative preference. It is the practical consequence of a broad statutory waiver and a hospice plan-of-care model in which the terminal prognosis often drives multiple body systems, medication needs, functional decline, pain management, psychosocial distress, and equipment requirements. CMS's hospice booklet states that once the hospice benefit starts, Original Medicare covers everything needed related to the terminal illness and related conditions, but the care must come from a Medicare-approved hospice provider. It lists doctor services, nursing care, medical equipment, medical supplies, prescription drugs for pain and symptom control, hospice aide and homemaker services, therapies, social worker services, dietary counseling, grief counseling, short-term inpatient care, respite care, and other Medicare-covered services needed to manage the terminal illness and related conditions. A provider seeking to route a service outside the hospice channel must therefore establish a clean unrelatedness theory, not merely a different billing preference.

Claims coding is the procedural tool used to enforce that distinction. CMS's Claims Processing Manual explains that an independent attending physician may bill Medicare Part B to the A/B MAC (B) for professional services related to the hospice patient's terminal illness when the physician is not employed by, and not paid under arrangement with, the hospice; such services use modifier GV, meaning the attending physician is not employed or paid under agreement by the hospice provider. (CMS) The same manual states that A/B MACs use Common Working File hospice entitlement information to validate hospice coverage dates and to examine and adjudicate professional services coded with GV or GW modifiers. (CMS) The Managed Care Manual further distinguishes hospice care, meaning Original Medicare items and services related to the terminal illness for which hospice was elected, from non-hospice care, meaning either services not covered by Original Medicare or services not related to the terminal condition. (CMS)

The residual liability channel for Medicare Advantage is therefore narrow but important. Under § 422.320, the hospice-electing enrollee remains enrolled in the plan unless disenrollment occurs and remains entitled to plan benefits other than those that are the responsibility of the Medicare hospice. (Legal Information Institute) The hospice booklet states that a person who was in a Medicare Advantage Plan before hospice may stay in that plan while paying plan premiums; the plan may cover medically necessary extra services such as dental or vision benefits, covered services for unrelated health problems, and, if drug coverage is included, drugs not related to the terminal illness. The Managed Care Manual adds that for covered non-hospice-care Part A and Part B services, the enrollee may use the MA plan or Original Medicare; if Original Medicare is used and plan rules are followed, the plan must pay the difference between Original Medicare cost sharing and plan cost sharing where applicable. (CMS) This residual channel is not a reinstatement of full Part C risk for hospice care. It is a continuation of non-hospice and supplemental responsibilities.

The administrative friction arises when providers, plans, hospice teams, and families disagree about relatedness. A claim submitted to the private plan for a service related to the terminal condition may be denied because the hospice election places that liability in the hospice or Original Medicare channel. A claim submitted to Original Medicare as unrelated may be reviewed because the hospice election creates a terminal-condition overlay in Medicare systems. A non-hospice physician may need the GV modifier when acting as the designated attending physician, while unrelated professional services may require the GW logic, and institutional claims for treatment of a non-terminal condition may require condition-code routing under Medicare claims guidance. (CMS) These technical codes matter because they are the language by which the federal system distinguishes hospice Part A, attending-physician Part B, unrelated Original Medicare, residual MA, and noncovered liability.

Improper routing can create illegal or premature household collections. If a hospice provider fails to file the Notice of Election on time, CMS states that noncovered days attributable to the late filing are provider liability and may not be billed to the beneficiary. (CMS) If a service is terminal-related but obtained from an independent physician who is not the designated attending physician and not arranged by the hospice, the Claims Processing Manual states that the physician or provider must look to the hospice for payment when the care is related to the terminal condition. (CMS)

If a service is genuinely unrelated, CMS materials permit continued coverage through Original Medicare or, for a continuing MA enrollee, through the MA plan subject to plan rules, cost sharing, and reimbursement obligations. The household's defensive task is therefore not only preserving receipts. It is classifying the claim correctly before billing pressure becomes collection pressure.

The Household Medicare Diagnostic Matrix must isolate this payer-reversion row with exact inputs. The matrix must record Part A entitlement, hospice election date, designated hospice program, attending physician status, terminal diagnosis, related conditions, unrelated-condition rationale, MA enrollment status, plan premium status, Part D status, supplemental-benefit status, Notice of Election timing, A/B MAC (HHH) filing status, GV or GW professional-claim logic where applicable, and any institutional unrelated-care coding pathway. It must also record whether a service is hospice care, non-hospice Part A or Part B care, non-hospice Part D care, supplemental benefit care, or excluded care. This is not redundant data entry. It is the financial map that determines whether Original Medicare, the hospice provider, the A/B MAC system, the MA organization, Part D, or the household ledger bears the immediate claim.

The final synthesis is that Original Medicare becomes the primary payer for hospice during Part C enrollment because federal law deliberately removes hospice from the ordinary managed-care risk pool. Section 1812(a)(4) creates hospice as a discrete Part A benefit, Section 1812(d) defines the hospice election and waiver of other terminal-condition payment rights, Section 1853(h) directs hospice payment to the elected hospice program by the Secretary, and 42 CFR § 422.320 reduces or eliminates ordinary MA capitation while preserving only residual rebate and prescription-drug payment components. (Social Security) The carve-out is a legal firewall. It protects terminal-illness-related palliative care from being forced through a private plan's ordinary capitation logic, while leaving unrelated services and supplemental benefits to be routed through the appropriate residual channels. Failure to understand this reversion exposes a retirement household to misrouted bills, denial notices, duplicated payment demands, provider collection errors, and unnecessary asset liquidation during the most fragile phase of medical care.

MODULE VI: SYSTEMIC CROSS-HOUSEHOLD FINANCIAL IMPACTS

Chapter 14: Household Dependency Separations and Market Re-Entry

14.1 The Individual-Only Nature of Medicare Entitlement

Medicare entitlement is fundamentally individual. It is not a household policy, family contract, spousal rider, dependent-benefit platform, or multi-person deductible ledger. The federal program identifies eligibility through the legal status of a particular person: age 65 or older, disability entitlement after the applicable waiting period, End-Stage Renal Disease, ALS, premium-free Part A entitlement through qualifying work history, or premium Part A and Part B eligibility through the relevant enrollment rules. CMS describes premium-free Part A eligibility as requiring entitlement based on the person's own earnings record or the earnings record of a spouse, parent, or child, with the underlying worker record built from quarters of coverage earned through FICA payroll taxes during working years. (CMS) Medicare & You 2026 likewise states that Part A usually has no monthly premium when the individual or spouse paid Medicare taxes for a sufficient period, while premium Part A in 2026 costs either $311 or $565 per month depending on work-tax history. The fact that a spouse's work record may help establish premium-free Part A for an eligible person does not convert Medicare into a joint account. It remains an entitlement assigned to the individual beneficiary's federal file.

This individual-only architecture collides directly with the commercial health-insurance architecture used by employers. Employer group health coverage commonly operates through employee, employee-plus-spouse, employee-plus-child, and family tiers; it can maintain a single contract relationship covering multiple household members under one payroll deduction, one employer subsidy arrangement, and one integrated open-enrollment decision. Medicare does not replicate that structure. There is no Medicare family plan, no dependent rider for a younger spouse, no child continuation inside the Medicare account, and no household Medicare deductible shared across spouses. Medicare & You 2026 describes Medicare enrollment in terms of individual Part A and Part B entitlement periods, including a seven-month Initial Enrollment Period tied to the person turning 65 and Special Enrollment Period rules tied to that person's own or family-member employment-based group health coverage status. The operational consequence is unbundling: a family previously insured through one employer plan must be separated into distinct legal accounts once one member moves into Medicare and other members remain outside Medicare eligibility.

The single-entitlement baseline is most disruptive when a primary wage earner reaches Medicare eligibility before a spouse or dependent child. A commercial employer plan may have covered the entire household because the worker was an active employee. Medicare covers only the Medicare-entitled individual. If retirement, termination of employment, reduction of hours, or a plan-status change causes the employer family contract to end, the younger spouse and dependent children do not migrate automatically into Medicare. They must be mapped into another legally available coverage pathway, such as continuing employer coverage if available, COBRA continuation, a spouse's employment-based plan, individual market coverage, Medicaid or CHIP where eligible, or another applicable source. Medicare eligibility itself does not normally terminate active employer group coverage; the Department of Labor explains that enrolling in Medicare while still employed generally does not result in loss of group health coverage, although rare plan-specific circumstances can cause a loss and trigger COBRA rights. (DOL) The sharper risk is therefore not Medicare enrollment alone. It is Medicare enrollment combined with the household's loss of the employer family coverage structure.

The spousal stranding phenomenon arises from this mismatch between a family coverage contract and an individual federal entitlement. A worker may enter Medicare smoothly while a younger spouse loses the employer-subsidized family premium tier that made household coverage affordable. A dependent child may lose eligibility through the employee's separation from employment, plan termination, or loss of dependent status under plan terms. COBRA can preserve access to the same employer plan benefits after a qualifying event, but COBRA is a continuation right, not a subsidy continuation right. The Department of Labor explains that COBRA qualified beneficiaries include the employee, spouse or former spouse, and dependent children who were covered under the group health plan on the day before the qualifying event; a qualifying event matters only if it causes the qualified beneficiary to lose coverage under the plan. (DOL) COBRA therefore can preserve the plan framework, but often converts the household from employer-subsidized coverage into a direct premium obligation.

The COBRA-Medicare intersection is one of the most misunderstood transition points. DOL guidance lists termination or reduction in hours as an event generally producing up to 18 months of COBRA coverage for the employee, spouse, and dependent child, while employee enrollment in Medicare can produce up to 36 months for the spouse and dependent child if it causes loss of coverage. (DOL) The same DOL guidance states that when an employee enrolls in Medicare while working and later experiences a qualifying event, COBRA can be available after the qualifying event even if Medicare enrollment occurred earlier; dependents may receive coverage measured as 36 months from the date the employee became entitled to Medicare or 18 months from the date coverage was lost, whichever is later. (DOL) This timing rule is the COBRA secondary qualifying-event trap: the spouse or dependent's continuation period can depend not only on the date employment ends, but also on the date the worker became entitled to Medicare.

The Medicare side adds another layer of risk. Medicare & You 2026 states that COBRA is not coverage based on current employment and does not count as current employer coverage for the Part B Special Enrollment Period; retiree coverage, VA coverage, individual Marketplace coverage, and severance-related former-employer coverage are likewise excluded from the current-employment category. Medicare & You further warns that COBRA may pay only a small portion of costs once Medicare eligibility exists, and that Medicare-eligible individuals may have to pay most costs if Medicare enrollment is mishandled. For dependents, COBRA may preserve coverage temporarily. For the Medicare-eligible worker, COBRA is not a Part B safe harbor. The household matrix must therefore separate the worker's Medicare enrollment obligation from the spouse's or child's continuation right.

The tax side is equally individualized. IRS Publication 969 defines an HSA-eligible individual as one covered by a high deductible health plan on the first day of the month, without disqualifying other coverage, not enrolled in Medicare, and not claimable as another taxpayer's dependent. (IRS) Publication 969 states the rule with absolute clarity: beginning with the first month of Medicare enrollment, the individual's HSA contribution limit is zero, and the rule applies to retroactive Medicare coverage, making contributions during a retroactive coverage period excess contributions. (IRS) This rule is person-specific. It bars the Medicare-enrolled spouse from contributing or receiving employer contributions into that spouse's HSA after Medicare begins, but it does not automatically bar a different spouse who remains HSA-eligible from contributing to that separate spouse's HSA.

Family HDHP coverage creates the tax-friction layer. Publication 969 states that for 2026, the HSA contribution limit is $4,400 for self-only HDHP coverage and $8,750 for family HDHP coverage, and it also states that an eligible individual age 55 or older receives an additional $1,000 catch-up contribution. (IRS) For married persons, Publication 969 states that if either spouse has family HDHP coverage, both spouses are treated as having family HDHP coverage, and if each spouse has family coverage under separate plans, the family contribution limit is split equally unless the spouses agree on a different division. (IRS) Critically, Publication 969 cautions that the married-person rules apply only if both spouses are eligible individuals, and separately states that each spouse who is an eligible individual and wants an HSA must open a separate HSA because a joint HSA is not permitted. (IRS)

The split-architecture household is therefore administratively demanding. A Medicare-enrolled spouse may remain covered under the other spouse's family HDHP as medical coverage, but that Medicare-enrolled spouse is no longer an HSA-eligible individual. The non-Medicare spouse may still be HSA-eligible if covered by an HDHP, not covered by disqualifying other coverage, not enrolled in Medicare, and not claimable as another person's dependent. Publication 969 permits HSA distributions for qualified medical expenses of the HSA beneficiary, spouse, and dependents, but contribution eligibility remains tied to the account holder's own eligibility status. The legal result is asymmetric: the account may still pay qualified family medical expenses tax-free if properly administered, but contributions must be computed only through the eligible individual's allowed limit.

The compliance hazard intensifies when Medicare Part A is retroactive. Medicare & You 2026 states that premium-free Part A can go back retroactively six months from Part A sign-up or Social Security or Railroad Retirement Board application, but not earlier than the first month of Medicare eligibility. Publication 969 then characterizes HSA contributions made during retroactive Medicare coverage as excess contributions. (IRS) A household that stops HSA contributions only on the visible application date can therefore overcontribute if Part A is backdated. This is not a minor payroll-entry issue. Excess HSA contributions can require corrective withdrawal, income inclusion, excise-tax analysis, and Form 8889 coordination.

The Household Medicare Diagnostic Matrix must treat Section 14.1 as the foundational row for employer coverage disconnect and dependent separation. The matrix must record the identity of each household member, Medicare entitlement date, Part A effective date, Part B status, employer coverage status, active employment status, COBRA qualifying event date, dependent eligibility, Marketplace eligibility, Medicaid or CHIP eligibility, HDHP coverage tier, HSA account owner, Medicare retroactivity exposure, employer HSA contributions, payroll-cafeteria elections, and whether each spouse is independently an HSA-eligible individual. The matrix must not allow the household to be analyzed as one insurance unit after one member becomes Medicare-entitled. The household may still share finances, prescriptions, dependents, and tax filings, but the legal coverage accounts split.

The final actuarial conclusion is that Medicare entitlement individualizes a previously bundled household risk structure. The Medicare-eligible worker may achieve stable federal coverage while a younger spouse or dependent child becomes stranded outside the Medicare system. COBRA may preserve the prior group plan temporarily, but its qualifying-event mechanics, premium obligations, Medicare coordination rules, and maximum-duration clocks require separate tracking. HSA eligibility fractures along individual lines: one spouse's Medicare enrollment can reduce that spouse's contribution limit to zero, while the other spouse may retain a family HDHP contribution pathway only if that spouse remains independently eligible under Publication 969. Failure to map these individualized accounts can produce uninsured dependents, duplicate premiums, missed COBRA elections, loss of Part B Special Enrollment Period protection, excess HSA contributions, retroactive tax exposure, and sudden liquidation of household assets for medical costs that were assumed to remain inside a single employer family contract.

14.2 Triggering the Dependency Special Enrollment Period

The dependency Special Enrollment Period is the statutory bridge between an employer-sponsored family coverage system and the individual health insurance exchange. Its legal foundation is 45 CFR § 155.420, which requires an Exchange to provide Special Enrollment Periods during which qualified individuals may enroll in qualified health plans and enrollees may change qualified health plans when specified triggering events occur. The regulation is expressly dependent-inclusive: it defines a dependent for these purposes and requires the Exchange, when specified, to allow a qualified individual, enrollee, and dependent to enroll or change coverage after a listed triggering event. (Legal Information Institute) The consequence for a Medicare transition household is direct. When a primary worker's transition into Medicare coincides with retirement, separation from employment, or loss of the employer-sponsored group family plan, the younger spouse or dependent child does not inherit Medicare. Instead, the dependent's legal pathway becomes an individual-market enrollment analysis under the loss-of-minimum-essential-coverage provisions of § 155.420.

The qualifying life event is the loss of minimum essential coverage, not the mere fact that another household member enrolled in Medicare. Section 155.420(d)(1) provides that a qualified individual or dependent has a triggering event when that person loses minimum essential coverage, and the date of loss is the last day the consumer would have coverage under the previous plan or coverage. (Legal Information Institute) Employer-sponsored group health coverage ordinarily constitutes minimum essential coverage, and IRS Form 8962 instructions likewise identify most employer-sponsored coverage as MEC. (IRS) Therefore, when dependent coverage under the employer family plan actually terminates because the worker retires, employment ends, coverage tier changes, or the employer plan ceases to cover dependents, the dependent's loss of MEC creates a legally protected market re-entry event. The Medicare entitlement of the worker is the surrounding fact pattern; the dependent's own coverage loss is the operative Exchange trigger.

The legal architecture prevents a dependent from being trapped until the next annual open enrollment period when employer family coverage disappears. Section 155.420(c) supplies the filing clock: the general rule allows 60 days from the date of the triggering event to select a qualified health plan, and the advanced-availability rule gives a person described in the loss-of-coverage provision 60 days before and, unless an Exchange option changes the post-event rule, 60 days after the triggering event to select a plan. (Legal Information Institute) HealthCare.gov's job-based-loss guidance operationalizes this rule by stating that a person who loses job-based insurance must apply for Marketplace coverage within 60 days of the loss, with coverage able to start the first day of the month after job-based coverage ends. (HealthCare.gov) HealthCare.gov's retiree page states the same rule for retirement-related loss of job-based coverage: a Marketplace application may be made with a Special Enrollment Period from 60 days before through 60 days after the separation date. (HealthCare.gov)

Effective-date mechanics make pre-loss action materially different from post-loss action. Section 155.420(b) generally requires coverage effective the first day of the month following qualified health plan selection, subject to special effective-date rules. For loss of coverage, the regulation states that if plan selection is made on or before the triggering event, coverage is effective the first day of the month following the triggering event; if the selection is made after the triggering event, the Exchange must ensure coverage effective under the regular rule or the first day of the following month, at the Exchange's option. The regulation also permits, at Exchange option, coverage effective the first day of the month in which coverage loss occurs if selection is made on or before the last day of the month preceding the triggering event. (Legal Information Institute) Thus, the dependency SEP is not merely a 120-day planning band. It is a calendar-placement problem. A dependent who selects coverage before the employer plan terminates can often avoid a gap; a dependent who waits until after coverage loss may encounter at least a short uninsured interval depending on the date of selection and Exchange implementation.

COBRA continuation coverage supplies the secondary choice trap. HealthCare.gov states that losing job-based coverage opens a Marketplace SEP and that COBRA can be compared with Marketplace options, but it also states that a voluntary early termination of COBRA outside Open Enrollment does not create a new Marketplace enrollment opportunity unless another life event occurs. (HealthCare.gov) HealthCare.gov's retiree guidance states the same rule: if COBRA runs out outside Open Enrollment, a Marketplace SEP applies, but a person cannot choose to drop COBRA outside Open Enrollment and enroll in a Marketplace plan instead; the annual Open Enrollment Period remains the ordinary escape route for voluntary early COBRA termination. (HealthCare.gov) The regulation's text supports the same conclusion by excluding loss caused by failure to pay premiums, including COBRA premiums before COBRA expiration, from the loss-of-coverage event, except in the special circumstance where employer contributions or government subsidies for COBRA completely cease. (Legal Information Institute)

The financial consequence of that trap is severe. A dependent who elects COBRA after the worker's Medicare transition may preserve continuity of the employer plan, but the premium often moves from employer-subsidized group economics to a direct continuation ledger. HealthCare.gov describes COBRA as temporary continuation coverage after job loss and states that the former employee usually pays the full premium, plus a small administrative fee. (HealthCare.gov) If COBRA is later judged unaffordable and voluntarily dropped after the 60-day Marketplace SEP has expired, the household may be locked out of Marketplace enrollment until the next Open Enrollment Period, unless COBRA exhausts or a different qualifying event occurs. The dependency SEP therefore requires a front-end election analysis. Waiting to test COBRA affordability after the SEP closes can convert a coverage bridge into a liquidity trap.

Premium tax credit re-entry depends on both enrollment status and tax eligibility. IRS instructions for Form 8962 state that the premium tax credit is available only for qualified health plans purchased through a Marketplace, and that Form 1095-A provides the information needed to compute the credit and reconcile advance credit payments on Form 8962. (IRS) The same instructions define the coverage family as individuals in the tax family who are enrolled in a qualified health plan and are not eligible for MEC other than individual-market coverage, and they state that PTC assists only with the coverage of individuals included in that coverage family. (IRS) When employer dependent coverage terminates, the dependent may move from an employer-MEC category into a Marketplace qualified health plan category, but premium tax credit eligibility still depends on household income, tax family status, lawful presence, premium payment rules, and absence of another disqualifying MEC offer.

Employer affordability rules are the central tax gate. IRS Form 8962 instructions state that employer-sponsored coverage is MEC, but a taxpayer or family member is considered eligible for employer-sponsored MEC for PTC purposes only if the offer is affordable and provides minimum value, unless the family member actually enrolls in that employer coverage. The instructions further state that if employer coverage is affordable for the employee but not affordable for other family members, PTC may be available for those family members if they enroll in a Marketplace qualified health plan. (IRS) HealthCare.gov states that for 2026 a job-based health plan is considered affordable if the share of the monthly premium for the lowest-cost plan offered by the employer is less than 9.96 percent of household income, and that an affordable spouse-employer offer can defeat Marketplace savings even if the offer is not accepted. (HealthCare.gov) The dependency SEP therefore opens the enrollment door, while the affordability and MEC rules determine whether the premium tax credit enters the household ledger.

COBRA has its own PTC classification. IRS Form 8962 instructions state that post-employment coverage, such as COBRA or retiree coverage, is not treated as available MEC unless the person actually enrolls in it. (IRS) This rule is decisive in a dependency transition. A dependent who declines COBRA and enrolls in Marketplace coverage may be tested for PTC without being treated as eligible for COBRA merely because COBRA was offered. A dependent who actually enrolls in COBRA, however, has coverage that can block Marketplace PTC during the months of COBRA enrollment because the dependent is no longer in the Marketplace coverage family for those months. The household must therefore classify COBRA before electing it, not after payment strain appears.

Cross-billing separation is the operational reality after the worker enters Medicare. The Medicare-entitled worker may owe Part B premiums, possible Part D premiums, income-related adjustments, Medicare Advantage or Medigap premiums where applicable, and separate drug or medical cost sharing. The dependent unit may owe Marketplace premiums, with or without advance premium tax credits, and may later reconcile APTC against actual household income on Form 8962. IRS instructions warn that APTC is based on Marketplace estimates and must be reconciled with actual PTC; excess APTC must be repaid subject to applicable limitations, while insufficient APTC may generate additional credit. (IRS) The family budget therefore splits into two regulated payment systems: Medicare premiums and claims for the worker, and Marketplace premiums, Form 1095-A reporting, and Form 8962 reconciliation for the dependent unit.

The Household Medicare Diagnostic Matrix must treat Section 14.2 as the primary operational row for dependency SEPs, qualifying life event verification, and 45 CFR § 155.420 market re-entry. The matrix must record each dependent's last day of employer-sponsored minimum essential coverage, the worker's Medicare effective date, the employment separation date, COBRA offer date, COBRA election deadline, Marketplace SEP opening date, Marketplace SEP closing date, plan-selection date, projected effective date, eligibility verification documents, other employer coverage offers, affordability percentage, household income estimate, expected tax family composition, Form 1095-A recipient, and Form 8962 reconciliation responsibility. Each variable changes either the enrollment right, the subsidy right, or the timing of coverage.

The final wealth-preservation conclusion is exact. A dependent Special Enrollment Period is not a discretionary courtesy; it is a statutory market-access mechanism triggered when a dependent loses minimum essential coverage. It allows the household to bypass annual open-enrollment limits, but only within the strict timing and evidentiary boundaries of § 155.420. It does not erase the COBRA choice trap, does not guarantee premium tax credits where affordable employer coverage remains available, and does not merge Medicare and Marketplace billing into one household account. Failure to coordinate these rules can leave younger spouses and dependent children uninsured, locked into unaffordable COBRA, excluded from premium tax credits, or exposed to point-of-service medical costs during a transition that appeared, at first glance, to involve only the worker's Medicare enrollment. Under the Household Medicare Diagnostic Matrix, the dependency SEP is a capital-protection mechanism: it converts a household coverage fracture into a dated, documented, and financially modeled market re-entry pathway.

14.3 Recalculating the Household Premium Tax Credit (PTC)

The Premium Tax Credit is not a flat public voucher assigned to a family health plan. It is a monthly federal tax calculation that compares the cost of qualified health plan coverage for the tax household's Marketplace coverage family against the household's statutorily required contribution. Under IRS Form 8962 instructions, the monthly credit amount is the lesser of the enrollment premiums for the month or the applicable second-lowest-cost silver plan premium for the coverage family, reduced by the monthly contribution amount. (IRS) This formula gives the Second Lowest Cost Silver Plan, commonly called the SLCSP or silver benchmark plan, its central role. The SLCSP is not necessarily the plan actually purchased. It is the statutory measuring stick used to compute the maximum premium assistance credit available for the people in the tax family who are enrolled in Marketplace coverage and not eligible for disqualifying minimum essential coverage. (IRS)

The governing regulation at 26 CFR § 1.36B-3 structures the premium-assistance amount around the taxpayer's applicable benchmark plan and monthly contribution amount. It treats the benchmark as a coverage-family calculation, not a household-gross-premium calculation. The regulation contains examples in which the applicable benchmark premium is assembled from the second-lowest aggregate cost of self-only policies or family policies needed to cover the members of the coverage family, including situations where family members live in different rating areas or cannot enroll under one policy. (Legal Information Institute) The administrative principle is exact: the benchmark follows the covered Marketplace lives, their ages, their locations, and the available silver-level plan options. It does not follow the Medicare-enrolled person once that person exits Marketplace eligibility for premium credit purposes.

The post-65 transition therefore produces a geometric subsidy change. When a primary tax filer or spouse becomes eligible for Medicare Part A or Part C, that individual generally has government-sponsored minimum essential coverage and is removed from the Marketplace coverage family for months of that eligibility. IRS Form 8962 instructions identify Medicare Part A or Part C as government-sponsored minimum essential coverage and state that an individual eligible for minimum essential coverage other than individual-market coverage is not in the coverage family for that month. (IRS) (IRS) The resulting recalculation is not optional. The applicable SLCSP premium must be recomputed for the remaining Marketplace coverage family, usually excluding the older Medicare-transitioning member's age-rated premium component. If the senior member had been one of the most expensive Marketplace lives, the benchmark premium can shrink sharply even though the household's gross income has not fallen proportionately.

This is the central distortion inside the household subsidy ledger. The household tax family may remain the same after Medicare begins, especially when spouses continue filing jointly and the Medicare-enrolled spouse remains in the same tax household. In that common case, the Federal Poverty Line percentage does not automatically rise merely because one spouse left Marketplace coverage; family size for Form 8962 is generally still based on the tax family, while the coverage family shrinks to only the Marketplace-covered members. The true inversion is therefore more precise than a simple household-size reduction. The expected contribution remains tied to household modified adjusted gross income and tax-family size, while the benchmark premium often falls because fewer people remain in the Marketplace coverage family. If the tax household itself also changes, such as through divorce, dependent status change, or separate tax filing rules, then the Federal Poverty Line percentage can change as well. IRS guidance separates these concepts by defining the coverage family as only those tax-family members enrolled in a qualified health plan and not eligible for other MEC, and by requiring monthly recalculation when that coverage family changes. (IRS)

The mathematical sequence after a Medicare transition is therefore a multi-column restructuring. First, the household must identify the month in which the Medicare-entitled person becomes eligible for disqualifying MEC. Second, that person must be removed from the Marketplace coverage family for the affected months. Third, the Marketplace or tax preparer must determine the applicable SLCSP premium for the remaining covered dependents or spouse in the relevant rating area. Fourth, the household's monthly contribution amount must be computed from household income and the applicable percentage table. Fifth, Form 8962 must compare the corrected benchmark minus the contribution amount against actual enrollment premiums and the APTC paid for each month. The IRS instructions expressly state that if the coverage family changed during the year and the Marketplace was not notified, the SLCSP premium reported on Form 1095-A may be missing or incorrect, requiring the taxpayer to determine the correct applicable SLCSP premium. (IRS)

The IRS examples make the Medicare-like correction visible even without using Medicare as the named fact pattern. In the Form 8962 instructions, when one member becomes eligible for minimum essential coverage partway through the year and the Marketplace is not notified, the coverage family changes, the SLCSP premium reported on Form 1095-A becomes incorrect, and the taxpayers must use monthly lines rather than annual totals to enter the corrected SLCSP amounts for the months after the change. (IRS) This same architecture applies when Medicare eligibility removes a senior from the coverage family. A full-year line 11 entry is generally inappropriate where the SLCSP changes midyear. Lines 12 through 23 become the monthly reconciliation corridor, allowing the tax return to show one SLCSP amount before Medicare and a different SLCSP amount after Medicare.

The 2026 contribution percentage environment intensifies the need for precision. IRS Revenue Procedure 2025-25 provides the applicable percentage table for taxable years beginning in calendar year 2026 under section 36B and § 1.36B-3(g). For 2026, the table ranges from 2.10 percent at less than 133 percent of the Federal Poverty Line, rises through multiple income bands, and reaches 9.96 percent for household income at least 300 percent but not more than 400 percent of the Federal Poverty Line; the required contribution percentage for employer-sponsored coverage affordability for 2026 is also 9.96 percent. (IRS) IRS's current Premium Tax Credit overview states that, for 2026, a taxpayer with household income above 400 percent of the Federal Poverty Line is not allowed a premium tax credit and must repay advance credit payments made on behalf of the tax family. (IRS) The household therefore cannot assume that the enhanced 2021 through 2025 subsidy environment continues unchanged into 2026.

Midyear reporting is the administrative protection against APTC overpayment. IRS guidance states that APTC eligibility is based on the Marketplace's estimate of the PTC and that changed circumstances, including income, family size, address, or eligibility for employer or government coverage such as Medicare, should be promptly reported to the Marketplace because unreported changes can make APTC substantially different from the actual PTC allowed on the tax return. (IRS) HealthCare.gov likewise instructs Marketplace enrollees to report income, household, and other changes, including changes affecting premium tax credit eligibility, through the Marketplace reporting process. (HealthCare.gov) The verified federal rule is prompt reporting rather than a universally stated statutory 30-day deadline for every Medicare transition. Separately, Marketplace verification processes can impose 30-day document submission deadlines after plan selection for certain Special Enrollment Period confirmations. (HealthCare.gov) The disciplined household file should therefore report the Medicare transition immediately and preserve Marketplace eligibility notices, plan-selection confirmations, and Form 1095-A corrections.

The tax clawback mechanism is neither discretionary nor informal. IRS Form 8962 is used to figure the Premium Tax Credit and reconcile it with advance payments of the Premium Tax Credit. (IRS) IRS instructions state that if APTC is more than the allowable PTC, the household has excess APTC and must repay the excess subject to applicable limitations; if APTC is less than the allowable PTC, the household may receive the difference as an additional credit. (IRS) IRS's Premium Tax Credit overview states that advance payments are reconciled on Form 8962 based on the income and family size reported on the tax return, and excess APTC is added to tax liability on the federal return. (IRS) If the Marketplace continued paying APTC based on a benchmark premium that included the Medicare-enrolled senior after that person ceased to be part of the coverage family, the excess subsidy becomes a spring filing liability.

This reconciliation risk is amplified by Form 1095-A dependence. The Marketplace reports monthly enrollment premiums, SLCSP premiums, and APTC on Form 1095-A, and the IRS instructions state that Form 1095-A is needed to complete Form 8962. (IRS) However, the form is not always self-correcting. The instructions warn that when the coverage family changed and the Marketplace was not notified, the reported SLCSP may be missing or incorrect. (IRS) A household that blindly imports Form 1095-A column B into Form 8962 can therefore compound the original reporting failure. The correct manuscript principle is that the tax return must reflect the lawful coverage family for each month, even when the Marketplace statement was generated from outdated application data.

Cross-billing separation completes the financial picture. After the senior member transitions to Medicare, the household may carry Medicare Part B premiums, possible Part D premiums, income-related adjustments, Medigap or Medicare Advantage premiums where applicable, and Medicare cost sharing for the senior. Simultaneously, the younger spouse or dependents may carry Marketplace premiums, deductibles, cost sharing, and APTC reconciliation exposure. Those charges arise from different legal systems and different monthly ledgers. Medicare premiums are not Marketplace premiums. Marketplace APTC does not offset Part B. A Medicare-enrolled person's exclusion from the Marketplace coverage family can lower the SLCSP benchmark even while Medicare premiums add a new household bill. The household's net liquidity may therefore deteriorate even if the senior's Marketplace premium disappears.

The Household Medicare Diagnostic Matrix must treat Section 14.3 as the controlling row for Silver Benchmark Plan restructuring, APTC recalculation, and Form 8962 reconciliation. The matrix must record the Medicare effective month, the Marketplace termination month for the Medicare-enrolled person, the remaining coverage-family members, rating area, ages of remaining enrollees, corrected SLCSP premium by month, actual enrollment premium by month, APTC paid by month, household MAGI, tax-family size, Federal Poverty Line percentage, applicable percentage, monthly contribution amount, Form 1095-A accuracy, and whether lines 12 through 23 of Form 8962 are required instead of annual line 11. It must also record whether any household member remains eligible for employer-sponsored MEC, because employer affordability and minimum value rules can defeat PTC eligibility independently of the Medicare transition.

The final actuarial conclusion is that Medicare integration can shrink the Marketplace benchmark faster than it shrinks household income. The age-rated senior may leave the Marketplace premium calculation, but the joint tax household's income may remain intact, producing a lower benchmark subsidy base and a persistent expected contribution. If the transition is not reported promptly, APTC may continue at an inflated level and later reappear as excess APTC on Form 8962. If the SLCSP is not corrected after a coverage-family change, Form 1095-A may mislead the filing process. If the 2026 applicable percentage table and 400-percent Federal Poverty Line boundary are ignored, the household may underprice repayment exposure. Under the Household Medicare Diagnostic Matrix, the Premium Tax Credit is not a side calculation; it is a monthly social-insurance integration ledger. Mastery of SLCSP restructuring, Medicare MEC exclusion, Form 1095-A review, and Form 8962 reconciliation is essential to prevent a post-65 household transition from becoming a concealed tax liability and a sudden drain on non-sheltered retirement assets.

Chapter 15: Ancillary Risk Management and Wealth Preservation

15.1 Structural Isolation of Lifestyle Care Costs

The statutory exclusion of routine lifestyle care from Original Medicare begins with a precise boundary in the Social Security Act. Section 1862(a)(7) bars payment under Part A or Part B for routine physical checkups, eyeglasses except post-cataract eyewear described elsewhere in Medicare law, eye examinations for prescribing, fitting, or changing eyeglasses, refractive eye procedures, hearing aids, and examinations for hearing aids. Strict statutory accuracy requires an additional clarification: the general dental exclusion is not housed in Section 1862(a)(7), but in Section 1862(a)(12), which excludes services connected with the care, treatment, filling, removal, or replacement of teeth or structures directly supporting teeth, subject to a limited inpatient hospital exception when hospitalization is required because of the underlying medical condition, clinical status, or severity of the dental procedure. (Social Security) These provisions form a statutory exclusion cluster. The legal architecture separates catastrophic medical insurance from ordinary maintenance events that are high-frequency, highly predictable, and usually subject to consumer timing, provider selection, and episodic cash budgeting rather than classical insurance pooling.

Original Medicare's beneficiary-facing materials mirror that statutory architecture. Medicare & You 2026 states that Part A and Part B do not cover everything and lists long-term care, eye exams for prescription eyeglasses and corrective contact lenses, routine physical exams, hearing aids and fitting exams, and most dental care, including routine cleanings, fillings, tooth extractions, and dentures, among the items and services generally outside Original Medicare coverage. The same official handbook notes that a Medicare Advantage Plan or Medicare Cost Plan may cover some extra benefits, including vision, hearing, and dental services, but that such coverage exists outside the ordinary Original Medicare Part A and Part B benefit floor. (Medicare) The operational conclusion is exact: a retirement household cannot treat routine dental, vision, and hearing expenses as automatically absorbed by federal major medical insurance merely because Medicare entitlement has begun.

The historical insurance logic behind the exclusion is actuarial rather than accidental. Federal social insurance was designed to protect the aged and disabled population against medical events whose magnitude could overwhelm household liquidity: hospitalization, physician treatment, skilled nursing facility care under defined conditions, home health care, durable medical equipment, preventive benefits specifically added by Congress, and other medically necessary services within the statutory benefit categories. Routine dental cleanings, ordinary dentures, eyeglass refractions, eyeglass frames, hearing aids, and routine hearing-aid fitting examinations have a different risk profile. They recur predictably, they often involve scheduled consumption, and they commonly produce costs that are painful but not always catastrophic in the same sense as inpatient admission, chemotherapy, dialysis, advanced imaging, surgery, or post-acute care. Section 1862 therefore functions as a benefit-boundary statute: it preserves the federal health-insurance core for medically necessary covered services while leaving lifestyle-maintenance costs to supplemental markets, personal budgeting, Medicaid where available, employer or retiree benefits, or private ancillary products.

The exclusion does not mean that dental, vision, and hearing conditions are clinically trivial. Untreated oral disease may affect nutrition, inflammation, infection risk, cardiovascular status, and quality of life. Vision correction may determine fall risk, driving capacity, medication management, and independence. Hearing impairment may alter social participation, cognitive load, caregiver communication, and adherence to clinical instructions. The exclusion means that Congress did not place routine forms of those services inside the basic Original Medicare entitlement. Medicare & You 2026 preserves narrow medical connections, noting that Original Medicare may pay for some dental services closely related to certain covered services, such as heart valve repair or replacement, organ transplant, cancer-related treatment, or dialysis services for End-Stage Renal Disease. (Medicare) These exceptions reinforce the boundary rather than dissolve it. When dental care becomes integral to another covered medical intervention, Medicare may enter; when dental care remains ordinary maintenance, the statutory exclusion generally controls.

Medicare Advantage creates the principal manufactured layer through which excluded services are reintroduced into the Medicare marketplace. The official 2026 handbook states that most Medicare Advantage Plans offer extra benefits Original Medicare does not cover, including vision, hearing, dental, and more. (Medicare) Under 42 CFR § 422.102, Medicare Advantage organizations may offer mandatory supplemental benefits, subject to CMS approval, and may use uniform dollar allowances for packages of supplemental benefits, including reductions in cost sharing or coverage of specified items and services, limited to the plan year. The same regulation permits optional supplemental benefits purchased at the enrollee's discretion and offered without regard to health status. (Legal Information Institute) CMS's Medicare Managed Care Manual further distinguishes mandatory supplemental benefits, which are covered for every person enrolled in the plan and may be paid through premiums, cost sharing, or rebate dollars, from optional supplemental benefits, which are separately elected and paid through additional premiums and cost sharing; rebate dollars may not be applied toward optional supplemental benefits. (CMS)

This Part C supplemental-benefit architecture is not equivalent to comprehensive risk transfer. It is a regulated benefit-manufacturing mechanism layered onto a private Medicare contract. A plan may embed preventive dental allowances, eyewear allowances, routine eye examinations, hearing exams, hearing-aid support, or related benefits into the plan's mandatory supplemental structure, or may offer certain ancillary benefits as optional riders where permitted. These benefits can be valuable, but they are typically bounded by plan-year allowances, service definitions, frequency limits, provider-network rules, reimbursement procedures, prior authorization requirements, or excluded categories. Section 422.102 expressly recognizes uniform dollar amounts as maximum plan allowances for supplemental benefit packages, and the 2026 Medicare Plan Finder display enhancements in the source packet show CMS attention to in-network and out-of-network cost sharing, authorization requirements, and plan limits for supplemental benefits, including hearing, preventive and comprehensive dental, and vision categories. The legal inference is that ancillary benefits must be modeled as finite allowances, not as unlimited major medical indemnification.

The financial variance trap arises when a household treats an embedded benefit label as a comprehensive benefit promise. A plan may advertise dental, vision, or hearing coverage in a generic sense, yet the actual Evidence of Coverage may impose an annual maximum, a per-period eyewear allowance, a hearing-aid cycle limitation, a specific vendor pathway, an in-network requirement, a prior authorization rule, or a service-code exclusion. A five-hundred-dollar or one-thousand-dollar annual dental allowance, where present in a particular plan design, may reduce preventive or minor restorative exposure but may be exhausted quickly by crowns, implants, periodontal therapy, dentures, oral surgery, or repeated diagnostic imaging. Such figures are plan-specific examples rather than federal statutory amounts. The governing principle is that Medicare Advantage supplemental benefits can subsidize lifestyle care, but their design is bounded by contract terms, CMS approval, and annual plan documents. They should not be conflated with the catastrophic medical protection supplied by core Part A and Part B coverage.

Standalone commercial ancillary policies and indemnity structures operate in a different legal and economic register. Dental preferred provider organization arrangements, dental health maintenance arrangements, discount programs, vision plans, hearing-discount programs, and specified indemnity products may cover some categories excluded from Original Medicare or partially addressed by Part C supplemental benefits. These arrangements are not Original Medicare benefits. Their underwriting, premiums, waiting periods, annual maximums, networks, reimbursement schedules, excluded procedures, replacement intervals, and coordination clauses must be evaluated separately. The source packet itself distinguishes dental, vision, and hearing products from Medicare products, stating that such products offer additional benefits for consumers seeking dental, vision, or hearing coverage and are not affiliated or connected to Medicare. That separation is analytically important. Ancillary products may support liquidity planning, but they should not be represented as Medicare entitlement.

The economic rationale for isolating lifestyle care costs is grounded in the distinction between predictable consumption and insurable risk. Insurance is most efficient when it pools uncertain, low-frequency, high-severity events across a large population. Routine dental cleanings, periodic eye exams, replacement lenses, frames, hearing-aid batteries, routine hearing checks, and scheduled maintenance services are more predictable. When high-frequency claims are blended into core medical insurance, premium structure absorbs the expected cost of those claims plus administrative loading, utilization management, broker or distribution expense where applicable, claims processing overhead, and margin or reserve requirements. For predictable care, prepayment through insurance can become economically similar to paying the same expected cost through premiums, but with added administrative load. That does not make ancillary coverage irrational. It means ancillary coverage should be evaluated as a budgeting, discount-access, and cash-flow smoothing tool rather than as a perfect substitute for catastrophic insurance.

The core protection firewall is the household-level application of that actuarial principle. Major medical coverage must remain focused on the risks that can destroy capital: hospitalization, physician care, surgery, oncology treatment, injectable therapy, dialysis, post-acute care, emergency care, Part D specialty-drug exposure, and chronic disease management. Routine dental, vision, and hearing costs should be assigned to a separate lifestyle-care reserve, supplemental-benefit ledger, or ancillary-policy analysis. Decoupling those categories prevents household decision makers from overvaluing a modest dental or eyewear allowance while undervaluing hospital network structure, drug formulary exposure, maximum out-of-pocket limits, Part B cost sharing, Medigap underwriting rules, or hospice and long-term-care exclusions. A retirement household can suffer financial harm when an attractive ancillary package distracts from weak catastrophic protection.

Dedicated ancillary vehicles may still serve an asset-preservation function when correctly positioned. A standalone dental network may reduce negotiated charges for routine and restorative procedures. A vision plan may smooth predictable costs for annual refraction and eyewear. A hearing arrangement may reduce the cash shock of amplification devices that Original Medicare generally excludes. A limited indemnity structure may deliver fixed payments tied to specified utilization. These devices can protect liquidity by converting lumpy, recurring expenditures into scheduled premiums, discounts, or capped reimbursement rights. Yet their design remains bounded. Annual maximums, waiting periods, missing-tooth clauses, frequency limits, noncovered implants, cosmetic exclusions, out-of-network balance exposure, and replacement-cycle limitations can leave substantial cash costs at the point of service. The analytical posture must therefore remain disciplined: ancillary products are risk buffers, not a statutory replacement for the excluded Original Medicare benefit.

The Household Medicare Diagnostic Matrix must treat Section 15.1 as the primary row for ancillary benefits, lifestyle cost isolation, and Section 1862 benefit-boundary analysis. The matrix must separately record Original Medicare exclusion status, Medicare Advantage supplemental-benefit availability, mandatory versus optional supplemental classification, plan-year allowance amount, network scope, authorization requirements, frequency rules, excluded procedures, standalone ancillary premium, waiting period, annual maximum, expected utilization, and cash-reserve target. The matrix should also distinguish medically necessary services that may fall within Medicare coverage from routine services excluded by statute. This distinction is especially important for dental services connected to covered medical procedures, ophthalmologic treatment for disease, post-cataract eyewear, diagnostic hearing and balance evaluation where medically indicated, and routine lifestyle services that remain excluded.

The final synthesis is that routine dental, vision, and hearing costs occupy a legally isolated and actuarially distinct zone. Section 1862(a)(7) excludes routine physical examinations, eyeglass-related eye exams, refractive eye procedures, hearing aids, and hearing-aid examinations; Section 1862(a)(12) supplies the parallel dental exclusion for care, treatment, filling, removal, or replacement of teeth and supporting structures. (Social Security) Medicare Advantage and ancillary markets may rebuild portions of that excluded zone through supplemental benefits, optional riders, allowances, networks, and commercial policies, but those structures remain finite, contractual, and plan-specific. A financial planner or advisory professional who collapses lifestyle maintenance into catastrophic medical insurance analysis misprices both categories. The result can be double exposure: inadequate protection against true medical catastrophe and inadequate liquidity planning for recurring ancillary costs. Under the Household Medicare Diagnostic Matrix, structural isolation of ancillary care is therefore not an aesthetic planning preference. It is a capital-balance strategy designed to protect non-sheltered retirement assets from slow dental, vision, and hearing cost erosion while preserving analytic attention for the medical risks capable of causing immediate household insolvency.

15.2 The Economics of Stand-Alone Ancillary Insurance Contracts

Stand-alone ancillary insurance contracts operate as specialized risk-transfer and liquidity-management instruments for categories of care that federal Medicare treats as outside the core medical entitlement. Original Medicare generally does not cover most routine dental services, routine eye examinations for eyeglasses or contact lenses, hearing aids, or exams for fitting hearing aids; Medicare's public coverage pages state that noncovered dental, routine vision, and hearing-aid costs are paid by the beneficiary unless another source of coverage applies. (Medicare) The stand-alone ancillary contract therefore enters where the federal program's statutory and operational benefit perimeter stops. It does not enlarge Original Medicare. It creates a separate commercial funding layer, governed by its own premium, network, reimbursement schedule, waiting period, annual maximum, frequency rule, exclusion list, and claims-administration protocol.

The actuarial structure of a stand-alone dental, vision, or hearing contract differs from both major medical insurance and simple consumer discounting. A pure discount arrangement reduces a provider's billed charge through a contracted schedule but does not necessarily transfer claim risk to an insurer. A true insurance or indemnity contract collects premium in exchange for a defined obligation to pay, reimburse, or indemnify specified covered services according to a contract schedule. A dental preferred provider organization contract may combine negotiated network charges with tiered benefit categories: preventive services paid at or near the highest reimbursement percentage, basic restorative services paid at a lower percentage, and major restorative services subject to coinsurance, waiting periods, annual maximums, or missing-tooth exclusions. A vision indemnity schedule may provide defined reimbursement for refraction, lenses, frames, or contact lenses. A hearing contract may provide an allowance or scheduled benefit toward testing, fitting, or amplification devices. In each case, the economic function is the same: unpredictable point-of-service cash demand is partially converted into a pre-funded premium line item and a known contract formula.

This conversion has portfolio value even where the contract is not perfectly comprehensive. A retirement household's balance sheet is most fragile when cash liabilities are sudden, lumpy, and medically urgent. Ancillary events often appear non-catastrophic in legal classification yet capital-intensive in household reality: periodontal scaling and root planing across multiple quadrants, crown replacement, oral surgery not tied to a Medicare-covered medical procedure, multifocal lens upgrades outside the covered benefit, specialty eyewear, or premium hearing technology. A stand-alone contract does not need to eliminate the entire claim to improve the household ledger. It may reduce negotiated charges, cap part of the exposure, distribute cost through premium funding, or preserve access to contracted providers whose charges are lower than retail schedules. The value is risk smoothing, not unlimited federal entitlement.

Medicare Advantage supplemental benefits occupy a different structural position. Medicare.gov states that Medicare Advantage plans may offer extra benefits Original Medicare does not cover, including vision, hearing, and dental services; federal Medicare Advantage regulations also permit mandatory and optional supplemental benefits subject to CMS rules. (Medicare) The Medicare Managed Care Manual explains that mandatory supplemental benefits are covered for all enrollees in a plan and may be funded through premiums, cost sharing, or rebate dollars, while optional supplemental benefits are separately elected and paid through additional premium and cost sharing, and rebate dollars may not be used to fund optional supplemental benefits. (CMS) Embedded Part C ancillary benefits may therefore be useful, but they remain plan-year contract features inside a managed-care product, not free-standing, portable, comprehensive ancillary risk transfer.

The financial variance trap appears when a modest embedded allowance is mistaken for an uncapped ancillary protection layer. A Medicare Advantage benefit labeled dental, vision, or hearing may be subject to annual dollar limits, service-code restrictions, network vendors, prior authorization, replacement cycles, frequency caps, coinsurance, excluded procedures, or reimbursement ceilings. CMS materials distinguish the Medicare Advantage maximum out-of-pocket limit as a limit on out-of-pocket costs for Part A and Part B covered services; Medicare's 2026 handbook states that once the plan's annual limit is reached, the beneficiary pays nothing for Part A and Part B covered services, not every supplemental or noncovered lifestyle service. (Medicare) The consequence is technical but decisive: routine dental, vision, and hearing costs can remain outside the core maximum out-of-pocket firewall, even when a plan offers some supplemental assistance.

Unmanaged and out-of-network ancillary care can therefore create uncapped cash exposure. In dental markets, a non-network provider may bill according to the provider's own charge schedule, while the contract may reimburse only the allowed amount, scheduled amount, or a percentage of a usual and customary calculation. The difference becomes the beneficiary's responsibility unless the contract or applicable law supplies a stronger protection. In vision and hearing markets, provider relationships may be even more heterogeneous because product selection, retail markup, fitting services, technology tiers, warranties, batteries, accessories, and replacement cycles may sit outside a major medical claims logic. The out-of-network risk is not only a higher copayment. It can be the entire economic spread between the provider's charge and the contract's reimbursement formula.

The absence of a maximum out-of-pocket firewall is the central structural distinction. Major medical modeling often begins with deductible, coinsurance, copayment, and maximum out-of-pocket values. Ancillary modeling cannot assume that architecture. Original Medicare generally excludes routine dental, routine vision refraction, eyeglasses except limited post-cataract circumstances, hearing aids, and hearing-aid fitting examinations; Medicare Advantage may add extra benefits, but the Part C maximum out-of-pocket structure is tied to Part A and Part B covered services, while Part D has its own separate drug cost architecture. (Medicare) A retiree who relies solely on the medical MOOP concept may discover that a large dental reconstruction, advanced hearing purchase, or vision product upgrade does not count toward the medical cap that seemed to protect the annual budget.

The portfolio effect is magnified by sequence-of-returns risk. During the decumulation phase, a retirement household may fund living expenses from a mixture of cash reserves, taxable brokerage assets, pensions, Social Security, annuity income, and qualified retirement accounts. A sudden five-figure dental or hearing expense can force liquidation from assets intended to remain invested. If the withdrawal occurs during a market decline, the portfolio loses both principal and the future recovery that principal would have produced. The household is not merely paying a bill. It is converting a transient healthcare need into a permanent reduction in compounding capital. Stand-alone ancillary coverage or a dedicated ancillary reserve does not eliminate sequence risk, but it can reduce the probability that routine or restorative wellness care forces emergency liquidation.

Qualified retirement account withdrawals can compound the damage through tax-bracket effects. Distributions from traditional IRAs and similar pre-tax accounts generally increase taxable income when withdrawn, unless a specific exclusion applies. Higher taxable income can increase marginal tax exposure and, through the Medicare income-related monthly adjustment amount structure, can affect future Medicare premium liability because Medicare uses modified adjusted gross income from a prior tax year to determine whether income-related adjustments apply. Medicare & You 2026 states that Medicare uses modified adjusted gross income from the IRS tax return filed two years earlier to determine IRMAA, and identifies the income-related surcharge structure for Part B and Part D premiums. (Medicare) Thus, an unplanned ancillary withdrawal may create a delayed premium aftershock if it raises the household's relevant income measure above an applicable IRMAA threshold.

This creates a destructive feedback loop. A noncovered dental, vision, or hearing bill may force a taxable distribution. The taxable distribution may raise annual adjusted gross income or modified adjusted gross income. That elevated income may later increase Medicare premium obligations through IRMAA. The higher premium obligation then reduces future monthly cash flow, increasing the probability of additional withdrawals. The original ancillary bill is no longer isolated. It becomes a capital event, a tax event, and a future-premium event. The wealth-management problem is therefore not only claim reimbursement. It is the prevention of cross-system contamination among healthcare bills, tax reporting, Medicare premium adjustments, and investment drawdown timing.

A disciplined ancillary contract analysis must compare premium cost against expected utilization, catastrophic ancillary exposure, provider access, reimbursement formula, annual maximum, and administrative flexibility. A low-premium contract with a narrow network and small annual maximum may be economically appropriate for preventive maintenance but inadequate for restorative dentistry. A richer dental PPO with higher premium and broader contracted provider access may protect better against recurrent restorative needs, but only if waiting periods, missing-tooth clauses, major-service coinsurance, and annual maximums are understood. A vision schedule may be efficient for predictable annual eyewear needs but weak against advanced disease-related care already governed by medical coverage. A hearing benefit may smooth the cost of amplification devices, but technology-tier limits can leave a large residual charge. The evaluation must be contract-specific rather than category-based.

The Household Medicare Diagnostic Matrix must therefore assign stand-alone ancillary insurance its own risk-pool architecture. The matrix should record Original Medicare exclusion status, Medicare Advantage embedded benefit amount, supplemental-benefit network rules, medical MOOP applicability, stand-alone policy premium, annual maximum, deductible, coinsurance tier, waiting period, provider network, out-of-network reimbursement schedule, projected utilization, major-restorative probability, hearing-device replacement cycle, vision-product replacement cycle, cash-reserve target, and tax source for residual payment. It should also distinguish between insured risk transfer and mere discount access. A discount plan may improve price discovery, but it may not provide the same indemnity value as an insurance contract.

The final synthesis is that stand-alone ancillary contracts are not decorative add-ons to Medicare planning. They are specialized financial instruments designed to manage excluded, high-frequency, and sometimes high-severity lifestyle-care liabilities that can bypass the medical maximum out-of-pocket firewall. Embedded Part C benefits may reduce exposure, but they often operate through finite allowances, plan-specific networks, frequency restrictions, and reimbursement limits. Unmanaged out-of-network dental, vision, and hearing costs can produce uncapped point-of-service charges, forced portfolio withdrawals, tax-bracket effects, and future IRMAA pressure. Under the Household Medicare Diagnostic Matrix, stand-alone ancillary insurance is a capital-protection row: it converts lifestyle-care volatility into a modeled premium, reimbursement, and reserve strategy. Mastery of these contract economics stabilizes household wealth during the decumulation phase by preventing routine wellness needs and restorative-care spikes from eroding non-sheltered assets, disrupting investment strategy, or triggering avoidable tax and Medicare premium consequences.

Appendix: The Primary Source Compliance Matrix (Statutory Cross-Reference Index)

Primary Source Compliance Matrix

Statutory Cross-Reference Index

The Primary Source Compliance Matrix functions as the legal audit rail for the Medicare, Marketplace, and tax-coordination architecture developed across the manuscript. Medicare administration is not located inside a single doctrinal chamber. Title XVIII of the Social Security Act establishes the statutory Medicare program, CMS administers Title XVIII, the Secretary's Medicare regulations are codified principally in Chapter IV of Title 42 of the Code of Federal Regulations, Social Security operational files determine many entitlement and premium events, and the Internal Revenue Code governs HSA eligibility, Premium Tax Credit computation, payroll tax records, and tax-return data used in income-related Medicare premium determinations. (Social Security)

The methodology of the matrix is deliberately conservative. Each entry separates the operational element from the primary statutory source, then identifies the regulatory enforcement mechanism and the actuarial consequence for household liquidity. Consumer handbooks can explain program behavior, but a compliance appendix cannot rest on paraphrase alone. The household exposure created by a missed Part B Special Enrollment Period, an excess HSA contribution after retroactive Part A, an inaccurate SLCSP benchmark, a Part D formulary denial, or a hospice-related misrouted claim can liquidate assets faster than an ordinary premium comparison model can detect. The matrix therefore treats statutory anchoring as a risk-management function: legal source validation becomes an asset-protection device.

Block A: Enrollment and Financing

Operational Element: Part A and Part B Enrollment Gates

Primary Statutory Source: Section 1837 of the Social Security Act, with premium Part A and Part B enrollment rules implemented through 42 CFR Parts 406 and 407.
Regulatory Enforcement Mechanism: Section 1837 states that enrollment occurs only in the manner and form prescribed by regulation and only during an enrollment period prescribed in or under that section. The Initial Enrollment Period begins three months before the month of first eligibility and ends seven months later; the General Enrollment Period runs January 1 through March 31; the current-employment Special Enrollment Period extends through months of qualifying group

health plan coverage based on current employment and ends with the last day of the eighth consecutive month in which the individual is no longer so covered. (Social Security) Implementing rules at 42 CFR § 406.21 identify the premium Part A Initial Enrollment Period, while 42 CFR Part 407 contains the Part B enrollment structure, including the Initial Enrollment Period, General Enrollment Period, automatic enrollment, and Special Enrollment Period provisions. (Legal Information Institute)

Actuarial Impact on Household Liquidity: Enrollment windows translate time into premium liability. A missed Part B window can create delayed coverage and a permanent premium surcharge, while a missed premium Part A window can create a time-limited premium increase. The Part B late-enrollment surcharge is enforced through 42 CFR § 408.22, which increases the standard monthly premium by 10 percent for each full twelve-month period in the delay interval. (eCFR) This rule converts a filing error into a lifetime annuity-like penalty stream. A household diagnostic file must therefore record entitlement date, Initial Enrollment Period boundaries, active-employment group health plan status, Special Enrollment Period proof, General Enrollment Period contingency, and penalty exposure.

Operational Element: IRMAA Surcharge Architecture

Primary Statutory Source: Section 1839(i) of the Social Security Act governs the income-related monthly adjustment amount for Part B.

Regulatory Enforcement Mechanism: Section 1839(i) increases the monthly premium when modified adjusted gross income exceeds statutory thresholds, defines modified adjusted gross income by reference to adjusted gross income with specified add-backs, and generally uses the taxable year beginning in the second calendar year preceding the premium year. (Social Security) 42 CFR § 408.20 supplies the standard Part B monthly premium framework, and 42 CFR § 408.28 implements the IRMAA increase by requiring Medicare beneficiaries to pay an income-related monthly adjustment amount in addition to the Part B standard premium when modified adjusted gross income exceeds the applicable thresholds. (eCFR)

Actuarial Impact on Household Liquidity: IRMAA turns tax planning into Medicare premium planning. The household does not merely pay a premium based on age or plan selection. It may pay an income-sensitive federal surcharge derived from IRS tax-return data transmitted into the Medicare premium system. The two-year lookback creates a delayed liquidity shock: a Roth conversion, asset sale, forced IRA withdrawal, capital gain, or one-time taxable event can inflate Medicare premiums in a later year. The matrix must therefore connect modified adjusted gross income, filing status, tax-exempt interest, life-changing event review, SSA premium notices, Part B IRMAA, and Part D IRMAA into a unified premium-risk ledger.

Operational Element: Trust Fund Separation Boundaries

Primary Statutory Source: Sections 1817 and 1841 of the Social Security Act.
Regulatory Enforcement Mechanism: Section 1817 creates the Federal Hospital Insurance Trust Fund, financed in significant part through payroll taxes imposed on wages and self-employment income and transferred through Treasury mechanisms into the HI account. (Social Security) Section 1841 creates the Federal Supplementary Medical Insurance Trust Fund, a separate trust fund that includes financing streams for Part B and the Medicare Prescription Drug Account. (Social Security)

Actuarial Impact on Household Liquidity: HI and SMI separation is not an accounting ornament. Part A's wage-tax financing logic differs from Part B and Part D's premium and general-revenue financing structure. The household sees a single Medicare card; the federal ledger sees different trust funds, different premium mechanisms, different solvency risks, and different annual rate-setting disciplines. A matrix entry that fails to separate HI from SMI will misclassify Part A entitlement economics, Part B premium exposure, Part D premium and subsidy exposure, and the relative policy risk of trust-fund financing stress.

Block B: Managed Care and Part D Drug Volatility

Operational Element: Non-Discrimination Formulary Mandate

Primary Statutory Source: Title XVIII Part D authority under the Social Security Act, implemented principally through 42 CFR Part 423.
Regulatory Enforcement Mechanism: A necessary technical correction controls the compliance index. 42 CFR Part 423 Subpart V is not the substantive formulary-design subpart; it is the Part D communication requirements subpart, covering definitions, CMS review and distribution of materials, communications standards, websites, required materials, and agent or broker requirements. (Legal Information Institute) The substantive formulary architecture is centered in 42 CFR § 423.120, which requires a Part D sponsor using a formulary to develop and review that formulary through a Pharmacy and Therapeutics Committee and to meet formulary adequacy requirements. (eCFR) Subpart V remains relevant as the disclosure and communication enforcement layer because plan materials must accurately describe formularies, tiers, restrictions, pharmacy access, and benefit terms.
Actuarial Impact on Household Liquidity: The formulary is the household's pharmaceutical balance sheet. Tier placement, prior authorization, step therapy, quantity limits, formulary exclusions, protected-class rules, specialty-tier placement, and pharmacy network terms determine whether prescription costs arrive as

predictable copayments, volatile coinsurance, denied claims, or exception appeals. The statutory compliance lesson is that a formulary cannot be treated as a marketing list. It is a regulated clinical-financial instrument, with Subpart C controlling access and Subpart V controlling the communications regime through which that access is disclosed.

Operational Element: Part D Exceptions, Coverage Determinations, and Five-Level Appeals Pipeline

Primary Statutory Source: Title XVIII Part D appeals authority, implemented through 42 CFR Part 423 Subparts M and U.

Regulatory Enforcement Mechanism: 42 CFR Part 423 Subpart M governs grievances, coverage determinations, redeterminations, and reconsiderations for Part D plan sponsors, Part D Independent Review Entities, and enrollee rights. (eCFR) The Part D appeals sequence begins with the plan's coverage determination, proceeds to Level 1 plan redetermination, then Level 2 reconsideration by the Part D Independent Review Entity, then Level 3 hearing or review at OMHA if the amount in controversy threshold is met, then Level 4 Medicare Appeals Council review, and finally Level 5 federal district court review if the judicial threshold is met. CMS describes the Part D process as beginning with a plan coverage determination and escalating through plan redetermination, IRE reconsideration, ALJ, Medicare Appeals Council, and federal judicial review. (CMS)

Actuarial Impact on Household Liquidity: Appeals timelines are liquidity controls. A denied specialty medication, refused formulary exception, failed prior authorization, or rejected reimbursement claim may require immediate cash payment unless the dispute is corrected within the administrative pipeline. For 2026, CMS states that the Part D ALJ amount in controversy threshold is exactly $200, and the proper OMHA request must be filed within 60 calendar days from the IRE reconsideration decision notice. (CMS) CMS's 2026 appeals flow chart and Medicare's public appeals guidance identify the federal district court threshold as exactly $1,960 for 2026. (CMS) The matrix must therefore track denial date, notice receipt, 65-day redetermination convention, 60-day IRE and ALJ windows, expedited versus standard status, amount in controversy, prescriber evidence, and household cash bridge for the disputed drug.

Block C: Transitions and Tax Crossovers

Operational Element: Hospice Managed Care Carve-Out

Primary Statutory Source: Section 1812(a)(4) and Section 1812(d) of the Social Security Act.

Regulatory Enforcement Mechanism: Section 1812(a)(4) establishes hospice care as a Part A benefit in lieu of certain other benefits, available during two 90-day periods and an unlimited number of subsequent 60-day periods when the individual makes a hospice election. Section 1812(d) governs the hospice election and provides that payment may be made only when the individual elects hospice care from a particular hospice program instead of certain other Medicare benefits; it also deems the individual to have waived Medicare payment for hospice care furnished by another hospice program, unless arranged by the elected hospice, and for services related to the terminal condition or equivalent to hospice care, subject to statutory exceptions. (Social Security)
Regulatory Enforcement Mechanism: 42 CFR § 422.320 supplies the Medicare Advantage capitation rule. A hospice-electing enrollee remains enrolled in the Medicare Advantage plan unless disenrollment occurs, but the enrollee is entitled through the plan only to benefits other than those that are the responsibility of the Medicare hospice. CMS does not make the ordinary MA capitation payment on behalf of the hospice-electing enrollee, except for the rebate portion and any monthly Part D payment. (eCFR)

Actuarial Impact on Household Liquidity: Hospice election shifts terminal-illness-related palliative liability away from the private MA risk pool and back into the Original Medicare hospice payment channel. This prevents the household from assuming that plan networks, ordinary Part C authorization rules, or MA cost-sharing charts govern hospice-related care. The household matrix must classify services as hospice-related, unrelated Medicare-covered, supplemental plan benefit, Part D unrelated-drug exposure, or excluded custodial cost. Misclassification can create denied claims, delayed payments, provider collection activity, and unnecessary asset liquidation during end-of-life transitions.

Operational Element: HSA Contribution Prohibitions After Medicare Enrollment

Primary Statutory Source: Internal Revenue Code Section 223.
Regulatory Enforcement Mechanism: Section 223 provides that the monthly HSA contribution limitation is zero for the first month an individual is entitled to benefits under Title XVIII of the Social Security Act and for each month thereafter. (Legal Information Institute) IRS Publication 969 states the operational tax rule in consumer-facing form: beginning with the first month of Medicare enrollment, the individual's HSA contribution limit is zero, and the same rule applies to retroactive Medicare coverage, making contributions made during the retroactive period excess contributions. (IRS)

Actuarial Impact on Household Liquidity: HSA error risk is retroactive and tax-sensitive. A worker delaying Medicare while remaining in an HDHP may contribute lawfully until Medicare entitlement begins. Once premium-free Part A is established, including retroactively, contributions during affected months can become excess contributions requiring correction and possible excise-tax exposure. The matrix must record Part A effective date, Social Security application date, HSA payroll deduction stop date, employer HSA contribution timing, spouse eligibility, family HDHP status, catch-up contributions, and corrective distribution deadline.

Operational Element: Dependency Premium Tax Credit Recalculation and SLCSP Restructuring

Primary Statutory Source: Internal Revenue Code Section 36B.
Regulatory Enforcement Mechanism: 26 CFR § 1.36B-3 governs computation of the premium assistance credit and defines the applicable benchmark plan. The applicable benchmark plan for family coverage is the second-lowest-cost silver plan that would cover the members of the taxpayer's coverage family; the regulation's examples show that when a family member becomes eligible for other minimum essential coverage, the benchmark may be recomputed for the remaining Marketplace coverage family. (eCFR) IRS Form 8962 is the federal tax form used to compute the Premium Tax Credit and reconcile it with advance payments of the Premium Tax Credit. (IRS)

Actuarial Impact on Household Liquidity: A Medicare transition can shrink the Marketplace coverage family while household modified adjusted gross income remains inside the same tax unit. The Second Lowest Cost Silver Plan benchmark may lose the age-rated premium component associated with the Medicare-enrolled adult, while the household's contribution amount remains based on income, family size, and statutory percentage rules. If APTC is not recalculated promptly, excess subsidies may flow for months and reappear as repayment liability on Form 8962. The matrix must record Medicare effective month, Marketplace termination month, remaining covered dependents, SLCSP by month, Form 1095-A accuracy, household MAGI, tax-family size, APTC paid, actual allowable PTC, and repayment exposure.

Compliance Integration and Methodological Close-Out

The Primary Source Compliance Matrix is the legal backbone of the Household Medicare Diagnostic Matrix. The front-facing household matrix identifies the operational event: retirement, delayed Part B, employer coverage loss, Marketplace re-entry, HSA cessation, Part D formulary denial, hospice election, IRMAA exposure, or dependent separation. The compliance matrix supplies the primary legal source that validates how that event must be processed. Without this back-matter apparatus, a planning system may appear organized but remain legally unstable.

The final methodological rule is that every household transition must be translated into four linked determinations: entitlement authority, payment authority, tax authority, and appeal authority. Entitlement authority determines whether Medicare, Marketplace, COBRA, employer coverage, or hospice applies. Payment authority determines whether the claim belongs to Original Medicare, a Medicare Advantage organization, a Part D sponsor, a hospice program, an Exchange plan, or private household cash. Tax authority determines HSA limits, Premium Tax Credit eligibility, IRMAA exposure, and excess subsidy repayment. Appeal authority determines whether a denial belongs in a grievance, coverage determination, plan redetermination, IRE reconsideration, OMHA hearing, Council review, or federal court.

The appendix therefore transforms retirement healthcare consulting from a preference-driven advisory exercise into a legally defensible discipline. Each row protects a different household asset: cash flow, tax position, prescription access, dependent coverage, Medicare premium stability, hospice coordination, and long-term capital preservation. The operative principle is uncompromising: Medicare literacy is not complete until the household can identify the governing statute, the implementing regulation, the administrative filing path, and the liquidity consequence of every transition. The Primary Source Compliance Matrix supplies that final firewall, stabilizing multi-generational family wealth against regulatory fragmentation, point-of-service billing failures, and unmodeled federal tax collisions.

Glossary of Federal Systemic Terms and Medical-Legal Nomenclature

Methodological Preface to Regulatory Nomenclature

Technical Medicare planning depends on linguistic precision because federal health insurance, private managed care, Marketplace subsidy law, and tax coordination rules do not use identical operational vocabulary. A term that appears plain in ordinary conversation can carry a specialized legal function inside Title XVIII of the Social Security Act, Title 42 of the Code of Federal Regulations, Title 45 Exchange regulations, or the Internal Revenue Code. The difference between a grievance and a coverage determination controls whether a drug denial enters the formal Part D appeals pipeline. The difference between Marketplace household size and Marketplace coverage family controls whether a silver benchmark premium is correctly computed. The difference between HSA family coverage and HSA eligible individual status controls whether contributions become lawful deposits or excess contributions. The difference between Medicare Advantage enrollment and Original Medicare hospice payment responsibility controls whether terminal-illness services are routed to a private plan, a hospice provider, or the federal fee-for-service channel.

This glossary establishes a controlled definitional baseline for the manuscript. Each entry identifies the operational meaning of the term, the primary legal or administrative source, and the actuarial relevance to household liquidity. Standard consumer explanations are useful for public education, but professional Medicare, Marketplace, and tax coordination analysis requires a source-anchored vocabulary. A single misunderstood term can produce a missed filing window, a denied claim, a delayed prescription, an excess HSA contribution, a Premium Tax Credit clawback, or an unplanned taxable distribution. The glossary therefore functions as a risk-management instrument: language becomes the first firewall against regulatory misclassification.

Advanced Premium Tax Credit (APTC)

The Advanced Premium Tax Credit is the monthly advance payment of the Premium Tax Credit made to an insurer to reduce the premium charged for a qualified health plan purchased through a Health Insurance Marketplace. IRS Form 8962 instructions describe APTC as a payment during the year to the insurance provider that pays part or all of the premium for a qualified health plan covering an individual in the tax family, with eligibility based on the Marketplace's estimate of the PTC available on the tax return. The same instructions require reconciliation of APTC against the actual PTC on Form 8962, with excess APTC repaid subject to applicable limits and underpaid PTC claimed as a credit. (IRS)

Actuarially, APTC is a liquidity-advance mechanism, not a final subsidy grant. It is sensitive to household income, tax family composition, Marketplace coverage family, rating area, age-rated premiums, and the applicable second-lowest-cost silver plan baseline. The risk arises when Medicare eligibility, employer coverage loss, dependent separation, marriage, divorce, dependent status change, or income movement is not reported promptly to the Marketplace. APTC may continue at an incorrect level for months, creating a deferred liability on the federal tax return.

Amount in Controversy (AIC)

Amount in Controversy is the minimum monetary value that must remain disputed before a Medicare appeal can escalate to designated higher levels of administrative or judicial review. For calendar year 2026, the verified AIC threshold for an Administrative Law Judge hearing at Level 3 is exactly $200, and the verified AIC threshold for judicial review in Federal District Court at Level 5 is exactly $1,960. CMS states that the ALJ threshold is recalculated annually and identifies the 2026 ALJ threshold as $200; federal notice materials identify the 2026 thresholds as $200 for ALJ hearings and $1,960 for judicial review. (CMS)

The AIC threshold converts claim value into procedural access. A low-dollar generic-drug dispute may terminate administratively before federal hearing jurisdiction becomes available, while a specialty-drug denial may cross the threshold immediately. In the Household Medicare Diagnostic Matrix, AIC is a gatekeeping variable that determines whether a denied drug, medical service, or payment claim can move beyond lower-level administrative review.

Capitation Exclusion (Hospice Carve-Out)

The Capitation Exclusion, in the hospice context, is the regulatory payment adjustment that removes hospice liability from the Medicare Advantage capitation stream once a beneficiary elects hospice care. Under 42 CFR § 422.320, no payment is made to a Medicare Advantage organization on behalf of a Medicare enrollee who has elected hospice care, except for the beneficiary rebate portion and any monthly prescription drug payment. (Legal Information Institute)

The actuarial function is a complete hospice risk carve-out. The Medicare Advantage plan may remain active for residual benefits and unrelated services, but terminal-illness-related hospice care is paid through the Original Medicare hospice mechanism. This prevents the terminal-care ledger from being embedded in the private plan's ordinary capitation risk rate. Household liquidity analysis must therefore classify services by relatedness to the terminal prognosis and by payer channel: hospice Part A, unrelated Medicare-covered care, residual plan supplemental benefit, Part D unrelated drug claim, or private household liability.

Coverage Determination

A Coverage Determination is the first formal Part D decision by a plan sponsor concerning receipt of, or payment for, a prescription drug, a formulary or tiering exception request, the cost-sharing amount owed, a quantity or dose limit, a step therapy requirement, or satisfaction of prior authorization or other utilization management requirements. CMS describes these categories directly in its Part D coverage determination guidance; 42 CFR § 423.566 requires each Part D sponsor to maintain procedures for timely coverage determinations regarding prescription drug benefits and enrollee cost sharing. (CMS)

A Coverage Determination is the legal ignition point for the Part D appeals sequence. Without a coverage determination, the dispute may remain a pharmacy rejection, inquiry, or grievance rather than an appealable benefit decision. The term therefore determines whether the household may move into redetermination, IRE reconsideration, OMHA review, Medicare Appeals Council review, and possible judicial review.

Excess HSA Contribution

An Excess HSA Contribution is a tax-disallowed deposit to a Health Savings Account that exceeds the contributor's statutory limit for the relevant tax period. Internal Revenue Code Section 223 provides that the monthly contribution limitation is zero beginning with the first month an individual is entitled to Medicare benefits under Title XVIII and for each month thereafter. IRS Publication 969 states that beginning with the first month of Medicare enrollment, the HSA contribution limit is zero, and that the rule applies to periods of retroactive Medicare coverage, making contributions during retroactive Medicare months excess contributions. (Legal Information Institute)

The household hazard is retroactivity. Premium-free Part A can be established before the visible application month in certain circumstances, and Publication 969 treats deposits during retroactive Medicare coverage as excess. The matrix must therefore track Part A effective month, Social Security application timing, payroll HSA deposits, employer contributions, spouse account ownership, and corrective distribution obligations.

General Enrollment Period (GEP)

The General Enrollment Period is the annual statutory Medicare enrollment window running from January 1 through March 31 for individuals who missed an earlier Part B enrollment opportunity and lack a qualifying Special Enrollment Period. Section 1837 of the Social Security Act states that the General Enrollment Period begins January 1 and ends March 31 each year. (Social Security)

The GEP is a remedial window with financial consequences. It allows late entry into Medicare Part B, and, where applicable, premium Part A, but it does not erase the late-enrollment penalty structure. Part B penalty rules can add 10 percent to the standard premium for each full twelve-month period of delayed enrollment without protected coverage. The GEP therefore functions as a liquidity-damage control point, not a penalty-free substitute for timely enrollment.

Income-Related Monthly Adjustment Amount (IRMAA)

The Income-Related Monthly Adjustment Amount is the income-based federal premium surcharge added to Medicare Part B and Part D obligations for higher-income beneficiaries. Section 1839(i) of the Social Security Act defines modified adjusted gross income for this purpose, generally using adjusted gross income with specified additions, including tax-exempt interest, and ordinarily uses the taxable year beginning in the second calendar year before the premium year. (Social Security)

IRMAA transforms tax events into Medicare premium events. A Roth conversion, capital gain, required distribution, sale of appreciated property, or other income spike can produce a delayed increase in Medicare premiums. IRMAA therefore belongs in both the tax and Medicare premium rows of the matrix. Its actuarial significance lies in the two-year lookback: a liquidity decision in one year can raise health-insurance premiums in a later year.

Minimum Essential Coverage (MEC)

Minimum Essential Coverage is the statutory baseline category of health coverage under Internal Revenue Code Section 5000A. The statute includes Medicare Part A, Medicaid, CHIP, eligible employer-sponsored plans, individual market coverage, grandfathered plans, and other recognized coverage categories within the MEC definition. It also identifies eligible employer-sponsored coverage as a group health plan or group health insurance coverage offered by an employer to an employee in the small or large group market. (Legal Information Institute)

MEC is a dependency-transition trigger. Under 45 CFR § 155.420, loss of qualifying coverage can open a Marketplace Special Enrollment Period, generally allowing plan selection within the regulatory SEP window. (Legal Information Institute) When a worker moves into Medicare and employer family coverage terminates for a younger spouse or dependent child, the dependent's loss of MEC, not the worker's Medicare card itself, becomes the Marketplace re-entry event.

Premium Tax Credit (PTC) Reconciliation

Premium Tax Credit Reconciliation is the annual federal tax process through which Form 8962 compares APTC paid during the year with the actual PTC allowed under the year-end tax return. IRS states that Form 8962 is used to figure the PTC and reconcile it with advance payments. IRS instructions further state that excess APTC must be repaid subject to applicable limitations, while insufficient APTC may produce an additional credit. (IRS)

The actuarial consequence is delayed settlement risk. Marketplace subsidies are estimated monthly but finalized annually. If Medicare eligibility removes a family member from the Marketplace coverage family, if income increases, or if a dependent loses eligibility, APTC can exceed the final allowable credit. The tax return then becomes the collection mechanism. Form 1095-A accuracy, SLCSP correction, and monthly Form 8962 entries become household liquidity controls.

Prior Authorization (PA) Override

A Prior Authorization Override is the clinical-administrative process used to obtain coverage for a drug or service subject to prior authorization criteria. In the Part D formulary context, the prescriber supplies clinical support showing medical necessity, contraindication to alternatives, failure of formulary therapy, adverse effects, dosage or quantity need, or other medically relevant facts. Section 423.578 requires the Part D exceptions process to evaluate medical necessity, allows the plan to require oral or written supporting statements and additional medical documentation, and treats exception decisions as coverage determinations. (Legal Information Institute)

The PA override is a documentation firewall. Without objective clinical support, a pharmacy rejection may remain a denial. With adequate documentation, the claim can become a formal exception request, then an appealable determination if unfavorable. The household liquidity impact is immediate because the drug may otherwise require full cash payment or remain unavailable.

Second Lowest Cost Silver Plan (SLCSP)

The Second Lowest Cost Silver Plan is the benchmark plan used to calculate the Premium Tax Credit under 26 CFR § 1.36B-3. The regulation provides that the applicable benchmark plan is generally the second-lowest-cost silver plan offered through the Exchange for the taxpayer's coverage family in the relevant rating area, and family benchmark computations are based on the members of the coverage family who must be covered. The regulation also defines the premium assistance amount as the lesser of enrollment premiums or the benchmark premium minus the monthly contribution amount. (Legal Information Institute)

The SLCSP is not always the purchased plan. It is the subsidy baseline. When a senior transitions to Medicare and leaves the Marketplace coverage family, the age-rated premium component associated with that senior may disappear from the benchmark. The household may still file one tax return, but the coverage family used for subsidy computation can shrink. This creates benchmark contraction, APTC recalculation, and Form 8962 reconciliation exposure.

Specialty Tier Threshold

The Specialty Tier Threshold is the CMS-established cost boundary used to determine whether a high-cost Part D drug may be placed on a specialty cost-sharing tier. Under 42 CFR § 423.104, a specialty tier is a formulary cost-sharing tier dedicated to high-cost Part D drugs with ingredient costs for a 30-day equivalent supply greater than the specialty-tier cost threshold. CMS uses Prescription Drug Event data to determine 30-day equivalent ingredient cost and the top-one-percent methodology, and generally approves specialty-tier placement when plan data show that more than 50 percent of the relevant 30-day equivalent claims exceed the threshold. (Legal Information Institute)

For the current threshold lineage, CMS's CY 2027 bidding instructions state that analyses for CY 2025 and CY 2026 exceeded the current $950 threshold but did not meet the 10 percent adjustment trigger, and that the CY 2027 threshold will increase to $1,080 because the calculation reached a 13.7 percent increase from the current $950 threshold. (CMS) Specialty-tier placement is actuarially important because it commonly shifts household exposure from flat copayments to percentage coinsurance, accelerating out-of-pocket accumulation and creating early-year cash-flow volatility.

Compliance Closing Integration

The glossary cross-couples directly with the Household Medicare Diagnostic Matrix. Each term functions as an operational variable. APTC and PTC Reconciliation govern Marketplace subsidy cash flow. AIC governs appeal escalation. Capitation Exclusion governs hospice payer reversion. Coverage Determination and PA Override govern Part D recourse. Excess HSA Contribution governs tax compliance. GEP governs late Medicare entry. IRMAA governs premium inflation. MEC governs dependency Special Enrollment Period access. SLCSP governs subsidy baselines. Specialty Tier Threshold governs drug-cost volatility.

A Medicare plan comparison without this vocabulary remains incomplete. The professional task is not merely selecting coverage. It is classifying federal status, payer channel, tax exposure, appeal right, documentation burden, and liquidity consequence. Mastery of this glossary transforms the manuscript's planning method into a legally defensible discipline. The final linguistic firewall is precision: the household's wealth is protected when each medical, tax, and coverage event is named accurately, sourced correctly, and routed through the proper federal mechanism.

Author Academic Profile & Institutional Disclaimers

Author Academic Profile

The author's professional identity rests at the intersection of financial economics, instructional leadership, federal benefits literacy, and systemic household risk analysis. The manuscript reflects a career architecture shaped by formal academic preparation, classroom-level pedagogy, insurance-market fieldwork, and the disciplined conversion of complex social-insurance rules into adult-learning systems. The author is a Doctoral Candidate in Education Management at Hampton University, with a PK-12 Administration focus and a research orientation centered on technology implementation, instructional leadership, and the organizational design required to make complex knowledge usable across diverse learner populations. That doctoral foundation gives the manuscript its structural emphasis on sequencing, scaffolding, cognitive load reduction, diagnostic frameworks, and institutionally coherent adult instruction.

The author's graduate training includes a Master of Arts in Teaching in Secondary Economics from Mercer University. That background supplies the manuscript's economic grammar: scarcity, incentives, household budgeting, intertemporal choice, risk pooling, marginal cost, price signaling, tax incidence, and liquidity management. Medicare is treated throughout the book not merely as a health benefit, but as a public-finance system that reshapes household consumption, taxation, insurance selection, portfolio withdrawal strategy, and dependent coverage continuity. The author's baccalaureate preparation, a Bachelor of Arts degree in Business Management and Corporate Finance from Morris Brown College, supplies the capital-structure orientation that appears throughout the text. Medicare enrollment, Part D formularies, HSA eligibility, Premium Tax Credit reconciliation, COBRA continuation, IRMAA exposure, and hospice carve-outs are analyzed as interconnected balance-sheet events rather than isolated consumer choices.

The author is also a licensed insurance professional in Georgia with applied field expertise in systemic risk management, asset protection, and multi-generational wealth preservation strategies. That licensure is not presented as a substitute for legal, tax, actuarial, or investment-advisory credentials. It is presented as a field-practice credential that grounds the manuscript in the operational realities households encounter when they translate federal rules into enrollment forms, premium bills, prescription claims, tax filings, continuation notices, and retirement cash-flow decisions. The author's distinctive contribution lies in integrating financial literacy, educator training, corporate finance, and regulated insurance analysis into a unified Medicare decision framework.

Pedagogical Philosophy and Workshop Alignment

The pedagogical philosophy underlying the manuscript is grounded in the belief that adult learners do not need diluted content; they need structured access to complex content. Medicare confusion often arises not because the underlying rules are impossible to understand, but because the rules are usually presented in fragmented channels: a Social Security enrollment page, a Medicare handbook, a plan Evidence of Coverage, an IRS publication, an employer benefits notice, a COBRA election packet, and a Marketplace eligibility screen. The author's instructional method converts that fragmentation into a matrix-based learning system. Each concept is placed into a visible operational lane: entitlement, payer order, tax coordination, prescription-drug exposure, appeal rights, household dependency, and portfolio liquidity.

The author's work as a Career, Technical, and Agricultural Education, Economics and Personal Finance public school teacher, reinforces this architecture. CTAE instruction requires translation between technical systems and performance-ready outputs. A student or adult learner must not merely hear a definition; the learner must know where the definition appears in a workflow, how it affects the next decision, and what error occurs when the definition is misapplied. That same instructional logic shapes this book. Dense federal rules are presented through repeated structures, cross-references, diagnostic rows, and source-mapped terminology. The result is a manuscript designed for serious reading, seminar instruction, professional reference, and household application.

The manuscript also functions as the theoretical foundation for specialized community financial workshops, including public-library seminar programming designed to move families "Beyond the Pension" into structured discussions of household liquidity, interest-rate arbitrage, infinite banking concepts, and retirement-risk containment. Such workshops are educational in character. Their purpose is to make institutional systems visible before families encounter a crisis point. Medicare is often the public doorway through which larger financial issues become unavoidable: when to claim Social Security, how to protect a spouse who is not Medicare-eligible, how to stop HSA contributions before retroactive Part A creates excess deposits, how to avoid a Premium Tax Credit clawback, how to read a formulary, and how to preserve non-sheltered capital when serious illness or ancillary care costs emerge.

Institutional Compliance and General Education Disclaimer

This text is structured as a general educational communication. It is designed to explain federal Medicare architecture, Marketplace coordination, tax-interaction principles, prescription-drug governance, serious-illness transitions, and household financial-risk patterns. It does not constitute individualized legal counsel, tax planning, investment advice, actuarial certification, fiduciary portfolio management, accounting advice, or medical advice. The analytical discussion of Title XVIII of the Social Security Act, 42 CFR Parts 422 and 423, Internal Revenue Code Section 223, Premium Tax Credit rules, hospice payment allocation, and Medicare appeals thresholds is presented for educational and institutional-literacy purposes.

CMS distinguishes communications from marketing in the Medicare Advantage and Part D context, explaining that communications provide information to current or prospective enrollees, while marketing is a subset that satisfies intent and content standards, including efforts intended to influence plan selection or retention and content addressing plan benefits, premiums, cost sharing, rankings, or rewards. (CMS) This manuscript is not plan-specific marketing material. It does not endorse, rank, solicit enrollment in, or promote any private Medicare Advantage organization, Medicare Prescription Drug Plan sponsor, pharmacy benefit manager, insurance carrier, provider network, or local plan. It does not present carrier-specific premiums, formularies, star ratings, service areas, supplemental allowances, enrollment applications, or comparative plan recommendations.

The author operates independently of private Medicare Advantage organizations, commercial pharmaceutical benefit managers, and local marketing networks for purposes of this manuscript's source analysis. The text is intentionally decoupled from carrier enrollment bias. Its method is institutional rather than promotional: it examines how federal rules allocate entitlement, payment, tax exposure, appeal rights, and household liquidity risk. Any use of examples, matrices, or hypothetical household structures is illustrative and educational. Actual enrollment, tax, legal, investment, or benefits decisions require review of current plan documents, official federal notices, employer benefit materials, tax records, and jurisdiction-specific professional guidance.

Actuarial Limitations and Independent Fiduciary Warnings

Federal health and tax parameters are temporally volatile. A figure that is accurate for one plan year may be indexed, superseded, recalculated, or procedurally revised in a later year. The manuscript's quantitative references should therefore be treated as plan-year specific unless the text expressly states a general rule. For example, CMS identifies the 2026 Amount in Controversy threshold for an Administrative Law Judge hearing as exactly $200, and the official Medicare Part D appeals flow chart identifies the 2026 Federal District Court judicial review threshold as exactly $1,960. (CMS) (CMS) The same CMS flow chart states that AIC requirements for ALJ hearings and Federal District Court review are adjusted annually in accordance with the medical care component of the Consumer Price Index. (CMS) Marketplace subsidy rules, by contrast, may depend on Federal Poverty Line metrics, household income, tax-family composition, rating area, and statutory contribution percentages.

The temporal volatility clause is not a formality. Medicare premiums, deductibles, Part D thresholds, IRMAA brackets, Marketplace affordability percentages, HSA contribution limits, appeal thresholds, and regulatory guidance can change. Plan-level formularies, provider networks, drug tiers, prior authorization requirements, supplemental benefits, and cost-sharing schedules can also change annually. The manuscript therefore establishes a decision method, not a permanent numerical guarantee. The responsible application of that method requires verification against the official materials governing the relevant year and the specific household fact pattern.

The fiduciary responsibility clause is equally central. A retirement household, financial planner, benefits advisor, attorney, tax professional, insurance professional, or institutional educator must verify current federal rules before executing high-stakes liquidity transitions, Medicare enrollment decisions, COBRA elections, HSA contribution strategies, Marketplace applications, Roth conversions, business-sale timing, trust distributions, pension elections, or employer benefits alterations. The manuscript does not replace consultation with qualified legal, tax, actuarial, medical, or investment professionals. It provides a rigorous conceptual map for identifying when such professionals should be engaged and what federal variables must be examined.

The final institutional position is that Medicare literacy is a wealth-preservation discipline. A household can lose capital through missed enrollment windows, improper COBRA sequencing, excess HSA contributions, unreported Marketplace changes, misclassified hospice claims, denied Part D prescriptions, unappealed formulary restrictions, unmanaged IRMAA exposure, and ancillary care costs outside statutory Medicare coverage. This manuscript is designed to reduce those risks by creating a legally grounded educational framework. Its disclaimers protect the integrity of the research and the financial position of the transitioning household by making the boundary clear: the text educates, organizes, and source-maps; actual execution belongs to verified documents, current federal rules, and appropriately credentialed professional judgment.

Institutional Resource Guide and Federal Document Registries

Methodological Preface to Systemic Data Retrieval

The Institutional Resource Guide functions as the manuscript's operational bridge between doctrinal analysis and active federal administration. Medicare, Marketplace coverage, and tax coordination cannot be administered safely from secondary summaries alone because federal benefit rules change through statutes, regulations, subregulatory manuals, plan filings, annual notices, tax forms, and electronic data systems. A household transition may require simultaneous reference to Social Security entitlement procedures, CMS plan data, Part D formulary files, OMHA appeal registries, IRS tax publications, Marketplace Form 1095-A records, and the Code of Federal Regulations. A professional analysis that relies only on abbreviated consumer summaries may miss a filing deadline, appeal threshold, HSA cessation rule, Part D formulary update, Marketplace subsidy correction, or hospice payment-routing instruction.

This directory is therefore a risk-management instrument. Its purpose is not merely to identify helpful websites. Its purpose is to isolate the authoritative institutional venues where operational decisions are actually validated. The methodology is source-hierarchical: statutory text controls legal entitlement; regulations control enforceable administrative structure; CMS and SSA manuals supply operational procedure; IRS forms and publications control tax execution; official federal portals supply case tracking, plan comparison, subsidy reconciliation, and filing instructions. This hierarchy protects household liquidity because the most expensive Medicare errors usually occur when a household treats a generalized explanation as though it were a final administrative determination.

Department of Health and Human Services, Centers for Medicare & Medicaid Services

Resource Registry: Medicare.gov Plan Compare and CMS Plan Finder Architecture

The official Plan Compare system on Medicare.gov is the federal consumer-facing plan comparison architecture for Medicare Advantage and Medicare drug coverage. It allows comparison of available Medicare health and drug plan options by location, premium, pharmacy, drug list, and related plan variables. Medicare.gov identifies this tool as the pathway to find Medicare health and drug plans in a specific area and compare costs. (Medicare) The system is not merely an informational brochure. It is a structured annual enrollment interface connected to plan filings, Part D drug data, pharmacy-network data, premium tables, and quality-rating information.

For actuarial household work, Plan Compare is a cash-flow modeling engine. It allows the household file to test whether a medication appears on a plan formulary, whether pharmacy selection changes annual drug cost, whether a plan's premium is offset by lower expected prescriptions, whether a drug requires utilization management, and whether plan quality ratings materially alter risk tolerance. CMS's public data environment separately maintains monthly prescription drug plan formulary and pharmacy network information for Medicare Prescription Drug Plans and Medicare Advantage plans; CMS identifies the dataset as monthly and sourced to the Centers for Medicare & Medicaid Services. (CMS Data) The operational discipline is straightforward: plan-comparison assumptions should be refreshed during the relevant plan year and rechecked before annual election decisions.

Resource Registry: CMS Internet-Only Manuals and Program Guidance

The CMS Internet-Only Manuals are the operational manual library used by CMS program components, contractors, Medicare Advantage organizations, state survey agencies, and other administrative actors. CMS describes the Internet-Only Manuals as replicas of the agency's official record copy and as day-to-day operating instructions based on statutes, regulations, guidelines, models, and directives. (CMS) This registry is crucial because many claims-processing, hospice, managed-care, appeal, and contractor procedures are not fully understandable from statutory text alone.

The actuarial relevance lies in claim routing and administrative causation. A hospice election, a Medicare Advantage encounter, a Part D claim, or an Original Medicare denial may turn on coding, contractor workflow, notice language, payer order, or operational definitions preserved in CMS manuals. The Household Medicare Diagnostic Matrix therefore uses the CMS manual library as a procedural verification layer: statutory text identifies the entitlement; regulations define the legal architecture; manuals explain how the file is actually processed.

Resource Registry: CMS Formulary Reference File and Part D Formulary Data Environment

The phrase "CMS Product No Defect (PND) and Formularies Registry" is not verified as an official public federal registry title in the primary sources reviewed. The accurate Part D public registry family consists of CMS formulary guidance, CMS Formulary Reference Files, and CMS data files containing prescription drug plan formulary, pharmacy network, and pricing information. CMS's formulary guidance page publishes annual and monthly Formulary Reference Files, including 2026 files and related pricing-data guidance. (CMS) The National Library of Medicine explains that the CMS Formulary Reference File is the listing of drugs that Part D plan sponsors must use when submitting Part D formularies to CMS for review. (National Library of Medicine)

This registry environment is the technical foundation for Part D drug volatility analysis. It supports verification of covered drug identifiers, formulary submissions, formulary changes, pharmacy-network data, and drug-plan comparison structures. A household that depends on high-cost drugs should not treat a printed annual formulary excerpt as the only evidence. Formulary status, tier placement, utilization restrictions, pharmacy networks, and pricing data can change under Medicare rules, so the formulary registry environment becomes the source-control layer for the prescription-drug rows of the matrix.

Department of Health and Human Services, Office of Medicare Hearings and Appeals

Resource Registry: OMHA e-Appeal Portal and ALJ Appeal Status Information System

The Office of Medicare Hearings and Appeals administers Level 3 of the Medicare appeals process. OMHA's e-Appeal Portal enables electronic submission of Medicare Part A and Part B appeal requests for hearing, documentation upload to existing appeals, and appeal-status checking. (hhs-ecape-portal.entellitrak.com) OMHA also maintains the ALJ Appeal Status Information System, or AASIS, which allows status checks for appeals filed with OMHA. (HHS.gov) The current OMHA public guidance clarifies that the e-Appeal Portal cannot accept Medicare Part C or Medicare Part D appeal requests at this time; that limitation must be respected when classifying managed-care or drug-plan disputes. (HHS.gov)

The 2026 amount-in-controversy threshold gives the OMHA registry immediate financial significance. CMS states that a request for an ALJ hearing must be filed within 60 days of receipt of the reconsideration decision, receipt is presumed five days after the decision notice unless contrary evidence exists, and the 2026 amount in controversy for an ALJ hearing is $200. (CMS) The Federal Register confirms the 2026 thresholds as $200 for ALJ hearings and $1,960 for judicial review. (Federal Register) For household planning, OMHA access is not merely a legal appeal stage. It is the point at which claim value, documentation quality, filing timeliness, and liquidity reserves determine whether a dispute can be heard by an independent federal adjudicator.

Social Security Administration

Resource Registry: Social Security Administration Program Operations Manual System (POMS)

The Social Security Administration's Program Operations Manual System is the agency's operational policy database. SSA describes the public POMS as a primary source of information used by Social Security employees to process Social Security benefit claims; the public version is identical to the employee version except for internal data-entry and sensitive content instructions. (Social Security Administration) SSA's POMS help page further describes POMS as the operational reference used by SSA staff to conduct daily business. (Social Security Administration)

For Medicare planning, POMS is indispensable because Part A and Part B enrollment are often processed through SSA systems rather than CMS consumer channels alone. POMS contains operational treatment of Special Enrollment Periods, group health plan coverage based on current employment, premium increases, effective dates, evidence requirements, and penalty computations. SSA's POMS provision on Part B late enrollment states that the Supplementary Medical Insurance premium is increased by 10 percent for each full twelve-month period in which the person could have been enrolled but was not. (Social Security Administration) POMS also explains the eight-month Special Enrollment Period after group health plan coverage based on current employment ends. (Social Security Administration) In liquidity terms, POMS verifies whether a household's Part B delay is protected or penalty-bearing.

Office of the Federal Register and Government Publishing Office

Resource Registry: Electronic Code of Federal Regulations and GovInfo

The Electronic Code of Federal Regulations is the continuously updated online version of the Code of Federal Regulations. The official eCFR page states that the CFR is the official legal print publication, while the eCFR is a continuously updated online version and is not an official legal edition. (eCFR) GovInfo explains that the annual CFR is published by the Office of the Federal Register, National Archives and Records Administration, and that the eCFR is an editorial compilation produced by the Office of the Federal Register and the Government Publishing Office, updated daily. (GovInfo)

This distinction matters because the eCFR is the most practical current regulation research venue, while the official legal edition and Federal Register history may be required for formal legal audit. The registry controls citations to 42 CFR Parts 406, 407, 408, 422, and 423, and to 26 CFR § 1.36B-3. It also prevents a common source error: the eCFR is not a CMS database, even when it contains CMS regulations. It is an Office of Federal Register and Government Publishing Office regulatory publication environment.

Department of the Treasury and Internal Revenue Service

Resource Registry: IRS Forms, Publications, and Internal Revenue Code Guidance

The IRS forms and publications archive is the tax execution registry for Medicare-adjacent household planning. IRS Publication 969 explains Health Savings Accounts, Archer MSAs, Medicare Advantage MSAs, health flexible spending arrangements, and health reimbursement arrangements. IRS Publication 969 states that beginning with the first month of Medicare enrollment, an individual's HSA contribution limit is zero, including retroactive Medicare coverage periods. (IRS) IRS Form 8962 is the tax form used to figure the Premium Tax Credit and reconcile it with advance payments of the Premium Tax Credit. (IRS)

The operational relevance is direct. HSA overcontributions, Marketplace subsidy overpayments, Form 1095-A discrepancies, and Form 8962 reconciliation liabilities are tax events with medical-insurance causes. The IRS archive supplies the governing execution forms and instructions, while the Internal Revenue Code supplies the statutory authority. A household file that does not connect Medicare effective dates to Publication 969 or Marketplace coverage records to Form 8962 may produce avoidable excess-contribution penalties or APTC repayment exposure.

Resource Registry: Marketplace Form 1095-A, Form 8962, and the CMS Data Services Hub Environment

There is no verified public federal portal formally titled the "Federal Marketplace Form 8962 Data Hub." The accurate public-facing structure is the Marketplace account and Form 1095-A record, followed by IRS Form 8962 reconciliation. HealthCare.gov instructs Marketplace enrollees to retrieve Form 1095-A from the Marketplace account and use its information, including the second-lowest-cost silver plan premium, to complete Form 8962. (HealthCare.gov) IRS states that Form 1095-A reports information about individuals enrolled in qualified health plans through the Marketplace and allows individuals to take the Premium Tax Credit, reconcile advance credit payments, and file an accurate tax return. (IRS)

The backend eligibility-verification environment is the CMS Data Services Hub. CMS describes the Hub as a routing tool that helps Marketplaces make accurate and timely eligibility determinations by verifying data against secure federal and state databases. (CMS) The distinction is essential: the Hub supports eligibility verification; Form 1095-A and Form 8962 support annual tax reconciliation. Household liquidity depends on both systems, because Marketplace eligibility errors can distort APTC during the year, while IRS reconciliation captures the excess or shortfall after year-end.

Technical Compliance and Methodological Close-Out

The Institutional Resource Guide cross-couples directly with the Household Medicare Diagnostic Matrix. Each registry is an execution venue. SSA POMS resolves entitlement, Special Enrollment Period, and late-enrollment penalty questions. Medicare.gov Plan Compare and CMS formulary data resolve plan, premium, pharmacy, drug-tier, and network questions. CMS manuals resolve claims-processing and payer-routing questions. OMHA and AASIS resolve Level 3 hearing status and procedural access. The eCFR and GovInfo resolve regulatory citation and annual legal-edition verification. IRS publications and forms resolve HSA and Premium Tax Credit execution. Marketplace Form 1095-A and the CMS Data Services Hub environment resolve subsidy eligibility and tax-reporting inputs.

The final methodological principle is source discipline. The household matrix identifies the risk; the registry supplies the evidence. A Part B penalty row points to POMS. A formulary volatility row points to CMS formulary data. A Part D denial row points to plan notices, CMS appeals guidance, and, where appropriate, federal appeals systems. A Medicare-Marketplace crossover row points to HealthCare.gov, Form 1095-A, Form 8962, and 26 CFR § 1.36B-3. A hospice carve-out row points to CMS manuals and Title 42 regulations. The resource guide therefore serves as the operational firewall of the manuscript: it converts policy knowledge into verifiable administrative action and stabilizes multi-generational household wealth against regulatory fragmentation, filing errors, and point-of-service financial breakdown.

Questions About This Book or Medicare Education Seminars?

Visit www.medicareigetitnow.com

to submit a general question, request information about an upcoming Medicare educational seminar, or inquire about hosting a seminar for your library, church, community, employer, or organization.

www.ingramcontent.com/pod-product-compliance
Lightning Source LLC
LaVergne TN
LVHW080026210926
848481LV00011B/3109

* 9 7 9 8 9 9 7 2 0 2 5 0 7 *